PRIMARY
CARE
MANAGEMENT

Notice

In preparing this book, the author and publisher have made every attempt to ensure that the guidelines presented follow accepted practice and standards. Because patient care entails a constantly evolving quest for knowledge, however, the health care provider is advised to rely on experience, current product inserts and other literature, and knowledge of the patient to determine the best treatment for each individual case, especially with respect to new drug and nutritional therapies. The author and publisher cannot be resposible for misuse or misapplication of the information in this work. Discrepancies or errors should be brought to the attention of the publisher.

PRIMARY CARE MANAGEMENT
Cases and Discussions

Goutham Rao

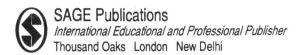

SAGE Publications
International Educational and Professional Publisher
Thousand Oaks London New Delhi

For information:

SAGE Publications, Inc.
2455 Teller Road
Thousand Oaks, California 91320
E-mail: order@sagepub.com

SAGE Publications Ltd.
6 Bonhill Street
London EC2A 4PU
United Kingdom

SAGE Publications India Pvt. Ltd.
M-32 Market
Greater Kailash I
New Delhi 110 048 India

Library of Congress Cataloging-in-Publication Data

Rao, Goutham.
    Primary care management: Cases and discussions / by Goutham
Rao.
        p.   c.m.
    Includes bibliographical references and index.
    ISBN 0-7619-1204-5 (cloth: acid-free paper)
    ISBN 0-7619-1205-3 (pbk.: acid-free paper)
    1. Family medicine—Case studies.   I. Title.
    RC66 .R36 1998
    616′ .09—ddc21   98-25307

This book is printed on acid-free paper.

99 00 01 02 03 04 05 7 6 5 4 3 2 1

Acquiring Editor:	Dan Ruth
Editorial Assistant:	Anna Howland
Production Editors:	Sherrise M. Roehr/Wendy Westgate
Editorial Assistant:	Lynn Miyata
Book Designer:	Rose Tylak
Typesetter:	Christina M. Hill
Cover Designer:	Candice Harman

Contents

Preface   vii

Introduction: How to Use This Workbook   ix

1. Evaluation of Involuntary Weight Loss: Mr. Joseph Drumdonald   1

2. Insomnia: Mr. Raffi Olefsky   27

3. Dizziness and Falls: Mrs. Enza Ianonne   46

4. Headache: Ms. Shannon Stapleton   55

5. Type II Diabetes: Mr. William Hodge   72

6. Hyperlipidemia: Mr. Nigel Waugh   94

7. Outpatient Management of Heart Failure: Mr. Stewart Ross   109

8. Gastroesophageal Reflux Disease: Mr. Roger Edstrom   123

9. Infantile Diarrhea: Francine St. George   138

10. Failure to Thrive, or Growth Deficiency: Lindsay Clarke   153

11. Management of Asthma: Ms. Liane Webber   176

12. Smoking Cessation: Ms. Liane Webber   195

13. Management of Early HIV Infection: Mr. Adam Moore   211

14. Menopause: Ms. Esmerelda Gutierez   226

15. Acute Low Back Pain: Mr. Thomas Ishigawa   237

Index   247

About the Author   251

Preface

Case studies have played an important role in medical education for many years, and there is considerable evidence that case-based learning is an effective educational medium. The traditional format for oral or written cases, widely used in inpatient medicine, was developed in the days of William Osler a century ago. It remains a clear, rational, and comprehensive way to convey medical information about a patient, but there is a consensus that it is unable to effectively capture the psychosocial aspects of a case. This has led to the development of a number of different formats for case studies, including the one I have designed for this book. It is a format that integrates medical, social, and psychological data into a detailed story that is meant to be innovative and entertaining.

Development of a new educational tool, such as a new format for case studies, has little impact without a practical application. For this reason, I have used the new format in this workbook of 15 case-based exercises, each written to develop the reader's knowledge of a particular core problem in primary care medicine. The workbook has been specifically designed to be used in the setting of group discussions, but its content and style make it a versatile product that I hope will find many different applications.

I would like to acknowledge the support, guidance, and encouragement of the fellowship faculty at the University of Pittsburgh Medical Center—St. Margaret and, in particular, Dr. Joel H. Merenstein, without whose help this project would have remained half completed, gathering dust in my basement.

— Goutham Rao, MD, CM, CCFP
Pittsburgh, Pennsylvania

Introduction:

How to Use This Workbook

A family physician at a dinner party was asked by an elderly woman sitting at his table what he did for a living.

"I'm a doctor. A family physician."

The woman, who had little knowledge of the complicated architecture of the medical profession, responded, "That's nice. What part of the body do you deal with?"

"I don't deal with any part in particular. We family physicians use the biopsychosocial model and the family-centered approach to medicine."

Slightly embarrassed by her inability to understand the family physician's terminology, she turned to the young lady next to her and started a conversation about gardening.

It is no secret that the specialty of family medicine continues to evolve and struggles to define itself. The terms commonly used to describe its uniqueness, such as *biopsychosocial model,* are sometimes intangible and obscure to physicians outside the specialty, let alone members of the general public. A simple way of explaining the uniqueness of family medicine is to consider what special skill family physicians possess.

A respirologist's range of skills includes bronchoscopy. This is his or her undisputed domain. An occasional thoracic or ENT surgeon may trample on this territory, but it is well known that respirologists perform bronchoscopy and perform it well. What about family practitioners? Like all good physicians, they obtain a history from a patient and perform a physical examination to make decisions. Their unique and often close relationship to patients, however, allows them to better incorporate a patient's life circumstances into an approach to management. This is their special skill. They are able to integrate a patient's living conditions and financial status, as well as his or her occupational, educational, and family history, with the presenting history and physical examination to derive a comprehensive management plan. If family physicians are *skilled integrators of a wide variety of information,* should there not be some way to evaluate and develop this skill? This idea is the basis for the case studies in this workbook.

Each case study comprises not only a thorough history of the present illness and physical examination but a very detailed social history and past medical history as well. In other words, the reader of the case has virtually all the information about the patient at his or her disposal and is asked to make decisions based on this information. The intent is not to simulate the actual office setting; it is impossible to gather the amount of information contained in each case in a reasonable period of time. Furthermore, the cases are written in the form of fictional stories. Authenticity is not the objective.

Each case study consists of a profile of the patient, which includes his or her social and past personal and family medical history. Readers are first to "absorb" and reflect upon this section before tackling the patient's presenting problem. "The Problem" is divided into several parts, each describing a new development in the patient's illness—a new chapter in the story. Each part of the problem is accompanied by one or more questions, the suggested responses to which are included immediately thereafter. As noted, the idea of each exercise is to incorporate the patient's social and psychological circumstances into the management of his or her problem. There are no right or wrong ways to go about this task, and participants are encouraged to be creative in their use of the patient profile. The focus of the "Discussion," therefore, is on the medical aspects of each case. Suggested responses are founded on the latest evidence-based practice guidelines, consensus statements, and research studies. Whenever possible, the viewpoint of several different organizations is presented.

The focus of each case study is one particular core problem in primary care medicine. The problems included are those that have traditionally presented challenges from a management perspective to medical students, residents, family physicians, and others involved in primary health care delivery. They are not necessarily, therefore, the most commonly encountered problems in practice. There is no case study on the "common cold," for example, because management of this disease is not sufficiently complex.

The emphasis is indeed on the management rather than the diagnosis of particular problems. The diagnosis of diabetes, for example, is relatively straightforward. Management of diabetes, on the other hand, encompasses patient education, pharmacologic and nonpharmacologic therapy, prevention of complications, and so on. The emphasis of the case study on diabetes is on these issues.

Critics of the workbook will no doubt point out that many complex problems in primary care medicine are not included. The workbook is not intended to be an exhaustive review of every complex problem encountered in practice. It is, rather, a tool for developing important decision-making skills while familiarizing the reader with the latest information on several important core topics. The core topic of each case is by no means the only medical problem addressed. The case on failure to thrive, for example, includes a section on cystic fibrosis. Indeed, though the list of core subjects for case studies is short, the entire workbook does cover much of the breadth of primary care medicine. This fact, together with the workbook's unique emphasis on the social and psychological aspects of medicine, makes it a fairly comprehensive primary care medicine resource.

The workbook has been specifically designed to be used in the setting of small-group discussions led by a discussion leader. He or she should be thoroughly familiar with the case study to be discussed beforehand, especially the goal and specific objectives of the exercise, as outlined in the "Guide for Discussion Leader." This preparation is extremely important. The discussion leader need not be an expert in the core topic of the case. Most of the cases have been introduced to participants in trial exercises over the past 3 years. Though the cases studies vary in length, each case discussion exercise can be easily completed in approximately 90 min.

A suggested three-part format for these group discussions is shown below.

1. *Review of Patient Profile.* The discussion participants are given 10 min to read "The Patient" section of the case study only. They should then be encouraged to express their

thoughts on this patient profile. The discussion leader could ask, for example, "What do you think about this patient and his family?" "Does this patient resemble someone in your practice?" This is the process through which the participants become familiar with a patient who exists only on paper. Part 1 should take a total of about 20 min.

2. *Tackling "The Problem."* The patient's presenting problem is presented in several parts, each accompanied by one or more questions, which the discussion leader can introduce in sequence. Participants should be encouraged to offer answers spontaneously to the questions rather than referring immediately to the suggested responses in the "Discussion." In leading the discussion, the discussion leader may or may not wish to rely entirely on these suggested responses. This is the bulk of the group discussion exercise. It should be interactive and not overly structured, but it should not consume more than 1 h.

3. *Review of Goal and Objectives.* An excellent way to end the exercise is for participants to determine if they can meet the goal and objectives outlined in the "Guide for Discussion Leader." This self-assessment should take no more than 10 min.

Group discussions based on the exercises in the workbook could constitute a regular curriculum in family medicine for senior medical students or junior family practice residents.

Flexibility will certainly contribute to the success of this workbook. There is, of course, no need to follow the format for group discussions outlined above. There is, in fact, no need to use the workbook only in group discussions. It is meant to be a versatile product. It can be used, for example, for individual study. Though the primary target audience consists of trainees in the field of family medicine, a number of other groups will find the workbook useful. These include trainees in other areas of primary care, practicing physicians who wish to use the workbook as a continuing medical education resource, physicians and educators involved in the development of evaluative resources such as oral and written examinations, and nurse practitioners involved in the delivery of comprehensive primary care.

1. EVALUATION OF

INVOLUNTARY WEIGHT LOSS

Mr. Joseph Drumdonald

*Goal: The goal of this exercise is to provide participants
with a rational approach to the problem of involuntary weight loss
and to the detection and treatment of major depression.*

Specific Objectives: Upon completion of this exercise, each participant should be able to accomplish the following:

1. List the most common causes of weight loss in the elderly.
2. Describe the classification of mood disorders according to *Diagnostic and Statistical Manual of Mental Disorders (DSM)* criteria.
3. Conduct an interview of a patient to detect the presence of major depression.
4. In general terms, describe the major forms of therapy for depression.
5. Classify the different medications used to treat depression.
6. Describe the side effects of the most commonly used antidepressant medications.

PART I

The Patient

Social History

Mr. Joseph Drumdonald is a 76-year-old retired dairy farmer who lives alone in a large home along a country road near Fairfield, Iowa. Joseph was born, raised, and has spent most of his life on a dairy farm. Indeed, the Drumdonald family had operated a farm for more than 120 years when Joseph retired in 1988. The patient is extremely proud of this heritage. In his words, "It was good honest work that kept you in touch with the land and put food on people's tables. I wouldn't have given up that life for anything." Despite the family's dedication to farming, Joseph's father, Zachary Drumdonald, insisted that his children receive a good education. Joseph completed high school just as World War II was beginning in Europe. Like many young men of his generation, he enlisted happily with the military. With the United States Navy, he joined the campaign against the Japanese in Southeast Asia. It is this period of his life that

Joseph remembers best. "A lot of people talk about the war. They talk about how they did heroic things and how they suffered. I was no hero. I was a scared young man. I did my duty. I made some great friends and then lost a lot of them."

Young Joseph Drumdonald returned to the United States in 1945 to all the fanfare that accompanies conquering war heroes. His only ambition, however, was to return to the farm and continue to help his family prosper. This help came at an appropriate time, as his father was severely ill. Zachary died in 1946, leaving the dairy farm in the secure hands of his two sons, Joseph and Henry.

In 1948, Joseph met Beatrice Poulson, a young schoolteacher, whom he courted enthusiastically. Beatrice was fond of Joseph, but her parents objected to the relationship. She had been previously pursued by a wealthy banker, and her mother, in particular, insisted that she marry someone with "proper standing in life." Eventually, against strong resistance from the Poulsons, Beatrice and Joseph were married in 1950. The couple had three children: Victoria, born in 1951; Samuel, born in 1954; and James, born in 1955. Tragedy struck the family in 1975, when Beatrice was diagnosed with ovarian cancer. She died in 1977 at the age of 49.

All three of Joseph's children are ambitious and well educated and had little interest in taking over the family farm. For this reason, an aging Joseph sold it in 1988 to a large corporation and bought a nice home close to his daughter and her family.

Joseph is a very soft-spoken gentleman with very few friends. He does not enjoy traveling far from home. He is visited frequently by his daughter Victoria, her husband Ted, and their four children. He enjoys gardening and fishing. Joseph also visits several dairy farms in the area, acting as an unpaid, informal "consultant"—an activity that gives him more of an opportunity to socialize than to contribute to the success of the farms. Samuel, a married financial consultant, lives in Des Moines and visits his father every couple of months. James Drumdonald is a divorced gynecologist affiliated with the University of Chicago Medical School. He makes infrequent visits to Iowa to visit family and friends.

Joseph's family is of Welsh and Scottish extraction. The Drumdonalds are Roman Catholics, but Joseph describes himself as "not overly religious." He attends church infrequently.

Past Personal and Family Medical History

Joseph does not know if he had any serious health problems as a child. "I had the usual stuff—measles, chicken-pox, but nothing devastating." While in the Philippines during the war, Joseph contracted a severe case of malaria and was placed in an army field hospital for several weeks.

Apart from numerous minor occupationally related injuries over the years, Joseph has been essentially healthy. He was seen for a periodic health examination 10 months ago. A random total cholesterol level drawn at that time was slightly high, and Joseph was given appropriate dietary advice. Joseph smoked cigarettes heavily until 1975, when he promised his wife, who worried that her husband would develop lung cancer, that he would quit completely. He has not touched a cigarette since. The patient drinks a couple of glasses of wine on occasion, usually at Victoria's house. He presently uses no medications and reports no allergies.

According to Joseph, his father Zachary died of "blood cancer." His mother Mary died in 1981 of a pulmonary embolism. She was 84 years old. Joseph's older brother Henry, 79, lives in a nursing home in Iowa City. He is in extremely poor health, suffering from heart failure, dementia, and chronic malnutrition. Joseph has two younger sisters. Isabella, 75, is a widow who lives in a retirement community in Green Valley, Arizona. Elaine, 73, is married and lives with her husband in Lincoln, Nebraska. Joseph does not know whether his sisters have any serious health problems.

To the best of his knowledge, Joseph's three children and eight grandchildren are in good health.

The Problem

You are the only physician in a small community in southeastern Iowa. There is a community hospital approximately 40 miles (70 km) away, where a limited array of diagnostic facilities and specialist services is available. Mr. Joseph Drumdonald has been your patient for 2 years. You last saw him 10 months ago for a periodic health examination, upon which you uncovered mild hypercholesterolemia but no other significant health concerns.

Joseph comes to your office accompanied by his daughter, Victoria. When asked what brings him in, Joseph shrugs his shoulders indifferently. His daughter, with a look of intense concern, replies, "Well, Doctor, I'm really worried about my dad. He's become so damn thin. He's just skin and bones. I can't believe this is happening to him. He's just wasting into nothing! He would never come in on his own! He never tells me anything!"

Your physician's assistant recorded a weight of 55.6 kg at this visit. Ten months ago, Joseph's weight was 64.3 kg.

Questions

1. Has Joseph lost a significant amount of weight?
2. What are the most common causes of involuntary weight loss in an elderly patient?
3. Excluding laboratory investigations, how would you approach this problem?
4. What initial screening laboratory investigations, if any, would you order in all patients with involuntary weight loss?

Discussion

1. Clearly, the loss of 1 or 2 kg of body weight should not raise a great deal of concern. An involuntary weight loss of 5% or more of body weight in a 6- to 12-month period, on the other hand, generally merits thorough evaluation (Robbins, 1989). Joseph has lost 8.7 kg, or 13.5% of his original body weight.

2. Morley (1990) categorizes the major causes of weight loss in the elderly as *social* (isolation, poverty, lack of transporta-

tion, etc.), *psychiatric* (secondary to dementia, depression, anxiety, etc.), *medical* (secondary to heart failure, thyroid disease, diabetes, etc.) and *age related* (secondary to impaired olfactory and taste sensitivity, etc.). The prevalence of these various causes of weight loss is a question, however, that has received limited attention. Marton, Sox, and Krupp (1981) prospectively evaluated 91 patients with involuntary weight loss at a Veterans

Administration (VA) hospital. In 26% of patients, no apparent cause was detected. In the remainder, a wide variety of causes became apparent. Weight loss was attributed to cancer in 20% of patients. Other medical illnesses, including gastrointestinal, cardiovascular, and pulmonary diseases, contributed to weight loss in another 50%. In 9% of patients, a psychiatric disease was deemed responsible. The obvious shortcoming of this study is the selective patient population—elderly males in a VA hospital, many of whom were smokers. A study by Rabinovitz, Pitlik, Leifer, Garty, and Rosenfeld (1986) of hospitalized patients in Israel with involuntary weight loss revealed a similar prevalence of psychiatric and undetermined causes but a higher (36%) prevalence of cancer. The mean age of patients in this study was 64.2 years, with a range of 27 to 88 years, and the ratio of males to females was 1.2:1. The patients studied were therefore somewhat more representative of the general population. For the purposes of this case discussion exercise, despite the small number of patients involved, the study by Thompson and Morris (1991) is of considerable value. Involuntary weight loss in 45 *ambulatory* elderly patients was evaluated. One third of the study participants were male. The mean age was 71.9 years. Depression was found to be the most common single cause of weight loss. Cancer accounted for only 16% of attributable causes. Hyperthyroidism was detected in 9% of patients. As in the other studies, no cause of weight loss was identified in a significant number of patients (24%).

3. The evaluation of involuntary or unintentional weight loss is by no means a simple matter. It is complicated by several factors (Drossman, 1995). In roughly 50% of patients who complain of weight loss,

significant loss of weight cannot be substantiated (Marton et al., 1981). At times, weight loss may not be clinically significant—as in the patient who begins to pursue a healthier diet or lifestyle without weight loss as an immediate goal. The etiology of unintentional weight loss is sometimes multifactorial, secondary to the interplay of medical, social, and behavioral factors, making assessment difficult. Finally, as noted above, despite extensive evaluation, no apparent cause may be found in a large number of subjects. This can be frustrating for both clinicians and patients.

Despite these difficulties, a number of rational approaches to the problem of involuntary weight loss are available. The first task is substantiation of the complaint. This has been done in Joseph's case, as a previous medical record is available. Nevertheless, discussion participants should be reminded of this seemingly obvious yet crucial first step so that patients are spared expensive evaluation when there is doubt as to whether weight loss has occurred.

Once it has been determined that significant weight loss has occurred, it is of value to identify patients in whom a physical cause is likely (Goroll, 1995). Once again, this avoids further unnecessary medical evaluation. In this context, based on their study, Marton et al. (1981) developed a linear discriminant rule to identify historical and physical factors upon which the likelihood of a physical cause of weight loss can be estimated. This estimate is based on an assigned score to each of six factors. These include *less than 20 pack-years smoking, no decrease in activities due to fatigue, nausea/vomiting, improvement in appetite, cough that has recently changed, and an abnormal physical exami-*

nation. Although it would be valuable to identify patients with a physical cause of weight loss, the applicability of this rule is limited by the selective population from which it was derived.

Robbins (1989) describes "The Nine D's" of weight loss in the elderly. These include the following: **dentition, dysgeusia, dysphagia, diarrhea, disease (chronic), depression, dementia, dysfunction, and drugs.** Though the nine Ds do not by themselves constitute an approach to involuntary weight loss, they do give some idea of how to gather historical information and perform a physical examination.

Wise and Craig (1995) describe a rational approach to weight loss that begins with obtaining the patient's past medical history, habits, and medication use. This information has already been provided in the patient profile. This should be followed by a thorough review of systems. The physical examination should include assessment of the patient's mood and affect. The skin and lymph nodes should be examined. A thorough cardiovascular, respiratory, muskuloskeletal, abdominal, and genital/prostate examination should be included. Finally, neurologic and mental status exams complete the physical assessment. That such a comprehensive initial evaluation is recommended (Wise & Craig) is an indicator of how difficult it can be to make a correct diagnosis in the patient with involuntary weight loss. Clearly, at some point in obtaining the history, one or more causes of weight loss may become apparent, and a thorough physical examination may seem unnecessary. As noted, however, involuntary weight loss can have multiple causes, increasing the yield of a comprehensive history and physical.

Based on the information above, a reasonable initial approach includes a thorough history and physical examination, with special emphasis on screening for depression, as this is very prevalent among elderly, ambulatory patients with involuntary weight loss. Detecting depression is discussed in greater depth in the next part of this exercise. The nine Ds can be incorporated into this initial assessment. They are self-explanatory except for **dysfunction,** by which Robbins (1989) refers to the social causes of weight loss secondary to decreased intake, such as inability to prepare meals or inability to obtain food due to lack of transportation, fear in unsafe neighborhoods, and so on. An inquiry into how Joseph's meals "get on the dinner table" is a useful approach to social causes.

4. In the study by Marton et al. (1981), subjects underwent a number of simple screening laboratory investigations, some of which were found to be useful in determining the cause of weight loss. The most useful examination was chest radiology. In the study of ambulatory elderly patients by Thompson and Morris (1991), patients were evaluated retrospectively through chart review, and laboratory tests were ordered at the discretion of each patient's physician. In this study, laboratory investigations were unlikely to be ordered purely as "screening" measures without direction from the history and physical examination. Several tests, including thyroid function, occult fecal blood, and sigmoidoscopy, were found to have diagnostic value. Wise and Craig (1995) advocate a conservative approach to the use of screening laboratory studies that, **when the history and physical examination fail to provide clues to the cause of weight loss,** would include cell blood count (CBC), erythrocyte sedimentation rate (ESR), urinalysis, liver enymes, albumin, calcium, phosphorus, electrolytes, blood glucose, thyroid-stimu-

lating hormone (TSH), chest film, and HIV testing in high-risk patients. In addition, they recommend routine cancer screening, according to the guidelines of the American Cancer Society, which in male patients includes fecal occult blood testing at age 40 or older, flexible sigmoidoscopy at ages 50, 51, and every 3 to 5 years thereafter, and prostate-specific antigen in men over 50. These additional recommendations are certainly controversial. Joseph may have

had some of these cancer screening tests as part of his periodic health examination. In any case, **at this time, the focus of the evaluation should be the history and physical examination, after which specific laboratory tests, if indicated, can be performed.** In other words, there is no universal screening battery of tests that should be employed in all patients presenting with involuntary weight loss.

The Rest of the Story

You explain to both Victoria and Joseph that the evaluation of involuntary weight loss is often difficult and that you would like to begin by asking several important questions. Victoria seems anxious to begin, but her father sits quietly, expressionless. You direct all your questions to Joseph, but his daughter sometimes jumps in to answer. You ask her politely to let her father provide all the necessary information.

Joseph denies any fever, cough, shortness of breath, chest pain, palpitations, or swelling of his extremities. He denies dysphagia, dysgeusia, nausea, vomiting, diarrhea, or change in bowel habits or stool. He denies abdominal pain, heartburn, or jaundice. He does admit to a greatly decreased appetite in recent months and states that much of the time he has no desire to eat. When asked about fatigue, Joseph tells you in a quiet voice, "Doctor, I guess I just feel kind of worn out all the time. Don't have the energy to do much at all."

Joseph denies polyuria, nocturia, or urinary frequency, urgency, incontinence, or other urinary symptoms. He denies muscle or joint pains or stiffness. He reports no headaches, numbness, tingling or "pins and needles," or other neurologic symptoms. Joseph reports no heat or cold intolerance, excessive sweating, or any excessive thirst or hunger. He reports no dental or oral pain or difficulty chewing.

You ask Joseph how often he eats and how food gets "on his table." Victoria interrupts you again and tells you she drops off groceries at his house every week. Joseph appears a little annoyed with his daughter. "Victoria, let me tell the doctor! OK?"

Victoria looks a little embarrassed and allows her father to explain. "Doctor, Victoria does bring me groceries. I'm not much of a cook, though. I used to eat three square meals a day. Now I just don't feel like it, I guess. I can make bacon and eggs and toast. Victoria does make some great meals and brings them over quite often. I also go over to her place for dinner a couple of times a week, mainly to play with the grandkids. I haven't felt like getting out of the house lately."

Joseph tells you he normally eats a good variety of foods, including plenty of chicken and red meat, carrots and potatoes, and canned fruit. He tells you he has been relying on toast and canned foods to satisfy the little hunger he has had in recent months.

You decide that it is impossible, due to time constraints, to complete your initial evaluation at this visit. You have already decided to evaluate Joseph for depression and dementia, and you ask him to return in 2 days for a further work-up and a physical exam. He agrees.

PART II

The Problem

Joseph returns to your office as scheduled. He tells you, "Victoria drove me here, but I insisted that she not come in with me. She worries about me too much, doctor. I thought it would be best that she wait outside."

Questions

1. You have yet to rule out depression and dementia as causes of weight loss. How common is depression in elderly persons?
2. Why is it often difficult to make a diagnosis of depression?
3. How are mood disorders categorized?
4. How would you assess Joseph for depression?
5. How would you assess Joseph for dementia?

Discussion

1. There are various estimates of the prevalence of depression in the elderly. The prevalence of depressive symptoms in community residents over age 65 is approximately 15% (NIH Concensus Development Panel on Depression in Late Life, 1992). The prevalence of major depression among elderly persons living in the community is approximately 3%. Depressive illness is more common in elderly patients in hospitals and nursing homes.

2. Depression at any age is poorly diagnosed and treated by family physicians, as pointed out by Lemelin, Hotz, Swensen, and Elmslie (1994), who also suggest that several specific factors make the diagnosis difficult. Depressed patients who present to primary care physicians may not always be obviously depressed, and they frequently have physical rather than psychiatric complaints. Physicians tend to focus on such somatic symptoms and neglect the possibility of depression. They usually work within a tight office schedule and in an environment that does not provide substantial remuneration for diagnosing and treating psychosocial problems. Moreover, many patients in the setting of primary care do not meet the "official" diagnostic criteria as outlined in the *Diagnostic and Statistical Manual of Mental Disorders* (*DSM-IIIR* or *DSM-IV*) (American Psychiatric Association [APA], 1987, 1995a) for depression, a limitation that further complicates diagnosis. A recent "primary care" edition of the manual *(DSM-IVPC)* (APA, 1995b), although still using *DSM-IV* crite-

ria for depression, does take into consideration the manner in which patients with depression present in the primary care setting.

3. The simplest description of mood disorders as categorized by *DSM-IIIR* divides them into **major depressive disorder; dysthymia,** a less severe but more chronic form of depression; **bipolar disorders, characterized by episodes of "mania"** as well as depression; and **depression not otherwise specified,** a residual heterogeneous category. A more specific description of major depressive disorder is discussed later. The particular elements of the other disorders are beyond the scope of this exercise.

4. The Agency for Health Care Policy and Research (AHCPR) has prepared an impressive evidence-based guideline on the detection and diagnosis of depression in the primary care setting (U.S. Department of Health and Human Services, 1993b), which forms the basis for much of the following discussion. In it, the detection and treatment of depression is described as a stepwise process that begins with **maintaining a high index of suspicion and assessment of risk factors.** Joseph presents with involuntary weight loss. The fundamental breakdown of the causes of involuntary weight loss by Morley (1990) includes psychiatric disorders, and the possibility of depression has been noted throughout the preceding discussion. The primary risk factors for depression are the following: prior episodes of depression, family history of depressive disorder, **prior suicide attempts, female gender, age of onset under 40, postpartum period, medical comorbidity, lack of social support, stressful life events, and current alcohol or substance abuse.** Joseph does have a history of sub-

stance abuse. He has no history of disabling medical illnesses. The patient profile makes no mention of personal or familial psychiatric illnesses of any kind, but it is worthwhile to question Joseph or his daughter specifically about this. Other potential risks include stressful life events and lack of social support. The nature of any stressors on Joseph's life are unclear. The loss of his wife many years ago must certainly have been a difficult experience. Joseph has significant contact with Victoria and her family but has few friends. Whether he "lacks" social support should be explored further.

Upon evaluation of depressive risk factors, the next step is the detection of depressive symptoms. In this context, the AHCPR has found patient self-report questionnaires to be of great value (USDHHS, 1993b). These are brief questionnaires that can be easily completed in a few minutes by selected patients. They are able to identify nearly every patient with depression (high sensitivity) but have a very high false-positive rate of 25% to 40% (low specificity). They are effective, therefore, as a case-finding tool, rather than as a general screening tool. In other words, such questionnaires should only be administered to patients in whom depression is suspected, like Joseph. Furthermore, the diagnosis of depressive illness should never be made on the basis of such questionnaires alone but in conjunction with a formal clinical interview for depressive symptoms. There are a number of these questionnaires, including one, designed specifically for detection of depression in older patients, known as the **Geriatric Depression Scale** (Yesavage, 1992; see appendix). In the short form, 5 to 9 of 15 possible positive responses is associated with a high likelihood of depression. A score of 10 or more means that the patient is almost certainly depressed.

The essential step, regardless of whether self-report questionnaires are used, is the clinical interview and history to determine which, if any, mood disorder is present. Valuable information can be gathered from close relatives or friends. Victoria may serve as a valuable resource. In the clinical interview, Joseph should be asked about symptoms that constitute the *DSM* criteria for **major depression** (see Appendix). This should be the priority because the evidence for the effectiveness of various treatments for major depression is strong. The effectiveness of treatments for other depressive illnesses, such as dysthymic disorder, has yet to be studied extensively.

The assessment of suicide risk is obviously of extreme importance. Risk factors for suicide include Caucasian race, male gender, advanced age, and living alone (USDHHS, 1993b)—all of which apply to Joseph.

The presence of 5 out of 9 of the *DSM* criteria confirms the diagnosis of *major depression.* This number of positive criteria, along with a prior history of mania, characterized by elevated mood or elevated mood and increased energy, is defined as *bipolar illness.* The lack of the requisite criteria for major depression, but a persistently depressed mood for 2 or more years with at least two other symptoms including appetite disturbance, sleep disturbance, fatigue, low self-esteem, hopelessness, and poor concentration, is consistent with *dysthymia.* Other patients with depressive symptoms can be categorized as having *depression not otherwise specified.* The importance of the clinical interview and determining the presence of major depression should be emphasized to all partici-

pants rather than the specific criteria for other mood disorders.

5. This is a question of extreme importance. It was originally raised when considering the causes of weight loss. Dementia, through progressive impairment of olfaction, blunted thirst and hunger, impaired swallowing and other physiological mechanisms, leads to decreased intake and weight loss (Robbins, 1989). In the context of evaluation of depression in an elderly person, the possibility of early dementia must be considered. Distinguishing between depression and early dementia is often extremely difficult, as many patients with dementia may present only with depressive symptoms. Furthermore, depressed elderly patients may present with symptoms of cognitive impairment, a condition known as *pseudo dementia.* To complicate matters further, depression and dementia often coexist. Roughly 17% to 30% of Alzheimer's patients, for example, suffer from both dementia and depressive illness (Alexopoulos & Chester, 1992).

Dementia is a disease characterized by a decline from previously attained intellectual levels, in which memory; other cognitive capacities such as language, orientation, and abstract thought; and general adaptive behavior are progressively affected. There are a number of sophisticated formal screening tools for detection of dementia in the elderly. The use of these is beyond the scope of this exercise. A simple mini–mental status exam has been advocated as part of the evaluation of involuntary weight loss and is useful in detecting dementia (Folstein, Folstein, & McHugh, 1975; see Appendix). Victoria herself, in addition to being a valuable witness to her father's possible depressive symptoms, may have noted cognitive deficits that Joseph is either unable or unwilling to recognize. Such help from a family member may not be enough to detect early dementia, but the AHCPR (USDHHS, 1993b) guideline has made it clear that focusing the evaluation on the detection of depression, whether it be isolated or coex- istent with dementia, and treating it promptly should be the priority. Often, the best way to detect dementia in the elderly is to treat depressive illness and reassess the patient for cognitive deficits once that treatment is successful.

The Rest of the Story

You tell Joseph that you would like to continue with the evaluation of his weight loss. You begin with a physical examination, the results of which are summarized below:

Gen: Pleasant, quiet, thin elderly gentleman, with slightly flat affect.

  Wt. = 55.6 kg, BP = 120/75, P = 72/min, RR = 18/min

HEENT: dentures—upper and lower jaw/good fit/no oral infections or other abnormalities

Skin: no rashes or lesions, discoloration, or other abnormalities

Lymphatics: No cervical, axillary, epitrochlear, or inguinal lymphadenopathy

Resp: within normal limits

CVS: within normal limits

Abdomen: within normal limits

MSK: within normal limits

Rectum/prostate: within normal limits

Neurologic exam: Gait, strength in extremities, deep tendon reflexes, and plantar responses all within normal limits. Romberg test negative.

Upon completion of your physical examination, you decide to perform a *mini–mental status examination* (see Appendix). You explain to Joseph that the questions you will ask him will help detect problems with memory and thought that may indirectly be related to his loss of weight. Joseph responds, "No problem. Go ahead, Doctor."

Joseph scores 28 out of 30, incorrectly calculating two "serial 7s" in the assessment of attention and calculation, which he attributes to "having trouble concentrating."

You tell Joseph that he has done fairly well on the mental status exam. You mention to him that depression often leads to decreased appetite and that you would like to evaluate him further for this. He agrees, and you ask him to complete a **Geriatric Depression Scale** questionnaire. You ask him for permission to call Victoria and ask her about his mood and any possible problems with thought and memory. Joseph responds, "Victoria worries about me too much. Yes, I've been quite down lately. Please go ahead and call her, but she may have a tendency to exaggerate because she's so worried about me."

You leave the room to make your call while Joseph completes the questionnaire. Victoria is at work and has only a couple of minutes to talk. You ask her if she has noticed a change in her father's mood recently. "Oh yes, Doctor. No doubt about it. He mopes around the house all day. He doesn't like to get outdoors. That's not like him at all. He never complains to me about being down. He just says he's worn out, but I think he's depressed. I've never seen him

Choose the best answer to describe how you have felt over the past week:

1. Are you basically satisfied with your life?	Yes	(No*)
2. Have you dropped many of your activities and interests?	(Yes*)	No
3. Do you feel that your life is empty?	(Yes*)	No
4. Do you often get bored?	(Yes*)	No
5. Are you in good spirits most of the time?	Yes	(No*)
6. Are you afraid that something bad is going to happen to you?	Yes*	(No)
7. Do you feel happy most of the time?	Yes	(No*)
8. Do you feel helpless?	Yes*	(No)
9. Do you prefer to stay at home, rather than going out and doing new things?	(Yes*)	No
10. Do you feel you have more problems with memory than most?	(Yes*)	No
11. Do you feel it is wonderful to be alive now?	Yes	(No*)
12. Do you feel pretty worthless the way you are now?	Yes	(No)
13. Do you feel full of energy?	Yes	(No*)
14. Do you feel your situation is hopeless?	Yes	(No)
15. Do you feel that most people are better off than you are?	Yes	(No)

SOURCE: Adapted from Yesavage (1992, p. 256).
NOTE: * Responses are indicative of depression. Five to nine of the asterisked responses indicates the possibility of depression. Ten or more is virtually diagnostic of depression.

Figure 1.1 Geriatric Depression Scale: Joseph's Answers

like this. It started about three months ago and has been getting worse." You ask Victoria if Joseph has ever had episodes of elevated mood and energy accompanied by unusual behavior. She does not recall any episodes of that type. To the best of her knowledge, Joseph has never expressed suicidal thoughts nor made any suicide attempts. Victoria does not know of anyone in her and Joseph's family with a previous history of depression.

You inquire about Joseph's social supports. Victoria tells you, "Well, he's got us, of course. We live only a couple of miles away, and he comes over about once a week. I visit him a couple of times a week, usually. Lately I've been going more often because I'm worried about him. He really doesn't have a lot of close friends, Doctor. I mean, he goes out to the farms once in a while, but most of them have been sold to companies, and they don't want him around. He belongs to a seniors social club in town. He rarely goes there."

When asked about stressful events in her father's life, Victoria tells you, "Well, he's really quite a simple man. Nothing has changed in his life for many years. I think giving up the farm was stressful a few years back, but he got used to that. I can't think of anything stressful going on his life right now. My dad is very fond of my brother's son, Keith, who applied for medical school recently but wasn't accepted anywhere. I think Dad was disappointed. Keith lives in Chicago but loves to come out to Iowa to visit. I can't see that as being a major stress for Dad, though."

You ask Victoria whether her father appears to have difficulty with memory or thought processes. She tells you that although Joseph has been complaining recently about trouble concentrating, in her view, he has been "razor sharp" as usual over the past few months. He always arrives for dinner at Victoria's house right on time. He has not forgotten any of his grandchildren's birthdays and always sends gifts. In Victoria's words, "I hope I'm like that when I'm his age!"

PART III

The Problem

Joseph fills out the **Geriatric Depression Scale** questionnaire as shown in Figure 1.1.
You decide to conduct a formal interview for depression. Your account of that interview is represented by the dialogue shown below:

I glanced at the questionnaire Mr. Drumdonald had completed. He asked me almost
   immediately, "Doctor, are you saying that I'm depressed?"
Doctor: Well, that is a possibility, Joseph. I need to ask you some more questions. Do you
   think you're depressed?
Joseph: I have been feeling really down in the dumps lately. No doubt about it.
D: How long have you been feeling this way?
J: I would say at least 3 or 4 months. It wasn't bad at first. I feel really down right now.
D: Do you feel down every day?
J: Well, some days are better than others, but yes, I feel down most of the time.
D: Do you find that you have less interest in usual activities, or in things you especially
   enjoy?
J: I don't feel like doing very much at all, Doctor. I mean, I like getting outdoors. Victoria
   will tell you now I just feel like staying at home by myself. I like to drive around and
   visit farms. I haven't done that for quite a while.
D: Have you been sleeping well?
J: No, Doctor. Just awful, actually. I don't have much trouble falling asleep, but for some
   reason, I wake up at 4:00 a.m. every morning and can't fall asleep again. I just lie there
   feeling miserable. It wears me out the whole day.
D: How would you describe your energy level?
J: It's as if the energy has been zapped right out of me. I don't feel like I have any energy at
   all. I actually feel sluggish all the time.
D: How is your appetite?
J: Well, it's just not there, Doctor. I don't know why. I thought maybe I have some illness.
   I just don't feel like eating. I used to eat three square meals a day. Now, I just eat a little
   now and then, and only when I'm really hungry. It's no wonder that I'm just skin and
   bones.
D: How do you feel about yourself and the future?
J: I don't understand what you mean.
D: Well, do you ever have feelings of worthlessness or guilt?
J: Well, I have those sorts of feelings. I don't think I want to get into that right now. I don't
   feel really bad about the future.

D: That's fine, Joseph. If you're uncomfortable with certain questions please let me know.

J: Don't take it the wrong way, Doctor. I mean, we've all got guilty feelings. I just don't feel like talking about that.

D: You told me earlier that you had difficulty concentrating.

J: Yes, that's right. I just can't seem to focus. I mean, I don't think I'm going senile or anything. I love reading, Doctor. I can finish a novel in a week or so. Now I have so much trouble paying attention to what I'm reading sometimes.

D: I need to ask you, Joseph, if you have had thoughts of suicide or made any attempts.

J: Oh no, Doctor. I don't believe in that sort of stuff at all. It pains me to see so many young people throwing their life away that way. No, I've never been suicidal at all.

D: That's reassuring to hear, Joseph. Has anyone in your family had trouble with depression or made suicide attempts?

J: No, Doctor. No one that I know of.

D: How do you normally spend your time, Joseph? Do you spend it with friends?

J: I don't have too many, Doctor. The social club in town is full of World War II vets, and I used to go there. I don't know, they're really not my kind of people. They complain about everything. They all head to Florida come November and complain about getting sunburnt. I just never felt I belonged there. I mostly keep in touch with Victoria, Ted, and the kids. That's all, Doctor.

D: Do you ever get lonely?

J: I miss Beatrice terribly, Doctor.

At this point, Joseph looks as if he is about to cry. He lowers his head and covers his face with his hands for a few seconds. He returns to his previous posture with a calm, composed expression.

D: I do miss her a lot, Doctor. She was taken from me when she was far too young. Three months ago was the 20th anniversary of her death.

D: Losing your wife must have been a terrible experience for you, Joseph. I'm truly sorry.

J: Thank you, Doctor. Life has its ups and downs, I guess.

Questions

1. Is Joseph depressed?
2. The loss of his wife appears to be a very traumatic episode in Joseph's life. Could it be responsible for his present condition?
3. Laboratory investigations were discussed earlier. Would you like to obtain any tests now?

Discussion

1. There is no doubt that Joseph suffers from a depressive disorder. The focus of the interview is on determining the presence of major depression. Though Joseph is not all that forthcoming on certain issues, he does provide a convincing history of major depression. He has had depressed mood for more than 2 weeks. He

complains of lack of interest in usual activities. He has compromised sleep. He complains of fatigue and sluggishness. He complains of inability to concentrate. It is already known that he has lost weight. He has met the requisite number of criteria for major depressive illness. The dialogue above is clearly somewhat of an idealized clinical interview. Many elderly patients may not be as informative. Furthermore, as pointed out earlier, symptoms may not so neatly fit the *DSM* guidelines for major depression. This, as pointed out earlier, is extremely common in the setting of primary care and in some ways represents a shortcoming of *DSM* criteria for depression (Lemelin et al., 1994).

2. No training in family medicine is needed to realize that traumatic events, such as the unexpected death of a spouse, are associated with profound grief and often with persistent effects on outlook and behavior. Depression in its most severe forms is not regarded as a simple reaction to life circumstances but rather as a serious and treatable disease. Nevertheless, as noted previously, stressful life events are risk factors for major depression. The depression that immediately follows death of a spouse, regardless of its severity, is classified by *DSM-IIIR* as "uncomplicated bereavement" (APA, 1987). Zisook and Shuchter (1991), in a prospective study of recent widows and widowers, found that a substantial number suffer depressive symptoms of sufficient severity to meet the criteria for major depression. The prevalence of such major depression decreased from the time of death of the spouse. Of the 250 patients followed, 24% reported symptoms consistent with major depression at the end of 2 months of bereavement. Even at 13 months, 16% of patients had depression severe enough to be called major depres-

sion. Follow-up was not continued beyond 13 months.

Did Beatrice's death precipitate Joseph's present depression? Uncomplicated bereavement rarely begins more than 2 to 3 months after the loss. It is possible that the recent 20th anniversary of Beatrice's death was the precipitant. It is also possible that Joseph's depressed state has brought painful memories of the loss of his wife to the surface. In short, there is no easy answer to this question, and for practical purposes, there may be no need to answer it at this time from the point of view of diagnosis and management. Joseph has major depression, and treating it should be the priority.

3. The next step in the evaluation of depressed patients is a complete medical history and physical examination to search for one or more causes or factors associated with major depression. Roughly 10% to 15% of cases of major depression are caused by medical illnesses such as thyroid disease or other conditions such as substance abuse (USDHHS, 1993b). This evaluation has been completed, albeit without a confirmed diagnosis of depression, in conjunction with the evaluation of involuntary weight loss. A renewed consideration of laboratory investigations is appropriate at this time. Laboratory tests may be used to screen for medical causes of depression and to confirm the diagnosis by detecting abnormalities characteristic of the disease (USDHHS, 1993b). Respecting the latter, the search for biological correlates of depression in the elderly has revealed no tests of sufficient sensitivity and specificity to aid in the diagnosis. There is some indication that impaired dexamethasone suppression of the hypothalamic-pituitary-adrenal axis, for example, occurs in elderly depressed

patients, but this information has yet to be used to develop a useful test to support the diagnosis of depression (NIH, 1992).

Blazer (1989) emphasizes the utility of a battery of screening tests, including a CBC, serum B12, and folate and thyroid function studies, to find associated medical conditions. The AHCPR, on the other hand, advocates a conservative approach to ordering laboratory investigations to identify medical causes of depression. No universal screening panel is recommended. Laboratory tests produce higher yield in older patients, in patients in whom the first depressive episode occurs after age 40, in patients unresponsive to routine treatment, and in those in whom the review of systems reveals signs and symptoms uncommonly encountered in routine cases of depression (USDHHS, 1993b). Thyroid function tests, for example, can be ordered in depressed patients with symptoms of thyroid disease but should not be performed on all depressed patients. Joseph has no signs or symptoms of any serious medical illnesses. It is best, once again, to forgo laboratory testing at this time.

PART IV

The Problem

Upon conclusion of your interview, you decide that Joseph Drumdonald is suffering from major depression. You inform the patient of this. "Well, Doctor, I have been very down—no doubt about it. You're not going to send me to a shrink, are you?"

You tell Joseph that most cases of uncomplicated major depression can be adequately treated by a family physician and that at this time there is no need for him to see a psychiatrist. You acknowledge that the idea of seeing a psychiatrist does not seem to appeal to him.

"I've got nothing against psychiatrists, Doctor," Joseph says. "I trust you. If you can help me, I'd greatly appreciate it."

Questions

1. In broad terms, which categories of therapy are available for depression?
2. What form or forms of therapy would you recommend for Joseph?
3. You have informed Joseph that he suffers from major depression. What more would you like to tell him about this illness?

Discussion

1. The AHCPR (USDHHS, 1993c) classifies the treatments of major depression into four large categories that include **medication, psychotherapy, a combination of medication and psychotherapy, and electroconvulsive therapy** (ECT). In addition, Shearer and Adams (1993) describe other nonpharmacological aids in the treatment of depression, including environmental management, prescribed pleasurable activity, and exercise. Environmental management involves avoiding

circumstances in which depressive symptoms are made worse. Spending time indoors, for example, if it exacerbates depression, should be avoided by spending more time outside. Shearer and Adams recommend the "prescription" of one pleasurable activity each day, such as listening to music, regardless of whether such activities provide pleasure to the depressed patient. These types of nonpharmacologic interventions were not evaluated by the AHCPR, and the evidence for their efficacy is scant. Nevertheless, there is an obvious intuitive basis for many such activities, such as exercise, which is known to improve well-being. Moreover, such nonpharmacologic interventions are unlikely to be detrimental in any way. Discussion participants, therefore, may wish to incorporate environmental management, pleasurable activity, and exercise into the overall management plan.

2. The goals of therapy for major depression are to reduce or eliminate signs and symptoms, restore occupational and psychosocial function, and prevent relapse (USDHHS, 1993c). There is evidence of varying persuasiveness for the efficacy of medications, psychotherapy, combination therapy, and ECT in different circumstances for the treatment of depression. ECT is generally reserved as first-line therapy for extremely severe forms of depression or for depression complicated by psychotic features (USDHHS, 1993c).

Various forms of psychotherapy have been popularized recently as effective forms of therapy for depression. These include cognitive **behavioral therapy, brief dynamic psychotherapy, and interpersonal psychotherapy.** Most trials designed to assess the efficacy of these forms of psychotherapy have enrolled patients with mild or moderate depressive symptomatology. Such studies have recently been subjected to considerable criticism. Hartman and Lazarus (1992) point out, for example, that the assessment of outcome in studies of psychotherapy has been questionable. Furthermore, many trials of psychotherapy have used a so-called *waitlist* control. A treatment group receiving psychotherapy is compared to a control group that receives no treatment during the trial. Patients with more severe symptoms may refuse to be waitlisted, making the control and treatment groups incomparable at the outset.

Hartman and Lazarus (1992) also point out that the results of many trials of psychotherapy have been difficult to explain. In a study by Thompson and Gallagher (1987), the effectiveness of three completely different forms of short-term psychotherapy for depression (brief cognitive therapy [BCT], behavioral therapy, and psychodynamic therapy) was evaluated. All three therapies produced similar high rates of positive outcomes compared to waitlisted controls. This leads one to question what specifically about psychotherapy influences outcome. There is the possibility that simple contact with a supportive therapist, regardless of the specifics of the therapy, is sufficient to produce a positive outcome. In this context, the results of the National Institute of Mental Health (NIMH) Treatment of Depression Collaborative Research Program (Elkin et al., 1989) are important to consider. Random assignment to one of four treatment groups was made for 250 patients. The treatment groups involved (a) imipramine plus clinical management, consisting of weekly 20- to 30-min sessions with a blinded qualified professional who reviewed symptoms and side effects and offered support; (b) a placebo group that received placebo medication and the same clinical management; (c) a group that received interpersonal psychotherapy; and (d) a group that received cognitive behavioral therapy. The placebo group in this trial was therefore not a waitlist group or a "no treatment" group, as patients did receive some contact and support from a qualified mental health professional. Overall, for patients with "mild" depressive symptoms, there was no significant difference in outcome among the four groups. For more severely depressed patients, imipramine plus clinical management was the superior treatment. The two psychotherapies were less effective, with interpersonal therapy slightly better than cognitive behavioral therapy. The placebo treatment was significantly less effective than the other three among more severely depressed patients.

The NIMH results should not be presented to discussion participants as "gospel" or the final word on the value of psychotherapy but rather as a study in which some of the methodological concerns raised by many critics have been addressed. What is the final word on psychotherapy for depression? The AHCPR (USDHHD, 1993c) has found that in general, there is evidence for the efficacy of various forms of psychotherapy as the sole treatment in patients with milder forms of depression. There are various ways to measure the severity of depression that are beyond the scope of this exercise. It is fair to say that Joseph, who has been depressed for some time and has lost a significant amount of weight as a consequence, suffers from moderate to severe depression.

Combination psychotherapy and medication is helpful for patients with a partial response to either therapy alone but is not known to have any specific advantage in the initial treatment of uncomplicated depression (USDHHS, 1993c).

The preceding discussion clearly points to medication as the most appropriate form of therapy for Joseph Drumdonald. There is a large body of evidence supporting the efficacy of antidepressant medication. The evidence is compelling enough that the AHCPR (USDHHS, 1993c) recommends that all patients with moderate to severe major depressive disorder be treated initially with medication, whether or not psychotherapy is used. The ultimate choice of antidepressant therapy, of course, should respect the patient's own preference. Some patients are wary of taking medications, others of receiving psychotherapy.

3. Obviously, even medication treatment of depression should be accompanied by appropriate counseling and support, as was the case in the NIMH trial (Elkin et al., 1989). Patient education should include certain key points; education is known to positively influence the patient's compliance with treatment (USDHHS, 1993a). Joseph should be told that depression is a medical illness. He should be told that the vast majority of patients recover, and that there are many effective treatments. He should be informed that the aim of treatment is complete symptom remission but that a large number of patients experience relapse (roughly 50% after treatment is discontinued). He and his family should be informed that it is important to seek help as soon as possible, should signs and symptoms of depression reappear after successful treatment. Shearer and Adams (1993) also emphasize that the patient, his or her family, and the physician should develop a plan to assure the patient's safety should suicidal tendencies appear.

PART V

The Problem

You inform Joseph that depression is a curable medical illness, with a number of effective treatments available. You tell him, however, that recurrence is extremely common and that it is important once treatment is successful to inform you of any signs or symptoms of relapse, such as depressed mood, poor sleep or appetite, or feelings of guilt or worthlessness. Joseph has no suicidal ideation, but you emphasize the importance of developing a plan to ensure his safety if such tendencies appear. Joseph has no weapons, medications, or other obvious suicide tools in his home. He agrees to call Victoria should he at any time feel suicidal. Furthermore, with Joseph's permission, you call Victoria and ask her to bring Joseph to her home should he express any suicidal thoughts or should she suspect suicidal intentions on his part. She agrees to this plan.

You discuss the two main commonly employed initial modes of therapy for major depression, namely psychotherapy and medications. You have no formal training in any form of psychotherapy, so you inform the patient that he would probably have to see another health care professional to receive it. You also tell Joseph that medications have a long, proven track record in treating moderate or severe depression.

Joseph responds in a quiet, somber tone, "Doctor, as I said, I do trust you. I don't think psychotherapy is for me. I mean, I don't know much about it, but I can't see myself enjoying it very much. I'm really down, and I need help. I don't need anyone messing within my mind."

You tell Joseph that psychotherapy can be effective, but that you respect his decision to decline it.

Questions

1. What are the main types of medications used to treat depression?
2. What would you prescribe for Joseph?
3. When would you like to see the patient again?

Discussion

1. Several categories of medications are used to treat depression. The **tricyclic antidepressants** have been available for many years and are known to be effective and inexpensive. The **heterocyclic antidepressants** include bupropion and trazodone. The **monoamine oxidase inhibitors** (MAOIS) include isocaboxacid and tranylcypromine. The relatively new **selective serotonin reuptake inhibitors** (SSRIs) include the original fluoxetine and the newer fluvoxamine, paroxetine, and sertraline. Finally, **anxiolytic medications,** including alprazolam, buspirone, diazepam, and chlordiazepoxide, are uncommonly used in the treatment of depression.

2. Of the medications commonly used to treat depression, no one medication is significantly more effective than any other. The choice of antidepressant, therefore, should not be made on the basis of efficacy

but rather on a number of other factors (USDHHS, 1993c), which include the following: **side effects; prior response to a particular medication, either by the patient or by a first-degree relative; concurrent medical illnesses and medication use; type of depression; and cost, convenience, practitioner's experience with a particular medication, and other factors.**

Neither Joseph nor, to the best of his knowledge, anyone in his immediate family has been treated for major depression in the past. Joseph has no known concurrent medical illnesses nor does he take any medications at present. The selection of an antidepressant medication depends therefore on other variables—most important, side effects.

The side effects of antidepressants can be classified as **anticholinergic** (i.e., dry mouth, blurred vision, urinary hesitancy, constipation), CNS (principally drowsiness or insomnia), **cardiovascular** (mainly orthostatic hypotension or cardiac arrhythmias), and **gastrointestinal** (e.g., bloating, abdominal cramping, and increased appetite and weight gain).

In general, the tricyclic antidepressants are associated with anticholinergic side effects, significant orthostatic hypotension, drowsiness, weight gain, and cardiac arrhythmias in predisposed patients or with overdose. The SSRIs are generally safer but are often associated with insomnia, agitation and GI discomfort. The MAOIs have a mix of side effects and are commonly used to treat depression that has proved resistant to other antidepressants or depression presenting with atypical features, such as weight gain or increased sleep rather than weight loss and insomnia. It is best to review Joseph's circumstances now, prior to selection of an agent. He is an elderly man without any serious medical problems, including no history of cardiac arrhythmias or other heart disease. He presents with typical major depression characterized by profound loss of appetite and weight and early-morning awakening. An antidepressant should be chosen that has minimal adverse effects, but the side-effect profile of a medication can be an advantage. The side effects of increased appetite and drowsiness may help Joseph restore his weight and sleep pattern. The side-effect profiles of the major antidepressants are shown in Figure 1.2.

An excellent choice for Joseph is a tricyclic antidepressant of the secondary amine variety, such as nortriptyline or desipramine. These medications have fewer anticholinergic side effects than other tricyclics of the tertiary amine variety (USDHHS, 1993a). Moreover, rather than aggravating insomnia or weight loss, as is often the case with SSRIs, nortriptyline and similar medications are associated with drowsiness and moderate weight gain. The tricyclics, unlike the SSRIs, are inexpensive. They lack the convenience of some SSRIs, however, whose starting dose is often the effective therapeutic dose. Most tricyclics require gradual dosage increases (Zisook, 1996). The initial starting dose of nortriptyline is 10 mg per day, administered as a single dose at bedtime. It can be adjusted at a frequency of q3 days to a standard therapeutic dose of 20 to 100 mg/day (Zisook, 1996).

3. The initiation of treatment begins the **acute phase** of management of depression. Joseph should be seen frequently during this period, roughly weekly for 6 to 8 weeks (USDHHS, 1993c), not only to review his symptoms but to monitor medication side effects, make dosage adjustments, and provide ongoing support.

| Drug | Anticholinergic[b] | Central Nervous System | | Cardiovascular | | | Other |
		Drowsiness	Insomnia/ Agitation	Orthostatic Hypotension	Cardiac Arrhythmia	Gastrointestinal Distress	Weight Gain (Over 6 kg)
Amitriptyline	4+	4+	0	4+	3+	0	4+
Desipramine	1+	1+	1+	2+	2+	0	1+
Doxepin	3+	4+	0	2+	2+	0	3+
Imipramine	3+	3+	1+	4+	3+	1+	3+
Nortriptyline	1+	1+	0	2+	2+	0	1+
Protriptyline	2+	1+	1+	2+	2+	0	0
Trimipramine	1+	4+	0	2+	2+	0	3+
Amoxapine	2+	2+	2+	2+	3+	0	1+
Maprotiline	2+	4+	0	0	1+	0	2+
Trazodone	0	4+	0	1+	1+	1+	1+
Bupropion	0	0	2+	0	1+	1+	0
Fluoxetine	0	0	2+	0	0	3+	0
Paroxetine	0	0	2+	0	0	3+	0
Sertraline	0	0	2+	0	0	3+	0
Monoamine oxidase inhibitors (MAOIs)	1	1+	2+	2+	0	1+	2+

Side Effect[a] spans the Central Nervous System and Cardiovascular headings.

SOURCE: USDHHS (1993a, p. 14).
NOTES: a. 0 = absent or rare; 2+ = in between; 4+ = relatively common.
    b. Dry mouth, blurred vision, urinary hesitancy, constipation.

Figure 1.2   Side-Effect Profiles of Antidepressant Medications

PART VI

The Problem

You prescribe nortryptiline for Joseph at a dose of 10 mg at bedtime for 3 days and then 20 mg for 4 days. You explain the benefits and side effects of this medication. You ask him to return in 1 week and to call should he have any questions or concerns in the interim.

Joseph returns to your office for follow-up. He tells you he has been sleeping better. He no longer reports early-morning awakening, and he actually reports some daytime drowsiness. He says he continues to feel down, with no improvement in his mood. His appetite remains poor. He has had little interest in engaging in previously enjoyable activities, such as visiting his daughter and son-in-law. Joseph reports no dry mouth, blurred vision, urinary hesitancy, or constipation. He reports no dizziness or weakness upon standing.

Questions

1. Would you increase the dose of nortryptiline?

Discussion

1. Joseph is responding to a relatively low dose of nortryptiline (20 mg qHS), as evidenced by the improvement in his sleep. Dosage adjustments can be made on the basis of side effects, which in Joseph's case are not present except for some daytime drowsiness. Side effects are likely to diminish with time. There are well-established minimal therapeutic blood levels for nortriptyline, desipramine, imipramine, and amitriptyline. Toxic blood levels have also been established for some antidepressants. Blood-level monitoring is not recommended for all patients, but it is recommended for certain groups including, among others, *patients who respond poorly to treatment or who develop signs of toxicity; patients with concurrent medical illnesses or medication use; and elderly patients.* Conditions such as age or specific illness can affect the metabolism of antidepressants in the body, making it difficult to predict what a therapeutic dose would be (USDHHS, 1993c). There is no need to increase Joseph's dose at the present time, especially without a serum nortryptiline level. A treatment failure is generally considered to have taken place if the serum level of antidepressant is within the therapeutic range for 2 to 4 weeks and the patient shows little or no symptomatic improvement.

At this visit, in addition to offering ongoing support and encouragement, Joseph should be told that the drowsiness and consequent improvement in his sleep are to be expected with nortryptiline. A nortryptiline level can be obtained at this visit. Joseph's physician should be available by telephone should Joseph have any questions or concerns. He should continue to be seen frequently during this acute phase of management.

PART VII

The Problem

You tell Joseph that the improvement in sleep and slight daytime sleepiness are both effects of the medications and that his mood and energy levels should improve in the coming weeks. You obtain a serum nortryptiline level at this visit, which returns 2 days later as considerably subtherapeutic.

You gradually increase Joseph's dose of nortryptiline to 40 mg po qHS over the next 2 weeks. You continue to see him weekly and monitor his nortryptiline levels, which remain in the low therapeutic range, biweekly. Joseph gradually reports improving mood and energy. He begins to pursue many of his usual activities, especially spending time with his family. His appetite improves dramatically, such that 4 weeks after beginning treatment, Joseph has gained 6 kg. His sleep normalizes within 3 weeks.

With Joseph's permission, you call Victoria, who tells you she's delighted with the change in her father's condition. "Dad is back to his usual self! He loves playing with the kids. He's talking about making plans for the holidays. It's wonderful." Victoria repeatedly expresses her gratitude for your help.

Six weeks after beginning treatment, Joseph returns to your office. You realize immediately that he behaves quite differently than at your first encounter. Joseph is engaging, softspoken but cheerful. Excerpts from your encounter are represented below.

Doctor: So, Joseph, it looks like things are going pretty well.
Joseph: I certainly can't complain, Doctor. I can't thank you enough. Victoria was so worried about me. I was so miserable. I feel just fine, Doctor.
D: You would say your mood is back to normal?
J: Definitely. I mean, I get upset once in awhile, just like the next guy. I don't feel down any more. It's a miracle what those pills can do for you.
D: How is your energy level?
J: It's great, Doctor. I'm outside most of the time. We've got a barn out back that I've been meaning to fix up for quite a while. I finally feel like I can do it.
D: How is your concentration?
J: It's been pretty good, I guess. I mean, I'm no spring chicken. I realize that. I love reading, and I'm getting back to that now.
D: I know you've gained plenty of weight recently. How would you describe your appetite?
J: Bit too much of an appetite if anything, Doctor!

For the first time in your encounters with Joseph, he laughs, after exercising his wit.

J: So doctor, now that I'm cured, can I stop taking the nortryptiline?

Questions

1. How would you answer Joseph's question?

Discussion

1. The acute phase of treatment ends upon recovery from the episode of major depression, which appears to have taken place. Roughly 25% of patients will relapse into an episode of depression upon discontinuation of treatment at this point (USDHHS, 1993c). For this reason, **continuation treatment** in the form of medication at the same dosage for 4 to 9 months is recommended for patients who respond completely to acute-phase medication (USDHHS, 1993c). Continuation treatment significantly reduces the likelihood of relapse. Patients who have frequent, recurrent episodes of depression that respond to treatment are sometimes prescribed long-term **maintenance therapy.** Fortunately, Joseph does not yet fall into this category.

Conclusion

You explain to Joseph that, although he has recovered from his episode of major depression, the likelihood of relapse remains high, and continuing his medication for 4 to 9 months is a way of preventing this.

He tells you, "Well, I'm not big on taking pills, but I've gotten used to it. I don't want to feel that miserable again. I'll continue taking the medication. You've helped me so much, Doctor. You've helped me get so far. I don't want to fall back into a depression."

You acknowledge Joseph's gratitude. You review the signs and symptoms of depression and ask Joseph to contact you should these recur. You tell Joseph that you continue to be available for help and advice, and you ask to see him in 1 month to continue to monitor his symptoms, nortryptiline level, and any side effects.

References

Alexopoulos, G. S., & Chester, J. G. (1992). Outcomes of geriatric depression. *Clinics in Geriatric Medicine, 8*(2), 363-376.

American Psychiatric Association. (1987). *Diagnostic and statistical manual of mental disorders* (3rd ed., Rev.). Washington, DC: Author.

American Psychiatric Association. (1995a). *Diagnostic and statistical manual of mental disorders* (4th ed.). Washington, DC: Author.

American Psychiatric Association. (1995b). *Diagnostic and statistical manual of mental disorders: Primary care version* (4th ed.). Washington, DC: Author.

Blazer, D. (1989). Current concepts: Depression in the elderly. *New England Journal of Medicine, 320*(3), 164-166.

Drossman, D. A. (1995). Approach to the patient with unexplained weight loss. In T. Yamada (Ed.), *Textbook of gastroenterology* (2nd ed.; pp. 717-730). Philadelphia, PA: J. B. Lippincott.

Elkin, I., Shea, M. T., Watkins, J. T., Imber, S. D., Sotsky, S. M., Collins, J. F., Glass, D. R., Pilkonis, P. A., Leber, W. R., & Docherty, J. P. (1989). National Institute of Mental Health Treatment of Depression Collaborative Research Program: General effectiveness of treatments. *Archives of General Psychology, 46*, 971-982.

Folstein, M. F., Folstein, S. E., & McHugh, P. R. (1975). Mini-mental state: A practical method for grading the cognitive state of patients for the clinician. *Journal of Psychiatric Research, 12*, 189-198.

Goroll, A. H. (1995). Evaluation of weight loss. In A. H. Goroll, L. A. May, & A. G. Mulley (Eds.), *Primary care medicine: Office evaluation of the adult patient* (3rd ed.; pp. 38-42). Philadelphia, PA: J. B. Lippincott.

Hartman, C., & Lazarus, L. W. (1992). Psychotherapy with elderly depressed patients. *Clinics in Geriatric Medicine, 8*(2), 355-362.

Lemelin, J., Hotz, S., Swensen, R., & Elmslie, T. (1994). Depression in primary care: Why do we miss the diagnosis? *Canadian Family Physician, 40*, 104-108.

Marton, K.I., Sox, H.C., & Krupp, J. R. (1981). Involuntary weight loss: Diagnostic and prognostic significance. *Annals of Internal Medicine, 95*, 569-574.

Menscer, D., & Leitch, B. B. (1993). Approach to the geriatric patient. In P. D. Sloane, L. M. Slatt, & P. Curtis (Eds.), *Essentials of family medicine* (p. 90). Baltimore, MD: Williams and Wilkins.

Morley, J. E. (1990). Anorexia in older patients: Its meaning and management. *Geriatrics, 45*(12), 59-66.

National Institutes of Health Consensus Development Panel on Depression in Late Life. (1992). Diagnosis and treatment of depression in late life. *Journal of the American Medical Association, 268*(8), 1018-1024.

Rabinovitz, M., Pitlik, S. D., Leifer, M., Garty, M., & Rosenfeld, J. B. (1986). Unintentional weight loss: A retrospective analysis of 154 cases. *Archives of Internal Medicine, 146*, 186-187.

Robbins, L. J. (1989). Evaluation of weight loss in the elderly. *Geriatrics, 44*(4), 31-37.

Shearer, S. L., & Adams, G. K. (1993). Nonpharmacologic aids in the treatment of depression. *American Family Physician, 47*(2), 435-441.

Thompson, L. W., & Gallagher, D. (1987). Comparative effectiveness of psychotherapies for depressed elders. *Journal of Consulting and Clinical Psychology, 55*, 385-390.

Thompson, M. P., & Morris, L. K. (1991). Unexplained weight loss in the ambulatory elderly. *Journal of the American Geriatrics Society, 39*, 497-500.

U.S. Department of Health and Human Services, Public Health Service, Agency for Health Care Policy and Research. (1993a). *Depression in primary care: Detection, diagnosis and treatment. Quick reference guide for clinicians* (AHCPR Publication No. 93-0552). Rockville, MD: U.S. Department of Health and Human Services.

U.S. Department of Health and Human Services, Public Health Service, Agency for Health Care Policy and Research. (1993b). *Depression in primary care: Vol. 1. Detection and diagnosis* (AHCPR Publication No. 93-0550). Rockville, MD: U.S. Department of Health and Human Services.

U.S. Department of Health and Human Services, Public Health Service, Agency for Health Care Policy and Research. (1993c). *Depression in primary care: Vol. 2. Treatment of major depression* (AHCPR Publication No. 93-0551). Rockville, MD: U.S. Department of Health and Human Services.

Wise, G. R., & Craig, D. (1995). Evaluation of involuntary weight loss: Where do you start? *Postgraduate Medicine, 95*(4), 143-150.

Yesavage, J. A. (1992). Depression in the elderly: How to recognize masked symptoms and choose appropriate therapy. *Postgraduate Medicine, 91*(1), 255-261.

Zisook, S. (1996). Depression in late life: Special considerations in treatment. *Postgraduate Medicine, 100*(4), 161-172.

Zisook, S., & Shuchter, S. R. (1991). Depression through the first year after the death of a spouse. *American Journal of Psychiatry, 148*(10), 1346-1352.

Appendix
Geriatric Depression Scale

Choose the best answer to describe how you have felt over the past week:

1. Are you basically satisfied with your life?	Yes	No*
2. Have you dropped many of your activities and interests?	Yes*	No
3. Do you feel that your life is empty?	Yes*	No
4. Do you often get bored?	Yes*	No
5. Are you in good spirits most of the time?	Yes	No*
6. Are you afraid that something bad is going to happen to you?	Yes*	No
7. Do you feel happy most of the time?	Yes	No*
8. Do you feel helpless?	Yes*	No
9. Do you prefer to stay at home, rather than going out and doing new things?	Yes*	No
10. Do you feel you have more problems with memory than most?	Yes*	No
11. Do you feel it is wonderful to be alive now?	Yes	No*
12. Do you feel pretty worthless the way you are now?	Yes*	No
13. Do you feel full of energy?	Yes	No*
14. Do you feel your situation is hopeless?	Yes*	No
15. Do you think that most people are better off than you are?	Yes*	No

SOURCE: Yesavage (1992). Used with permission.
NOTE: * Responses are indicative of depression. Five to nine of the asterisked responses indicates the possibility of depression. Ten or more is virtually diagnostic of depression.

Diagnostic Criteria for
Major Depressive Episode

A. Five (or more) of the following symptoms have been present during the same 2-week period and represent a change from previous functioning; at least one of the symptoms is either (1) depressed mood, or (2) loss of interest or pleasure. Note: Do not include symptoms that are clearly due to a general medical condition, mood-incongruent, delusions or hallucinations.

  (1) depressed mood most of the day, nearly every day, as indicated by either subjective report (e.g., feels sad or empty) or observation made by others (e.g., appears tearful). Note: In children and adolescents, can be irritable mood.

  (2) markedly diminished interest or pleasure in all, or almost all, activities most of the day, nearly every day (as indicated by either subjective account or observation made by others)

  (3) significant weight loss when not dieting or weight gain (e.g., a change of more than 5% of body weight in a month), or decrease or increase in appetite nearly every day. Note: In children, consider failure to make expected weight gains.

  (4) insomnia or hypersomnia nearly every day

  (5) psychomotor agitation or retardation nearly every day (observable by others, not merely subjective feelings of restlessness or being slowed down)

  (6) fatigue or loss of energy nearly every day

  (7) feelings of worthlessness or excessive or inappropriate guilt (which may be delusional) nearly every day (not merely self-reproach or guilt about being sick)

  (8) diminished ability to think or concentrate, or indecisiveness, nearly every day (either by subjective account or as observed by others)

  (9) recurrent thoughts of death (not just fear of dying), recurrent suicidal ideation without a specific plan, or a suicide attempt or a specific plan for committing suicide

B. The symptoms do not meet criteria for a Mixed Episode.

C. The symptoms cause clinically significant distress or impairment in social, occupational, or other important areas of functioning.

D. The symptoms are not due to the direct physiological effects of a substance (e.g., a drug of abuse, a medication) or a general medical condition (e.g., hypothyroidism).

E. The symptoms are not better accounted for by Bereavement, i.e., after the loss of a loved one, the symptoms persist for longer than 2 months or are characterized by marked functional impairment, morbid preoccupation with worthlessness, suicidal ideation, psychotic symptoms, or psychomotor retardation.

SOURCE: Reprinted with permission from the *Diagnostic and Statistical Manual of Mental Disorders*, Fourth Edition. Copyright © 1994 American Psychiatric Association.

Mini–Mental Status Examination

Scoring: 1 point per correct answer. Fewer than 24 correct strongly suggests dementia.

	Item	Score

Orientation

1-5	"What is today's date?" (ask specifically parts omitted)	1. Date	_____
		2. Year	_____
		3. Month	_____
		4. Day of week	_____
		5. Season	_____
6-10	"Can you tell me the name of the place where we are today? What floor are we on? What town are we in? What county are we in? What state are we in?"	6. Institution	_____
		7. Floor	_____
		8. Town (city)	_____
		9. County	_____
		10. State	_____

Registration

11-13	Ask if you may test memory. Use 3 objects: ball, flag, and tree. State them slowly and clearly. Ask for them to be repeated. The first repetition determines the score (0-3), but continue until repeated correctly (maximum 6 tries).	11. "Ball"	_____
		12. "Flag"	_____
		13. "Tree"	_____

Attention and calculation

14-18	"Begin with 100 and count backwards by 7." Stop after 5 subtractions (65). Score the total number of correct answers. If the subject cannot perform this, ask him to spell "world" backwards, scoring the number of letters in correct order.	14. "93"	_____
		15. "86"	_____
		16. "79"	_____
		17. "72"	_____
		18. "65"	_____
		alt. "dlrow"	_____

Recall

19-21	"Now recall the 3 words I asked you to remember"	19. "Ball"	_____
		20. "Flag"	_____
		21. "Tree"	_____

Language

22-23	Naming: Show and ask the names of: wrist watch, pencil	22. Watch	_____
		23. Pencil	_____
24	Repetition: "No ifs, ands, or buts"	24. Repetition	_____
25-27	3-stage command: Give the subject a blank sheet of paper and say "Take the paper in your right hand, fold it in half, and place on the floor"	25. Takes	_____
		26. Folds	_____
		27. Places	_____
28	Reading: Print "close your eyes" in large letters and have the subject read it. Score correct only if eyes close.	28. Reading	_____
29	Spontaneous writing: Ask the subject to write a sentence on a sheet of paper	29. Sensible sentence with subject/verb	_____
30	Copying: "Draw this figure." All 10 angles must be present and 2 intersect	30. Draws pentagons	_____
		TOTAL SCORE	_____

SOURCE: From Menscer and Leitch (1993).

2. INSOMNIA

Mr. Raffi Olefsky

*Goal: The goal of this group discussion exercise is
to assess and enrich the participants' understanding
of the evaluation and treatment of insomnia.*

Specific Objectives: Upon completion of this exercise, each participant should be able to accomplish the following:

1. Obtain a thorough history from a patient who complains of insomnia, taking into consideration possible medical, psychiatric, and substance-related factors.
2. Describe the essential elements of "good sleep hygiene."
3. Describe the way in which sleep disorders are classified, in general terms.
4. List the categories of pharmacologic agents used to treat insomnia.
5. Describe the indications for polysomnography.
6. Initiate and supervise a program of sleep restriction for a patient suffering from insomnia.

PART I

The Patient

Social History

Raffi Olefsky has certainly led an interesting life. Born in Moscow to a Jewish father and Armenian mother, both of whom were successful musicians, he began playing the violin at the age of 4 years. He exhibited enormous promise and was welcomed by the finest schools and instructed by some of the greatest violinists in the former Soviet Union. As a boy, he dazzled Nikita Khrushchev with his extraordinary gift during a special concert at the Kremlin. Raffi also toured the great concert halls of Europe with a prestigious youth symphony. At the tender age of 18, after years of having been showered with applause, having innumerable awards bestowed upon him, and being lauded as the greatest young talent in the country, Raffi was asked to join the Moscow Symphony. It was an opportunity that would take his career to even greater heights.

An international tour in 1977 brought Raffi, then just 22, and the rest of the orchestra to Montreal. It was in Canada, during the height of the Cold War, that Raffi and four other orchestra members decided to defect from the Soviet Union and start a new life. Raffi admits it was a poorly conceived plan. "We had no idea what to do or how to go about it. We saw Jaguars and Mercedes cars on the streets, fancy stores, and beautiful women. We thought this was our best chance to enjoy the good life." Raffi and his four comrades fled their hotel one night after the first of two concerts. Three of the five were soon caught and forced to return. Only Raffi and Vladimir Bykov, a brilliant cellist, escaped the reins of the symphony and its innumerable handlers and agents and presented themselves the next morning at a Canadian immigration office, seeking political asylum. It was a story that made headlines everywhere. The two musicians were allowed to stay in Canada, and Raffi had no difficulty in finding a position with the Orchestre Symphonique de Montreal.

The young violinist's career continued to flourish in the West until 1985, when a female member of the symphony accused Raffi of persistent sexual harassment. To this day, Raffi denies any wrongdoing. As he insists, "I never bothered anyone. I am someone who is easily misinterpreted." Several unsuccessful attempts were made, by the symphony's director and others, to resolve this matter discretely. Soon, three other female musicians came forward with similar complaints. Raffi was politely asked to leave the symphony in October 1985. His reputation tarnished, Raffi subsequently found it hard to find work. He performed briefly with symphonies in Cleveland, Winnipeg, and Houston. Despite his great talent, musical directors were reluctant to give Raffi a "starring role" or "special billing" for fear that too much attention would bring to light the ugly affair in Montreal and destroy their own symphony's reputation. Frustrated by these circumstances, Raffi gave up his career as a concert violinist in 1986 and returned to Montreal virtually penniless.

In the years that followed, Raffi made a living in a number of ways, some quite unusual. He started a violin repair business. He was neither a craftsman nor a technician and relied on his musical insight to "repair violins so that they sounded good." The business, catering to such a tiny market and with an inexperienced man at the helm, was a complete failure. Raffi then began earning small sums of money giving private violin lessons. He worked briefly in a music store. For a time he sold designer clothing door to door. He edited a newspaper catering to the Russian-Canadian community. He even worked for a dog-walking service, walking the dogs of those who dared not go outside in the dead of winter.

In 1988, he met Marie-Claude Bouchard, a biotechnologist, at a party thrown by a mutual friend. Raffi, who describes himself as "having a way with women," charmed the attractive Marie-Claude with his rare wit and the intriguing story of his life, omitting, of course, the accusations of sexual harassment. The two began a relationship and were married in 1991. It was a rocky marriage virtually from the start. With a hardworking wife who made a good living, Raffi no longer felt a need to struggle to support himself. He began to pursue several peculiar interests, including collecting exotic fish and birds, hobbies that put considerable strain on the family purse. Marie-Claude would often come home after a hard day at work to find a note from Raffi stating that he was out "having a drink with friends." She began to suspect that some of these "friends" were actually women with whom her husband was having extramarital affairs. In any case, for these and other reasons, the marriage fell apart. The couple was separated in 1994 and formally divorced in 1995.

Today Raffi lives alone in a one-bedroom apartment in downtown Montreal. He makes a fairly comfortable living as a violin instructor at a music school. He has adopted a more disciplined lifestyle and no longer spends his evenings out on the town. He is a charismatic and amicable person who has many friends from many walks of life. He enjoys reading, watching television, and playing chess. He spends roughly 3 to 4 hr a day playing the violin, an activity he still enjoys immensely.

Raffi belongs to a Russian community organization that sponsors social functions and assists new immigrants. He describes himself as "zero-percent religious."

Past Personal and Family Medical History

Raffi Olefsky has no recollection of any childhood health problems. He had an appendectomy at 19 years of age. He has never been hospitalized for any other reason or had any serious medical illnesses. Raffi smoked quite heavily from ages 18 to 33, when he met Marie-Claude, whose intolerance of cigarette smoke forced him to quit. He drinks approximately one to two beers daily. He has never used illicit drugs of any kind. The patient presently uses no medications.

The patient has had little contact with his family in Russia over the years. Raffi's father died in 1983 at the age of 61 after a long battle with lung cancer. His mother, 67, lives in Moscow and still works part-time as a music instructor. To the best of Raffi's knowledge, she is in excellent health. Raffi has an older brother, Daniel, 44, who works as an engineer in St. Petersburg. Daniel is perfectly healthy.

Both of the patient's maternal grandparents are still alive and living in Yerevan, Armenia, but Raffi is unfamiliar with their health status.

The Problem

You are an attending physician at a university-affiliated family medicine center in the heart of a large city. You have complete access to all diagnostic facilities and specialist services. Raffi Olefsky, a 41-year-old man, comes to your office and tells you he is in serious need of help in getting a good night's rest.

Doctor, I'll tell you what happened. I was driving to a friend's place in Drummondville. It was around 8:00 in the morning. I was very tired. I'm always very tired because I can't sleep at night. I guess I was feeling very drowsy. Pretty soon, I heard a police siren, and I was startled and pulled over. The policeman asked if I had been drinking. I told him no. He said I had been swaying between lanes and that I was very dangerous. The highway was quiet, but I could have hurt someone for sure. In any case, he was nice and told me to pull into a rest area and take a nap. I took his advice, but I have so much trouble sleeping. I could have died that day. I haven't had a good night's sleep for so long! I really need help!

Questions

1. Define "insomnia." How great a problem do you believe it is in a typical family practice?
2. What elements of the history would you initially like to obtain from Raffi?
3. What would you include as part of a physical examination?

Discussion

1. There are various definitions of insomnia. In general terms, insomnia is defined as insufficient or unsatisfying sleep despite adequate opportunity to sleep (Gillin, 1992). Estimates of its prevalence vary greatly. In a well-designed community survey of nearly 8,000 respondents (Ford & Kamerow, 1989), 10.2% reported insomnia. Insomnia was considered to be present in this study if a sleep disturbance lasting at least 2 weeks had occurred in the preceding 6 months. Other surveys using less strict criteria have revealed much higher rates of insomnia. In any case, it is clear that insomnia is an extremely common problem. Its consequences are profound and wide reaching. There is some evidence, for example, that prolonged insomnia is the cause rather than the result of anxiety and major depression (Ford & Kamerow, 1989). Furthermore, as poor sleep often leads to daytime fatigue and decreased alertness, as was the case in Raffi's hazardous driving, insomnia is often related to serious motor vehicle and occupational accidents (Dement & Mitler, 1993). Its economic burden is staggering by any standard.

Unfortunately, several studies indicate that family physicians inadequately detect, evaluate, and treat insomnia. In a study that compared the evaluation and treatment of insomnia by 501 family physicians and 298 nurse practitioners, the physicians were far less likely to elicit a sleep history and more likely to prescribe pharmacologic therapy, even to older patients, despite the known adverse effects of benzodiazepines and other medications in this population (Everitt & Avorn, 1990). A review of progress notes written on inpatients by psychiatric and nonpsychiatric physicians revealed that in only 12% of patients to whom benzodiazepines were prescribed by nonpsychiatric physicians did the record include any reference to sleep disturbance, suggesting that little effort had been made to evaluate this complaint (Shorr & Bauwens, 1992). Nonpsychiatric physicians in this study, however, included only internists and surgeons.

In summary, insomnia is an enormous societal problem with serious consequences, which in general is dealt with poorly by the medical community.

2. The inadequate assessment of insomnia by many family physicians is undoubtedly at least partly due to the inherent difficulty in evaluating this complaint. Insomnia has a vast number of causes, including medical and psychiatric disorders as well as the intrinsic "sleep disorders." What is needed is some framework for obtaining historical information in a thorough but efficient fashion. There are a number of sophisticated approaches used by sleep specialists and others (Douglass et al., 1994; Schramm et al., 1993). A simple way to begin is by determining the duration of disturbed sleep (Walsh & Mahowald, 1991), which can help pinpoint one or a set of causes. *Transient* insomnia, defined as 1 to several nights of disturbed sleep, is quite common and is usually due to short periods of stress, travel across time zones, or other similar situations. *Short-term* insomnia persists for up to 1 month and can have a variety of causes, including stressful or traumatic events such as divorce or the death of a loved one (grief reaction).

Chronic insomnia is sleep disturbance of more than 1 month's duration, and it has a vast number of possible causes. This is likely Raffi's problem, as he hasn't "had a good night's sleep" in recent memory. It is best, however, to clarify the duration of insomnia during the interview.

Unlike *inherent,* or primary, sleep disorders, chronic insomnia can be caused by a **medical** or **psychiatric** problem or can follow from the use of **illicit drugs, alcohol,** or certain **medications.** Among these possible causes, psychiatric disorders are most common, accounting for up to 50% of all causes of insomnia (Walsh & Mahowald, 1991). These include not only affective disorders, such as major depression, but personality disorders and acute psychoses. Medical problems that can cause insomnia include pain from any source (e.g., cancer); cardiovascular causes, such as orthopnea and angina; respiratory illnesses, such as COPD and sleep apnea; renal symptoms, such as urinary frequency; endocrine diseases, including hyperthyroidism; and delirium from any source. Gastrointestinal symptoms such as acid reflux can also disrupt sleep. A vast number of medications, illicit drugs, and excessive alcohol use can result in insomnia.

As the epidemiology of insomnia shows a preponderance of medical and psychiatric illnesses, a good starting point in the evaluation is to determine the presence of one or more of these. Clearly, investigating all possible causes, even so far as obtaining the relevant historical information, is an enormous task and highly impractical. It is best to review what is known about Raffi Olefsky at this point. He is an essentially healthy, relatively young patient. The profile reveals no serious medical illnesses such as COPD or hyperthyroidism. It is unlikely that a medical illness is responsible for his insomnia. Nevertheless, discussion participants may wish to incorporate a brief medical review of systems into the initial history to elicit complaints not discussed in the patient profile. This could include, for example, inquiry into renal, respiratory, and GI complaints as well as determining whether pain of any kind is disrupting Raffi's sleep.

An attempt should be made to identify the presence of one or more of the psychiatric causes of insomnia, although the patient profile makes no reference to any psychiatric disorders. Screening for depression is useful. Alexander (1993) describes a set of nine questions that can serve as a useful screening tool. Not all can be easily applied to Raffi's case, however. It is best to preface an inquiry into depressive symptoms with an explanation that includes why such a series of questions is important. Raffi could be told, for example, that sleep problems are often related to mood and that mood disorders are a serious but treatable condition whose presence should be determined. Raffi should also be asked whether he feels nervous or anxious much of the time. An affirmative response can be followed by another set of questions to qualify this complaint (see Figure 2.1; Alexander, 1993).

It is imperative to screen for drug and alcohol abuse in all patients with chronic insomnia (Walsh & Mahowald, 1991). Raffi has no history of illicit drug use. He does consume alcohol in moderation, but it may be wise to ask if he drinks heavily on occasion or feels he has any trouble with alcohol. Some participants may elect to use a more formal set of screening questions such as the CAGE questionnaire.

3. The physical examination is of considerably less value than the history in the routine evaluation of insomnia. It should be guided by any relevant information obtained from the history. Examination of the heart and lungs in a patient who complains of orthopnea as a cause of insomnia, for example, is certainly warranted.

1. Have you been feeling "blue" or "down in the dumps" lately?
2. Have you had changes in your appetite, sleep, sexual interest, or energy level?
3. Do you have difficulty concentrating?
4. How do you feel about yourself and your future?
5. How bad have you been feeling on a scale of 1 to 10, with 10 being the worst emotional pain you have ever experienced and 1 being not bad at all?
6. How long have you been feeling this way?
7. Have there been any recent significant losses in your life?
8. Have you felt like this before?
9. Is there a history of depression or antisocial behavior in your family?

SOURCE: Based on information obtained from Alexander (1993, p. 344).

Figure 2.1   Questions to Ask About Depression

PART II

The Problem

Raffi tells you that his difficulties with sleep began several years ago while he was a concert violinist, and they have persisted to this day. He saw a Dr. Bleaker 3 years ago for insomnia, and he prescribed lorazepam, 1 mg po qHS prn, but Raffi found the medication helpful only for a couple of weeks.

You decide to begin your evaluation by determining the likelihood of a medical or psychiatric cause for Raffi's problem. You ask him if he has any idea why he is unable to sleep. He tells you he is unaware of any specific cause.

Raffi denies pain of any kind that disrupts his sleep. He also denies cough, shortness of breath, heartburn, night sweats, polyuria, urinary frequency, or other nocturnal symptoms.

You ask Raffi if his pattern of drinking ever becomes heavy or if he feels he has trouble with alcohol. "Well, Doctor, I rarely drink more than three beers a day—even at parties. I do drink one or two beers sometimes just before bed. Sometimes it helps me fall asleep. That's why I do that. I've never had any trouble with alcohol. I don't drink hard liquor at all."

You tell Raffi that problems with sleep are often related to mood or feelings of anxiety. Raffi denies being a nervous or anxious person. "I don't think I'm nervous or anxious when I go to bed. I get frustrated. I try really hard to get to sleep so that I can feel well the next day."

Raffi denies feeling "down in the dumps." Apart from sleep disturbance, he denies any change in appetite, sexual interest, or energy. He says he gets irritable after a night of poor sleep and that this affects his concentration, particularly when he practices the violin. Raffi denies any great emotional pain or burden at the present time and any significant personal loss. He tells you that his divorce 2 years ago was not especially bitter and that he and Marie-Claude have remained on "friendly" terms. Raffi tells you that his sleep problem is a nuisance but that he feels somewhat optimistic about the future. "Look, I was a pretty well-known concert violinist, and now I teach teenagers in a school. They hardly know anything about me, but truly, I am really quite happy. I struggled to make money for so long, it's nice to be independent and have a good job. One day, I think I would like to play again with an orchestra. I feel pretty good about myself in general."

A very limited physical examination reveals that Raffi is a pleasant, slim man who looks his stated age. He is alert and displays normal affect. His vital signs are completely normal.

Questions

1. Where would you go from here?
2. How are sleep disorders classified?
3. Read "The Rest of the Story" in Part II. What are the most likely diagnoses in Raffi's case?
4. What is *sleep hygiene?* How can sleep hygiene be improved?

Discussion

1. The initial inquiry does not reveal any obvious medical, psychiatric, or substance-related cause of Raffi's insomnia that, if identified, would become the focus of further evaluation and treatment. These possible causes, however, should be kept in mind throughout the course of evaluation and treatment, as one or more may become apparent in the future. For the time being, the focus of the evaluation should be elsewhere, and the possibility that Raffi has an inherent sleep disorder should be assessed. This is a point at which discussion participants may feel uncertain of which path to follow. Walsh and Mahowald (1991) describe an extremely useful algorithm in such situations. It involves qualifying the sleep disturbance, then using this information to determine if a particular sleep disorder is present and to continue to rule out medical and psychiatric sources of insomnia. Walsh and Mahowald advocate determining the **duration, stability, description,** and **consequences** of the sleep complaint. This is done by asking four simple corresponding questions:

1. How long have you had insomnia?
2. Do you have this problem every night?
3. How would you describe your sleep complaint?
4. How does this affect your daytime functioning?

Raffi has already answered the first question in approximate terms. It is known that he has chronic insomnia. The fourth question has been partly answered as well. Raffi's insomnia had a near-fatal consequence. Further information on consequences is obviously needed.

The diagnostic value of determining the duration of insomnia has already been addressed. Transient and short-term insomnia are much more likely (due to obvious situational factors) than medical, psychiatric, substance-related, or inherent sleep disorders. The severity of insomnia is much more variable over time with medical and psychiatric causes than it is in intrinsic sleep disorders. In other words, there is a difference in **stability.** Patients who complain of insomnia that is caused by a medical or psychiatric complaint are less likely to have difficulty with sleep every night.

A **description** of sleep disturbance should include the specific pattern of insomnia. Difficulty in falling asleep, for example, is quite different from early-morning awakening, commonly associated with major depression. Some insomniacs, by contrast, have frequent awakenings throughout the night.

The effect of insomnia on **daytime functioning** is extremely important in helping to pinpoint a diagnosis and especially in assessing the severity of the problem and the urgency with which treatment should be instituted. Many insomniacs complain of daytime irritability and difficulty with concentration. Patients who complain of genuine daytime sleepiness are more likely to have a medical cause of insomnia. Raffi has suffered driving impairment as a consequence of insomnia, suggesting that this is indeed a very serious situation that necessitates prompt treatment.

2. There are several classification systems for sleep disorders. The most widely accepted is the American Sleep Disorders Association's International Classification, revised in 1990 (Pagel, 1994), which divides sleep disorders into four large categories: (a) those secondary to medical and psychiatric illnesses; (b) **parasomnias,** defined as disorders characterized by abnormal behavioral or physiological events during sleep, such as night terrors or sleep walking (*DSM-IV*, p. 553); (c) **dyssomnias,** disorders characterized by difficulty initiating or maintaining sleep, as well as those involving excessive sleepiness; and (d) a category of **proposed sleep disorders**—those that are not yet well characterized.

The dyssomnias are of greatest interest in Raffi's case. They are further divided into **intrinsic** and **extrinsic** sleep disorders as well as **circadian rhythm disturbances.** A discussion of all the disorders in each subcategory is beyond the scope of this exercise. A description of the most common is provided.

Psychophysiologic insomnia is the most common intrinsic sleep disorder. The patient associates cognitive arousal and anxiety with the bedroom and bedtime (Becker, Jamieson, & Brown, 1993). Such patients are the stereotypical insomniacs who worry about getting enough sleep and often unsuccessfully try to force themselves to sleep (Pagel, 1994).

Restless legs syndrome is a common intrinsic cause of insomnia characterized by a "creepy" feeling in the resting leg muscles that prevents sleep. Patients with **sleep-related myoclonus** exhibit periodic curling or jumping of limbs associated with brief awakenings. Both these disorders can be treated with pharmacotherapy.

Extrinsic sleep disorders include **poor sleep hygiene,** which will be addressed later, and **adjustment sleep disorder,** whereby a stressful life change leads to insomnia of variable duration and severity. Among common circadian rhythm disturbances is **delayed sleep phase syndrome,** in which patients report difficulty in falling asleep and in awakening at desired times. This occurs because the sleep phase of the sleep-wake rhythm begins well after the desired bedtime.

3. At this point in the discussion, it is best to review the information gathered. Raffi Olefsky is a relatively healthy 41-

year-old man who has been suffering from several years of insomnia that has adversely affected his daytime functioning by making him irritable, tired, and impairing his concentration and, on at least one occasion, his ability to drive. An inquiry into medical or psychiatric symptoms revealed nothing obvious. He does not use illicit drugs or medications but consumes alcohol in moderation. His pattern of sleep disturbance reveals difficulty in falling asleep on most nights.

As a medical, psychiatric, or substance-related cause is unlikely, the probability that Raffi has a primary sleep disorder is increased—more specifically, a dyssomnia. It is possible that Raffi has delayed sleep phase syndrome, but the time at which he falls asleep appears to be not only delayed but highly unpredictable. He appears to try to force himself to sleep. This behavior, as noted previously, is consistent with psychophysiologic insomnia.

An adjustment sleep disorder is unlikely in Raffi's case because his insomnia has persisted for so many years and he is unable to identify any precipitating stressful event. Raffi gives no history consistent with restless legs syndrome. It is usually difficult to determine the role of nocturnal myoclonus in insomnia by history, as the patient is usually unaware of the limb movements by which it is characterized. Poor sleep hygiene is a possible diagnosis for, or contributing factor to, Raffi's insomnia.

4. "Sleep hygiene" refers to the personal habits associated with bedtime and awakening and to specific behaviors that can influence the quality or quantity of sleep.

Good sleep hygiene encompasses a wide variety of daily activities that promote sufficient, restful sleep (Rakel, 1993). These include (a) avoiding spending too much time in bed waiting for the onset of sleep. Getting out of bed and pursuing another distracting activity until one feels drowsy is recommended in such situations. (b) Avoiding daytime naps and (c) not using the bed for activities other than sleep and sex, such as reading or watching television, are important components of good sleep hygiene as well. Patients should be (d) encouraged to wake up at the same time each day to maintain circadian rhythm. (e) Caffeine and other stimulants should be avoided late in the day. (f) Alcohol prior to bedtime should be avoided. Though it promotes the onset of sleep, it causes frequent awakenings, reducing the total sleep time (Hauri & Esther, 1990). Patients should (g) not go to bed feeling hungry. Foods containing tryptophan, such as milk, are thought to promote sleep.

(h) Cigarette smoking should definitely be avoided. (i) Late-afternoon or early-evening exercise is known to promote restful sleep, but patients should not exercise just prior to bedtime. Finally, (j) a quiet bedroom environment at a comfortable temperature is very important.

The Rest of the Story

Raffi tells you once again that he has been having sleep problems for a long time. He believes his troubles began about 6 or 7 years ago.

I remember it bothered Marie-Claude a lot. I would toss and turn and try to force myself to sleep and sometimes keep her up too. When we were married, I always envied her because she fell asleep so easily.

Raffi tells you he has trouble sleeping almost every night. More specifically, he experiences difficulty in falling asleep. He tells you,

I struggle so much to get to sleep. I keep my eyes shut and try not to move. I go to bed at 11:30 every night. It's so hard for me to tell when I will finally fall asleep—2:00 a.m., 4:00 a.m. If and when I do fall asleep, I don't wake up until morning. Sometimes I know I don't sleep at all. I feel just awful in the morning, but I have to go to work!

You ask Raffi to tell you more about how the lack of sleep affects his daytime activities.

Well, I feel like I'm not human sometimes. I feel so tired and I want to be still all the time. Everything I do in the day is a chore. I don't feel like brushing my teeth. I don't feel like driving to work. I don't feel like teaching. I have a very short temper with my students sometimes, and I know it is because my sleep is so bad. When I come home, I am exhausted, but I want to practice the violin. I have so much trouble concentrating. You know, I told you, I want to play with a symphony again some day. I need to practice. I need to stay in touch with the music. I have to work hard—but I can't. At 6:00 I am a vegetable. On days when I am dead tired and have not slept the night before, I still have some trouble falling asleep.

PART III

The Problem

After describing the effects of insomnia on his life, Raffi goes on to tell you he feels that sleeping well will have an important impact on his future.

It's not just how it affects me now. It affects how things will be 5 years from now. I have to practice; I have to send out resumes; I have to plan community events. I can't do that if I get home and feel miserable. I just can't. Dr. Bleaker once told me I should have a "sleep study" done—one of those things where they hook you up and watch you sleep. What do you think about that?

Questions

1. How would you answer Raffi's question?
2. Would you administer pharmacologic therapy?
3. Discuss the pharmacologic options for the treatment of insomnia.
4. What nonpharmacologic treatments would you prescribe for Raffi?

Discussion

1. The question refers to **polysomnography**—the method of quantifying sleep by measurement of a number of variables. These include EEG, heart rate, respiration, limb and eye movement, oxygen saturation, and sometimes other parameters. The specific details of the technique of polysomnography are beyond the scope of this group discussion exercise.

Sleep studies using polysomnography are usually performed by sleep specialists in specialized laboratories. They are extremely expensive and time-consuming. For these reasons, Reite, Buysse, Reynolds, and Mendelson (1995), in conjunction with the Standards of Practice Committee of the American Sleep Disorders Association, conducted an extensive review of literature on polysomnography published between 1966 and 1994 to determine which patients can benefit from this technique and how it can be used in a cost-effective manner. They concluded that there is **no evidence for the use of polysomnography in the routine evaluation of transient or chronic insomnia.** In other words, the diagnostic yield in the majority of cases is extremely low. In general, polysomnography is of greater value in older patients. It is valuable in the diagnosis of certain conditions. It is indicated if there **is a strong suspicion of a "sleep-related breathing disorder"** such as sleep apnea. It is also indicated for the **diagnosis of a periodic limb-movement disorder.** Both these conditions are quite rare causes of insomnia in a typical family practice. Sleep apnea is more common in overweight, middle-aged men who are prone to hypertension and complain of daytime sleepiness (Gillin & Byerley,

1990). Such patients also often complain of morning headache, irritability, or erectile dysfunction. Their bed partner often complains that the patient snores loudly (Rakel, 1993).

In general, Reite et al. (1995) recommend **an initial trial of either behavioral and/or pharmacologic therapy. Polysomnography can be considered in the event that such therapy fails.** There is, therefore, presently no need for polysomnography in Raffi's case. He should be told this.

2. It has already been noted that pharmacologic therapy for insomnia is often carelessly and excessively prescribed. Medications do not offer a long-term solution to the chronic insomniac. In general, pharmacologic therapy, particularly the benzodiazepine-type medications, should be prescribed only for short-term or transient insomnia; in other kinds of insomnia it should be prescribed only for brief periods of time.

The question of whether to prescribe "sleeping pills" for Raffi is debatable. Some participants may choose to offer Raffi a short course of pharmacologic treatment, as such therapy has a short onset of action and the patient's insomnia is particularly severe at present. Others may opt for nonpharmacologic therapy only.

3. There are a number of classes of medications used as sleeping or "hypnotic" agents. **Barbiturate** and **barbiturate-like** drugs were once commonly used for insomnia but, because of their serious side effects, they have virtually been abandoned for this purpose.

A number of over-the-counter hypnotic preparations contain **antihistamines,** such as diphenhydramine and hydroxyzine. They are only moderately effective and in some cases actually increase insomnia (Gillin, 1992).

Sedating antidepressants used in low doses at bedtime are often effective treatments for primary insomnia (Ware, 1983). Long-term use of these agents in chronic insomnia is of uncertain value. Many **antipsychotic** medications, such as haloperidol, have sedating properties but should not be routinely prescribed as hypnotics (Gillin & Byerley, 1990).

The most popular class of hypnotic medications is the **benzodiazepines.** This class includes a vast number of agents, all of which are effective and that vary in time of onset of action, half-life, and severity of side effects. Side effects include daytime somnolence; rebound insomnia upon discontinuation; tolerance; and withdrawal symptoms such as anxiety, amnesia, and (in the elderly) falls. Benzodiazepines can be classified according to duration of hypnotic effect as short, intermediate, and long acting.

Short-acting agents include midazolam and triazolam, seldom used for insomnia. The large variety of intermediate-acting agents includes lorazepam, oxazepam, and the newer temazepam (Gillin & Byerley, 1990).

Of particular interest is zolpidem, a new nonbenzodiazepine agent that, however, acts on the benzodiazepine receptor. It is associated with fewer side effects and no demonstrable tolerance, withdrawal, or rebound insomnia. It is also, unfortunately, very expensive (Hartmann, 1995).

4. Participants should be discouraged from carrying on a lengthy or detailed discussion of pharmacologic treatment of insomnia. As indicated, pharmacologic therapy is fraught with many problems, and the primary treatment of chronic insomnia involves other approaches. There are an enormous number of nonpharmacologic treatments, including everything from biofeedback to progressive muscle relaxation.

A general nonpharmacologic approach to the patient with insomnia, in whom a medical or psychiatric cause cannot be readily identified, involves **sleep-hygiene instructions and appropriate behavioral therapy** (Walsh & Mahowald, 1991). How to improve sleep hygiene has already been discussed. The question is, what sort of behavioral therapy should be recommended for Raffi?

The National Institutes of Health (NIH) recently convened a panel to examine the effectiveness of a wide variety of behavioral and relaxation approaches to chronic pain and insomnia (NIH Technology Assessment Panel, 1996). The panel reviewed therapies that include behavioral or cognitive components, appear in the scientific literature, and are commonly used in the United States. A number of evaluated therapies were found to be effective in insomnia, including biofeedback, meditation, and progressive muscle relaxation. The most effective treatments were **stimulus control, sleep restriction, and multimodal treatment.**

Stimulus control therapy involves the creation of a conditioned association between the bedroom and sleep. Activities in the bedroom are restricted to sleep and sex. It is often included as a component of sleep hygiene (Pagel, 1994). Multimodal treatment refers, of course, to the inclusion of more than one therapeutic modality in the management plan. As improving sleep hygiene already encompasses a variety of approaches to insomnia, this combined with a more sophisticated behavioral approach can be regarded as multimodal treatment.

Sleep restriction is a technique that limits the amount of time spent in bed to the amount of perceived sleep time; it involves progressively lengthening time in bed (TIB) as the *relative* amount of perceived or estimated sleep time increases. Many approaches to insomnia involve identifying one or more precipitating factors, such as depression or even poor sleep hygiene. Sleep restriction, on the other hand, attempts to modify one of the factors thought to *perpetuate* insomnia, namely, excessive time in bed, although it may not necessarily have been the cause of insomnia. An anxious patient, for example, may have difficulty sleeping because of his or her anxiety. That same patient quite likely spends much time in bed awake. Just as addressing the patient's anxiety may be beneficial, restricting time in bed may have a positive impact on sleep. The method is well described by Spielman, Saskin, and Thorpy (1987). Patients are first asked to maintain a 2-week **sleep log,** in which the time in bed each night and the amount of estimated sleep time is recorded. Time in bed is then restricted to the estimated sleep time only. For example, if a patient reports that she has spent an average of 8 hr a night in bed but feels she was asleep for just 4 hr, she is asked to spend only 4 hr in bed thereafter. The goal is to improve **sleep efficiency,** defined as

$$\frac{\text{estimated or perceived sleep time}}{\text{TIB}} \times 100\%.$$

(Spielman et al., 1987)

When the sleep efficiency over a period of 5 nights is 90% or more, the TIB is increased by 15 min. The process is continued until the patient reports subjective improvement in sleep quality and quantity. In a study using sleep restriction, Spielman et al. (1987) have compared patients' estimate of sleep time to that recorded through polysomnography. Patients with insomnia underestimated their total sleep time by an average of 58 min and overestimated their **sleep latency** (the time required to fall asleep) by 35 min. Sleep restriction therapy, therefore, initially causes some sleep deprivation, which may be quite uncomfortable for the patient. Patients should be told that they may "feel worse" early on but that things should improve as their total sleep time and sleep efficiency increase.

There are several other nonpharmacologic therapies from which Raffi may benefit and that the NIH panel did not specifically examine. "Light therapy," for example, which involves daily exposure to bright light, is of considerable benefit to those with delayed sleep phase syndrome: It can correct circadian disturbances. Guilleminault et al. (1995) have found that patients with psychophysiologic insomnia may also benefit from light therapy.

A suitable therapeutic plan for Raffi could involve thorough instructions on sleep hygiene and a well-monitored sleep restriction program. Such an approach is consistent with what is known to be most effective (NIH Technology Assessment Panel, 1996).

The Rest of the Story

You tell Raffi that "sleep studies" are usually only of immediate value when breathing problems or limb movements are suspected as a cause of insomnia. You inform him that a sleep study may be indicated later, if therapy for his problem fails.

You discuss sleep hygiene with Raffi at length. Specifically, you encourage him to set strict bed and wake times. You ask him to avoid spending more than 20 to 30 min in bed if sleep does not occur and to get up, leave the bedroom, and engage in another distracting activity until he feels drowsy.

Raffi consumes two cups of coffee each day, at variable times. You tell him to avoid coffee and other caffeinated beverages after noon. You tell him that although alcohol may help him fall asleep, the quality of sleep is adversely affected. You recommend that he stop using alcohol as a sleep aid.

You encourage Raffi to exercise regularly, avoid daytime naps, maintain a quiet bedroom environment at a comfortable temperature, and to use his bed only for sleep and sexual activity. Raffi seems very receptive to your recommendations.

> I guess most of things you talked about are good common sense. I'll definitely try to make some changes. I don't really exercise. I used to play soccer when I was younger. I have friends who still play on a team. If they're willing to take on an "old man," maybe I'll join in. I'll try to avoid coffee and beer close to bedtime. I do sometimes spend a lot of time lying in bed reading. I'll try to avoid that.

You explain the method of "sleep restriction" to Raffi. "I'm willing to try that," he says. "I just don't want to take any sleeping pills. I don't want to get hooked on those. They don't work for me very well anyway."

You tell Raffi that he is correct that some sleep medications promote dependence and are associated with tolerance, and you accept his decision to avoid them.

You ask Raffi to maintain a sleep log for the next 2 weeks, in which he is to record his total time in bed and estimated sleep time. He agrees and arranges a follow-up visit accordingly.

PART IV

The Problem

Raffi returns as scheduled. For the past 2 weeks, he has avoided alcohol and caffeine close to bedtime. He has tried to follow your other sleep hygiene recommendations to the best of his ability. He reports slight improvement in insomnia: "Well, it still takes me a long time to fall asleep. I still wake up feeling terrible. I do feel a little better. I think just talking to you helped a lot. What I needed was some guidance with this problem. Anyway, I made a sleep log as you asked."

Raffi's sleep log for the past 2 weeks is summarized in Figure 2.2. He has been going to bed around 11:30 each night but rising at more variable times depending on his class schedule at the music school.

Questions

1. What is Raffi's mean sleep time and efficiency over the past 2 weeks?
2. Apart from instituting a program of sleep restriction, would you make any other recommendations at this point?
3. How would you proceed?

Day	Hours in Bed	Estimated Hours of Sleep
1	7	3
2	9	7
3	7	2
4	7	5
5	7.5	6
6	9	3
7	7	5.5
8	8	5
9	7	3
10	7	6.5
11	8	4
12	7	6
13	7.5	7
14	7.5	7

Figure 2.2 Raffi's First Sleep Log

Discussion

1. Raffi's estimate of sleep time is 70 h/14 days, or 5 hr per night. Sleep efficiency is estimated sleep time/TIB × 100%. Raffi's mean efficiency is Σ [estimated sleep time/TIB × 100%]/14. In this case, mean efficiency is 66.4%.

2. Raffi's sleep log indicates relatively poor overall quantity of estimated sleep. His sleep appears to have improved in the past 3 days. He should be encouraged once again to maintain a constant wake time, regardless of what time he is scheduled to teach class at the music school. His knowledge of other sleep hygiene recommendations should be reinforced.

3. Raffi should be told to restrict his time in bed to just 5 hr a night and to return in a short period of time, perhaps 1 week to 10 days. He should be told that he may feel worse for a while but that restriction of time in bed is an essential component of the program.

PART V

The Problem

You begin a program of sleep restriction. You ask Raffi to spend only 5 hr per night in bed. You warn him that he may feel worse at the outset. Raffi agrees to follow the plan and returns in 10 days with an updated sleep log. He says he has had little trouble falling asleep over the past several days but finds it hard to climb out of bed in the morning. He has opted to remain awake late in the day for an extended period to reduce his time in bed. He has been spending considerable time watching late-night television. He says, "At least I have less trouble falling asleep. I don't think 5 hours is enough. Sometimes I cheat a little and catch a few extra minutes, but I have tried my best." His second sleep log is summarized in Figure 2.3.

Day	Hours in Bed	Estimated Hours of Sleep
1	7	3
2	9	7
3	7	2
4	7	5
5	7.5	6
6	9	3
7	7	5.5
8	8	5
9	7	3
10	7	6.5
11	8	4
12	7	6
13	7.5	7
14	7.5	7

Figure 2.3   Raffi's Second Sleep Log

Questions

  1. How would you assess Raffi's updated sleep log?
  2. Where would go from here?

Discussion

  1. Raffi's sleep efficiency has markedly improved. The calculated value works out to just over 90%, which is the threshold at which the time in bed can be lengthened. Raffi has not been absolutely compliant with the allotted time in bed. Failure to comply with sleep restriction is extremely common and represents one of the greatest difficulties with this method (Friedman, Bliwise, Yesavage, & Salom, 1991; Spiel-man et al., 1987). Some patients find the allotted time in bed intolerable (Friedman et al., 1991).

  2. A continued program of sleep restriction can be recommended, and Raffi's time in bed can be increased from 5 hr to 5 hr and 15 min. Raffi should be seen in a relatively short period of time, perhaps in 1 week.

PART VI

The Problem

You ask Raffi to increase his time in bed by 15 min a night and to return in 1 week with his updated sleep log. He returns as scheduled and tells you that he actually decided to increase his time in bed by half an hour. He is feeling considerably better.

Day	Hours in Bed	Estimated Hours of Sleep
1	7	3
2	9	7
3	7	2
4	7	5
5	7.5	6
6	9	3
7	7	5.5
8	8	5
9	7	3
10	7	6.5
11	8	4
12	7	6
13	7.5	7
14	7.5	7

Figure 2.4   Raffi's Third Sleep Log

I don't have too much trouble falling asleep. I am less irritable during the day. I can get more done in the evening. I think this program is working. I thought it would be better to go a little quicker, so I decided to add half an hour to my time in bed.

His updated sleep log is shown in Figure 2.4.

Questions

1. How would you assess Raffi's sleep log?
2. Where would you go from here?

Discussion

1. Raffi continues to exhibit high sleep efficiency. Most important, regardless of whether his self-reports of sleep time and TIB are accurate or whether he has been absolutely compliant with a program of sleep restriction, Raffi does indicate improvement in well-being, which is the ultimate measure of success.

2. Raffi appears to have gained considerable control over his insomnia. Although sleep latency is not recorded in his log, it is safe to say that prolonged sleep latency is no longer a problem, as his efficiency is very high. Raffi appears to understand the sleep restriction program very well and seems to be comfortable with self-management. He should be encouraged, therefore, to continue on his own. There is evidence that the beneficial effects of a sleep restriction program persist. Spielman et al. (1987) assessed subjects enrolled in a sleep restriction program at a mean of 36 weeks after the end of treatment and found that the average sleep efficiency remained high and that self-reports of sleep quality remained favorable. It is difficult to precisely gauge the success of the sleep restriction program in this case, as the relative contri-

bution of sleep hygiene instructions and education and the support and concern expressed by Raffi's physician are difficult to determine. In any case, the patient is now in control. Raffi could be followed up at a later date, assuming his insomnia continues to improve.

Conclusion

You congratulate Raffi on the success he has achieved in controlling his insomnia. You ask him to continue the sleep restriction program at his discretion. You review sleep hygiene recommendations once again and ask Raffi to return in 3 to 4 months for a general reassessment. You also wish him the best of luck with his musical career. He is very grateful for your help.

Raffi returns in 4 months and tells you he feels very well. He does experience trouble falling asleep from time to time for no apparent reason, but by practicing good sleep hygiene, he is soon able to get the problem under control. Raffi tells you he spends roughly 7 to 8 hr in bed and requires about 30 min to fall asleep. He reports greatly decreased daytime irritability and fatigue and reports increased energy in the early evening hours.

You congratulate the patient once again on his success and tell him you are available to provide help with insomnia or other medical matters in the future.

References

Alexander, M. (1993). Anxiety and depression. In P. D. Sloane, L. M. Slatt, & P. Curtis (Eds.), *Essentials of family medicine* (2nd ed.; pp. 339-347). Baltimore, MD: Williams and Wilkins.

Becker, P. M., Jamieson, A. O., & Brown, D. W. (1993). Insomnia: Use of a "decision tree" to assess and treat. *Postgraduate Medicine, 93*(1), 67-85.

Dement, W. C., & Mitler, M. M. (1993). It's time to wake up to the importance of sleep disorders. *Journal of the American Medical Association, 269*(12), 1548-1550.

Douglass, A. B., Bornstein, R., Nino-Murcia, G., Keenan, S., Miles, L., Zarcone, V. P., Jr., Guilleminault, C., & Dement, W. C. (1994). The sleep disorders questionnaire I: Creation and multivariate structure of SDQ. *Sleep, 17*(2), 160-167.

Everitt, D. E., & Avorn, J. (1990). Clinical decision-making in the evaluation and treatment of insomnia. *American Journal of Medicine, 89,* 357-362.

Ford, D. E., & Kamerow, D. B. (1989). Epidemiologic study of sleep disturbances and psychiatric disorders. *Journal of the American Medical Association, 262*(11), 1479-1484.

Friedman, L., Bliwise, D. L., Yesavage, J. A., & Salom, S. R. (1991, January). A preliminary study comparing sleep restriction and relaxation treatments for insomnia in older adults. *Journal of Gerontology, 46*(1), 1-8.

Gillin, J. C. (1992). Relief from situational insomnia. *Postgraduate Medicine, 92*(2), 157-170.

Gillin, J. C., & Byerley, W. F. (1990). The diagnosis and management of insomnia. *New England Journal of Medicine, 322*(4), 239-248.

Guiellleminault, C., Clerk, A., Black, J., Labanowski, M., Pelayo, R., & Claman, D. (1995). Nondrug treatment trials in psychophysiologic insomnia. *Archives of Internal Medicine, 155,* 838-844.

Hartmann, P. M. (1995). Drug treatment of insomnia: Indications and newer agents. *American Family Physician, 51*(1), 191-194.

Hauri, P. J., & Esther, M. S. (1990). Insomnia. *Mayo Clinic Proceedings, 65,* 869-882.

National Institutes of Health Technology Assessment Panel. (1996). Integration of behavioral and relaxation approaches into the treatment of chronic pain and insomnia. *Journal of the American Medical Association, 276*(4), 313-318.

Pagel, J. F. (1994). Treatment of insomnia. *American Family Physician, 49*(6), 1417-1421.

Rakel, R. E. (1993). Insomnia: Concerns of the family physician. *Journal of Family Practice, 36,* 551-558.

Reite, M., Buysse, D., Reynolds, C., & Mendelson, W. (1995). The use of polysomnography in the evaluation of insomnia. *Sleep, 18*(1), 58-70.

Schramm, E., Hohagen, F., Grasshoff, U., Riemann, D., Hajak, G., Weess, H. G., & Berger, M. (1993). Test-retest reliability and validity of the structured interview for sleep disorders according to *DSM-III-R. American Journal of Psychiatry, 150*(6), 867-872.

Shorr, R. I., & Bauwens, S. F. (1992). Diagnosis and treatment of outpatient insomnia by psychiatric and nonpsychiatric physicians. *American Journal of Medicine, 93*, 78-82.

Spielman, A. J., Saskin, P., & Thorpy, M. J. (1987). Treatment of chronic insomnia by restriction of time in bed. *Sleep, 10*(1), 45-56.

Walsh, J. K., & Mahowald, M. W. (1991). Avoiding the blanket approach to insomnia. *Postgraduate Medicine, 90*(1), 211-219.

Ware, J. C. (1983). Tricyclic antidepressants in the treatment of insomnia. *Journal of Clinical Psychiatry, 44*, 25-28.

3. DIZZINESS AND FALLS

Mrs. Enza Ianonne

*Goal: The purpose of this exercise is to evaluate and develop
the participants' knowledge of the causes of dizziness and falls,
diagnostic evaluation of dizziness, and prevention of falls among elderly persons.*

Specific Objectives: Upon completion of this group discussion exercise, each participant should be able to do the following:

1. List the major causes of falls among the elderly.
2. Take a focused history from an elderly person or from a witness when a fall has taken place.
3. Perform a focused physical examination to help determine the cause of a fall.
4. Know how to evaluate the complaint of "dizziness" in the elderly.
5. Know the basic strategies to prevent falls among the elderly that take into consideration medical, functional, and environmental factors.

PART I

The Patient

Social History

Mrs. Ianonne is an 81-year-old woman who lives with her daughter, Maria (56 years old); son-in-law, Michel (60); and grandson, Jean-Francois (20) in a large home in St. Leonard, Province of Québec.

Originally from Bologna, Italy, the patient is the eldest of three children, the daughter of a shopkeeper and his wife. Mrs. Ianonne attended school until age 16. She married Emiliano, a factory worker, in 1935. The couple left Italy for Montreal in 1937, where Emiliano found a job with the Imperial Tobacco Company. In 1950, he opened a small shoe repair business, which he managed until retirement in 1973. Mrs. Ianonne worked briefly as a seamstress in the early 1940s and, despite raising two children, also helped with the family business whenever possible.

Mrs. Ianonne's oldest child, Carlo (57), lives with his wife in Toronto. Her husband Emiliano passed away in 1978 from pancreatic cancer, after which she moved in with Maria, Michel, and their children.

The patient is part of a large and supportive family. Not only is she very close to Maria and Michel, she is frequently visited by Carlo and his wife. More recently, she has been visited by her grandson (Carlo's son) Peter; his wife, Alison; and their newborn daughter (Mrs. Ianonne's first great-grandchild), Amanda.

Mrs. Ianonne has a couple of close friends with whom she chats in a nearby park on pleasant summer afternoons. During the winter months, she stays in touch by phone. She also enjoys reading and playing cards with her grandson. She is a devout Roman Catholic and rarely misses Sunday service at her local church.

Past Personal and Family Medical History

Mrs. Ianonne was a healthy child who grew up to be a healthy young woman. Unfortunately, she did have a miscarriage in 1941. She cannot recall all the details but does remember that it was very psychologically traumatic.

The patient remained healthy until about age 60, when she developed degenerative changes in both hip and knee joints, producing painful arthritis. This has remained relatively stable and has not limited her usual activities.

Ten years ago, Mrs. Ianonne was diagnosed with Type II diabetes. This remained under quite good control with just dietary therapy until 3 years ago, when she was placed on glyburide. She does not perform home blood glucose monitoring. Her last fasting blood glucose was 4.5mmol/1 (81mg/dL) and was obtained 4 months ago.

About 6 years ago, Mrs. Ianonne began to develop a cataract in her left eye. This was extracted $4\frac{1}{2}$ years ago, and an artificial lens was inserted.

In 1992, Mrs. Ianonne presented to an emergency room with a 30-min history of inability to move her left arm. She also complained of diminished sensation over the same limb. This resolved shortly after presentation and was diagnosed as a transient ischemic attack. Carotid doppler studies arranged thereafter showed roughly 30% stenosis of both internal carotid arteries.

At the present time, Mrs. Ianonne takes glyburide 10 mg po qday, EC-ASA 325mg po qday, and Naprosyn 500mg po bid. She takes no other medications. She reports no drug or other allergies. She rarely drinks alcohol—she has one glass of wine on special occasions. She has never smoked.

Mrs. Ianonne's father died in 1950 in Italy at the age of 65, of what the patient believes was a heart attack. Her mother died in 1956 at the age of 68 of pneumonia.

The patient had two younger brothers. Alfredo was killed in action in 1940 during a military campaign in Greece. Giovanni died of a heart attack at the age of 61.

Both Mrs. Ianonne's children are relatively healthy, although Carlo has, as she puts it, "a touch of diabetes just like me." All her grandchildren are healthy.

The Problem

You are a family physician in a solo practice in the heart of the city, with easy access to special diagnostic facilities and specialists.

Mrs. Ianonne, an 81-year-old woman, has been your patient for 2 years. You last saw her 4 months ago for a periodic health examination and administration of influenza vaccine. She had no major complaints at that time and was relatively healthy.

On this occasion, Mrs. Ianonne comes to your office with her daughter Maria. The patient tells you that she has been experiencing episodes of dizziness for the past 2 months. Maria tells you that things have gotten worse in the past week, during which her mother has actually fallen four or five times while feeling dizzy. Just 1 week ago, the patient had a "spell" of dizziness while descending a flight of stairs at home. She stumbled over the last two steps, losing her balance and landing on her backside. The other falls took place while the patient was standing on level ground. These were unwitnessed, and the patient was found lying on her side. No significant injury was the result in any of these incidents.

When questioned further, Mrs. Ianonne tells you that she has "dizzy spells" roughly once a day, usually in the morning, during which everything she sees becomes dark and hazy. She feels faint, unsteady on her feet, and usually avoids falling by grabbing on to a secure object. The patient does describe a vague spinning sensation but cannot say whether she or her surroundings appear to be spinning. These episodes last about 5 to 10 min.

Mrs. Ianonne's symptoms occur within 3 to 4 hr after awakening. There is no consistent association with any particular activity. The spells, however, always come on when the patient is standing and has been standing for at least a few minutes. The patient reports no associated chest pain, diaphoresis, palpitations, or shortness of breath. There is no history of weakness of any limb, facial numbness, double vision, tremor, convulsions, loss of consciousness, or incontinence.

Mrs. Ianonne reports no recent visual disturbances or any pain or ringing in the ears. There has been no change recently in her hearing. Indeed, the patient tells you that she has been her usual self in between dizzy spells. She has no increased hip and knee pain. She has no complaints of increased thirst nor increased frequency or volume of urination. There is no history of fever, cough, nausea or vomiting, or change in appetite or weight.

Mrs. Ianonne denies any symptoms of depression or anxiety. There is no history of confusion or disorientation. Maria, however, tells you that her mother has not been her usual bright, cheerful self lately. She is able to perform her daily activities but refuses to leave the house for fear of suffering a nasty fall outdoors.

The patient tells you that she is not sure if anything can be done to help her. She believes that the dizzy spells are part of growing old and that as long as she has something to grab on to and is not too adventurous in her activities, everything will be just fine. Maria, on the other hand, is very concerned that her mother will eventually take a nasty tumble and suffer a serious injury. She tells you repeatedly that her mother never complained of dizziness in the past and that she is worried that this is a sign of something ominous.

Questions:

1. Before examining the patient, is there any additional historical information you would find useful?
2. What medical and functional risk factors for falls does Mrs. Ianonne possess?
3. On the basis of this history, what are some possible explanations for Mrs. Ianonne's dizzy spells?
4. How would you perform a focused physical examination of Mrs. Ianonne?
5. After reviewing the suggested physical examination provided, what further testing would you request? All laboratory results can be made available within 24 hr. Mrs. Ianonne is also able to return to your office the next day if you wish.
6. After reviewing the results of the suggested laboratory tests, how would you manage this patient's problem?

Discussion

1. Hindmarsh and Estes (1989) describe a "threshold" model for identifying the cause of falls in the elderly. In this model, no one factor can usually be identified that precipitates a fall. Rather, a fall is viewed as the result of a complex interaction between host and environment. In other words, a patient's medical and functional impairments permit a fall to take place when his or her environment is sufficiently hazardous. A change in any one medical or environmental factor may be enough to cross the threshold for falls.

A thorough diagnostic evaluation of falls begins with a careful history of the timing and circumstances of the events, together with associated symptoms. In Mrs. Ianonne's case, these include spinning, visual disturbance, and unsteadiness. A review of medications and concurrent medical illnesses is also invaluable and has been provided. We know that the dizziness is a fairly recent complaint and that there have been no previous episodes. The falls have taken place even more recently and have presumably triggered this medical consultation.

Mrs. Ianonne has been getting dizzy for reasons not immediately apparent. Consequently, she has fallen several times. What is missing from the history is a comprehensive description of the patient's home environment—the setting in which these falls have taken place. Though the patient has been dizzy for a couple of months, she has fallen only in the past week. One should ask about any change in the environment in the past week (see "The Rest of the Story"). In addition, it should be known whether the patient has engaged in any behavior in the past week that put her at increased risk of falling. For example, has she been climbing stairs more often than usual? Has she been wearing unsafe shoes or slippers?

One of the principal elements in fall prevention is a home safety assessment, which should be performed by either a physician or some other health care professional. Tinetti and Speechley (1989) have identified specific environmental factors that should be evaluated in a patient's home. These include lighting, floors, stairs, kitchens and bathrooms, footwear, and entrances.

2. Obviously, Mrs. Ianonne's dizziness is ultimately what causes her to fall, and this will be discussed in further detail. A thorough evaluation of falls should take into consideration all potential medical and functional factors, including other illnesses and medications.

Age by itself is a major risk factor for falls, for a number of reasons. Elderly persons have significantly less lower extremity strength than young adults (Rubenstein, Josephson, & Robbins, 1994). In general, gait impairment is much more common, including decreased gait velocity and step height. The elderly react more slowly to sudden environmental hazards and usually have decreased visual acuity and depth perception. All these factors contribute to Mrs. Ianonne's difficulties. Women fall more often than men until the age of 75, after which there is no difference (Campbell, 1981).

Joint-related problems, such as the osteoarthritis Mrs. Ianonne suffers, have been shown to predispose elderly persons to falls (Tinetti, Williams, & Mayewski, 1986).

The patient's medications deserve close attention. It has been shown that the risk of falls increases in elderly patients who take four or more different medications (Robbins et al., 1989). Mrs. Ianonne is below this level. Use of specific classes of medications is, however, associated with a greater risk of falling. These include sedatives, which presumably interfere with attention and sensory input, and also non-

steroidal anti-inflammatory drugs (Granek et al., 1989), which the patient does use.

3. **Dizziness** is a vague complaint used by patients to describe a variety of sensations, including "lightheadedness," "faintness," and true vertigo. Mrs. Ianonne provides a good description of her symptoms. It is safe to say that a sensation consistent with lightheadedness predominates. There is a history of "spinning," but it is hard to say whether she experiences true vertigo.

The patient's medication use provides a possible explanation for the dizzy spells, which, as mentioned at the outset, are the most obvious direct cause of the falls. Aspirin has been noted to cause vestibular dysfunction (Tinetti & Speechley, 1989). One of the most common side effects of the sulfonylureas is hypoglycemia, which often presents as episodes of dizziness (Field, 1989).

Cardiac disease in the form of dysrythmias, autonomic insufficiency, aortic stenosis, volume depletion, or carotid sinus hypersensitivity can account for that kind of dizziness most patients describe as lightheadedness. This sensation is worse soon after standing. There is little to support any of these conditions as a cause of Mrs. Ianonne's symptoms.

Mrs. Ianonne suffered a transient ischemic attack (TIA) that is likely to have involved the right carotid artery. Subsequent testing showed some atherosclerotic disease of both carotids. Though TIAs involving the carotid system rarely produce vertigo or any other form of dizziness, those involving the vertebrobasilar system often can. Vertigo is, however, rarely the sole manifestation of vertebrobasilar insufficiency. Furthermore, sequential ischemic attacks originating in the vertebrobasilar system rarely present in the same manner. All things considered, it is still best to be aware of this cause when assessing Mrs. Ianonne.

4. Essential components of the physical examination in this case include focused examination of the eyes and ears as well as the cardiovascular, neurological, and musculoskeletal systems. A suggested physical examination scheme is outlined in "The Rest of the Story," together with relevant findings.

Two special tests require further explanation. The "Get-up and Go" Test developed by Mathias, Nayak, and Isaacs (1986) has been shown to be an effective functional screening tool for detecting mobility problems in the elderly. It involves having the patient rise from a chair, walk toward a wall 3 meters away, turn around without touching the wall, and return to the original seated position. The test is graded on a scale of 1 to 5, with 1 indicating normal function and 5 indicating severe impairment and risk of falling.

As noted, it is unclear whether Mrs. Ianonne experiences true vertigo during her "dizzy" spells. One way to settle the question is to provide vestibular stimulation and ask if the patient experiences similar symptoms during her spells. The most benign way to do this involves the **Barany Maneuver.** The patient is first seated on a table with her head turned to the right. Next, she is lowered quickly to the supine position so that her head is approximately 30 degrees below the edge of the table. She is held in this position for 30 s. The maneuver is repeated two more times, once with the patient's head turned to the left and finally with the patient facing straight ahead. Any nystagmus and vertigo is recorded.

5. Further testing needs to be individualized. Baseline evaluation when the cause of falls and dizziness is not obvious includes a CBC to rule out anemia or an infectious process, serum electrolytes, fasting glucose, and TSH. Rubenstein et al. (1994) recommend electrocardiography to document arrythmia. They do not, however, recommend Holter monitoring in routine evaluation. Holter monitoring in elderly persons reveals a high rate of ventricular and supraventricular arrythmias, regardless of fall status (Rosado et al., 1989).

Mrs. Ianonne should return the next day if lab results warrant. She should refrain from risky behavior that might lead to falls in the interim. With or without abnormal laboratory results, the patient should be followed up soon for further evaluation and management.

6. The history, together with the very low fasting glucose level, strongly indicate that Mrs. Ianonne is suffering from episodes of hypoglycemia, probably from the use of glyburide.

Glyburide is second only to chlorpropamide as a cause of severe hypoglycemic episodes among sulfonylureas (Field, 1989). It is also the most commonly used sulfonylurea in the world. It has a half-life of 10 hr, but its effects last anywhere from 24 to 60 hr.

A suitable starting point in the management of this patient's problem is to discontinue the glyburide. The patient and her daughter should be educated thoroughly about fall prevention measures and should be encouraged to carefully inspect the home environment for potential hazards, making modifications as needed (see "The Rest of the Story").

The Rest of the Story

You are unable to do a home safety assessment due to time constraints. Instead, you ask Maria about Mrs. Ianonne's home environment.

Mrs. Ianonne lives in a large four-bedroom home with the rest of her family. Her room is located in the basement, which is accessible from the main floor by a flight of nine stairs. This staircase was the site of the patient's worst fall. Maria is not sure how high the steps are, but she tells you that her mother is usually able to negotiate the staircase without difficulty.

Most of the house, including Mrs. Ianonne's bedroom and separate washroom, is covered with plush carpet. The kitchen, located on the main floor, is covered with linoleum. The washroom is normally equipped; that is, there are no grab bars or other safety devices.

Maria admits that the basement is poorly lit and that light switches are located in awkward places. She is willing to call an electrician to solve the problem if it will help prevent her mother from falling.

The yard and entrances to the house are well maintained and kept free of ice and snow in the winter months.

Mrs. Ianonne received a new pair of house slippers a couple of weeks ago as a birthday gift from one of her friends. She has been wearing them daily since that time. Maria has never closely examined these. Mrs. Ianonne tells you that they are comfortable but a little slippery.

Suggested Physical Examination (corresponding results summarized)

Gen: Pleasant, well-groomed elderly woman

VS: P = 84, reg.; BP = 130/80, supine; BP = 125/80, seated; RR = 22/min

HEENT:

> Ears: Tms. (R & L) normal (Auditory acuity not formally assessed. Mrs. Ianonne had no difficulty hearing the examiner's questions and instructions)
>
> Eyes: Bifocal eyeglasses in good condition. VA: OD = 20/30 with correction; OS = 20/30 with correction. Mrs. Ianonne is able to read a newspaper at a distance of 30 cm without difficulty
>
> Conjunctivae: Normal (i.e., no pallor)
>
> Visual fields by confrontation: No deficits observed

Barany Maneuver: No nystagmus observed. Patient does experience a spinning sensation but indicates that this is not what she feels just prior to her falls

Respiratory exam: Within normal limits

Cardiovascular exam: No carotid bruits/Normal JVP/Normal heart sounds with no murmurs

Musculoskeletal exam:

> "Get-up and Go" Test: Completed slowly but without major gait or coordination difficulties; scored as 3—mildly abnormal
>
> Spine: Marked thoracic kyphosis
>
> Hips: Normal range of motion, but pain on internal rotation of both hip joints
>
> Knees: Flexion limited by app. 20 deg. bilaterally; pain on flexion beyond 90 deg.
>
> Ankles and feet: No significant abnormalities

Neurologic exam:

Romberg Test: Negative Romberg sign with minimal observed pronator drift

Motor: Normal strength in hip flexion, abduction and adduction; normal strength in knee flexion and extension; normal strength in ankle dorsiflexion and plantar flexion. No significant abnormalities in lower extremity bulk or tone. Rapid alternating movements of hands—within normal limits

Deep tendon reflexes: Normal

Babinski: Negative bilaterally

Sensory: Normal pain and vibration sensation in feet. Normal light-touch sensation in feet

Initial laboratory results (all values are in SI units unless otherwise specified; U.S. units are in brackets)

CBC: WBC = 7.8×10^9/liter; Hb = 7.5mM [12.2mg/dL]; Hct = 0.38; Plt = 272×10^9/liter

Electrolytes: Na = 139; K = 3.5; Cl = 103; CO_2 = 24; BUN = 6.4mM [17.9mg/dL]; Creat. = 91μmol/l [1.0mg/dL]

Fasting serum glucose: 1.6mM [29mg/dL]

sTSH: 1.92

EKG: normal

Conclusion

You see Mrs. Ianonne on the same day the lab results above become available. You decide to discontinue the glyburide, at least temporarily. The patient and her daughter are educated about fall prevention measures. Maria promises to look into getting the lighting fixed in the basement. Her mother promises to wear only good-quality footwear that provides reasonable stability and traction.

You tell the patient that falling is not a natural part of aging and can have serious consequences. You also tell her that her symptoms should improve upon discontinuing the glyburide and that she should be able to resume her usual activities without fear of falling.

You see the patient and her daughter in a follow-up visit 1 week later. The patient tells you that she has experienced no dizzy spells and consequently no falls. In fact, she tells you that she feels better than she has in months!

Mrs. Ianonne continues to report no increased frequency or volume of urination, no increased thirst, and no visual changes. You send her for another fasting glucose level, which returns as 7.0mM. You plan no further interventions in the short term.

References

Campbell, A. J. (1981). Falls in old age: A study of frequency and related clinical factors. *Age & Ageing, 10,* 264-270.

Field, J. B. (1989). Hypoglycemia. *Endocrinology and Metabolism Clinics of North America, 18*(1), 27-35.

Granek, E., Baker, S. P., Abbey, H., Robinson, E., Myers, A. H., Samkoff, J. S., & Klein, L. E. (1989). Medications and diagnoses in relation to falls in a long-term care facility. *Journal of the American Geriatrics Society, 35,* 503-511.

Hindmarsh, J. L., & Estes, E. H. (1989). Falls in older persons. *Archives of Internal Medicine, 149,* 2217-2222.

Mathias, S., Nayak, U.S.L., & Isaacs, B. (1986). Balance in elderly patients: The "Get-up and Go" Test. *Archives of Physical Medicine and Rehabilitation, 67,* 387-389.

Robbins, A. S., Rubenstein, L. Z., Josephson, K. R., Schulman, B. L., Osterweil, D., & Fine, G. (1989). Predictors of falls among elderly people. *Archives of Internal Medicine, 149*, 1628-1633.

Rosado, J. A., Rubenstein, L. Z., Robbins, A. S., Heng, M. K., Schulman, B. L., & Josephson, K. R. (1989). The value of Holter monitoring in evaluating the elderly patient who falls. *Journal of the American Geriatrics Society, 37*, 430-434.

Rubenstein, L. Z., Josephson, K. R., & Robbins, A. S. (1994). Falls in the nursing home. *Annals of Internal Medicine, 121*, 442-451.

Tinetti, M. E., & Speechley, M. (1989). Prevention of falls among the elderly. *New England Journal of Medicine, 320*, 1055-1105.

Tinetti, M. E., Williams, T. F., & Mayewski, R. (1986). Fall risk index for elderly patients based on number of chronic disabilities. *American Journal of Medicine, 80*, 429-434.

4. HEADACHE

Ms. Shannon Stapleton

*Goal: The goal of this exercise is to evaluate and develop
the participants' understanding of the assessment and treatment
of headaches in an adult patient.*

Specific Objectives: Upon completion of this exercise, each participant should be able to accomplish the following:

1. Obtain a comprehensive history from a new patient presenting with headaches.
2. Perform a focused physical examination of a new patient presenting with headaches.
3. List the signs and symptoms that distinguish benign from serious causes of headache.
4. List the common symptoms of migraine headaches.
5. Discuss nonpharmacologic and pharmacologic treatments for migraine headaches.

PART I

The Patient

Social History

Shannon Stapleton is a 20-year-old sophomore at Murray State University in Murray, Kentucky. The daughter of Bill and Mary Stapleton, Shannon presently lives in an off-campus apartment with her close friend, Jane. Shannon was born and raised in Myers, a small town in northeastern Kentucky, where her father works as a cabinetmaker. The patient is majoring in history and hopes to become a high school teacher. As Shannon is the first and only member of the Stapleton family to attend college, Bill and Mary are extremely proud of her. In Mr. Stapleton's words, "We're all hardworking folks, but none of us ever had the inclination to get a higher education. Shannon is the first, and I'm sure she'll do very well in life."

Shannon has two older sisters. Maggie, 25 years old, a hairstylist and divorced single mother of three, lives and works just outside Cincinnati. Alice, 22, a secretary, has been living with her boyfriend in Los Angeles for the past 3 years. The patient's maternal grandparents, Edmund and Hilary Brock, live only a short distance from the Stapleton home.

Shannon is an active and dynamic young woman. She is an average student who admits that she could do much better "if only I didn't socialize so much." The patient is a member of a college choral group and has, over the past 18 months, belonged to various other university clubs and organizations. She presently has a part-time job conducting tours of the Murray campus for prospective students and parents. She enjoys parties, attending sports events, singing, and country line-dancing. Shannon has a number of close friends in Murray, many of whom she knew back in high school in Myers. For the past year she has been seeing Todd McCardle, a mild-mannered fellow sophomore whose family lives in Murray. Todd's parents are very fond of Shannon and often involve her in their family's social activities.

The Stapletons are Methodists who attend church on a regular basis. Shannon attends a Methodist church in Murray but describes herself as "not all that religious." The Stapletons trace their ancestry to immigrants who came from England and Ireland in the 1830s.

Past Personal and Family Medical History

The patient was a healthy child and is unaware of any history of serious illnesses or hospitalizations. She began menstruating at age 13. She is sexually active with one partner and has been using *triphasil 28,* a triphasic oral contraceptive pill, daily for the past 3 years. The patient does not smoke or use any illicit drugs. She drinks alcohol in very small quantities, roughly one or two beers on an average of twice a month.

The patient's immunizations are up to date. She uses no medications apart from her birth control pill. She has comprehensive health insurance provided at a reasonable rate through her university.

Mary Stapleton, 48, is in very good health. She had a tubal ligation in 1988 and has no history of serious hospitalizations or other surgery. Bill Stapleton, 49, is fairly healthy. He has had a number of minor musculoskeletal injuries over the years, most of them acquired while working as a cabinetmaker. He is also significantly overweight and a voracious consumer of chewing tobacco.

Alice and Maggie, to the best of Shannon's knowledge, are in perfect health. Edmund Brock suffers from chronic stable angina. His wife Hilary, according to Shannon, is "slightly demented" but is otherwise healthy.

The Problem

You are a family physician working in a clinic that primarily serves a university community in a small town. There is a nearby community hospital with a nearly full complement of special diagnostic facilities. There are few specialists in town but many within a 100-km radius. Shannon Stapleton comes to your office one afternoon and tells you she has been having headaches.

Doctor, I'm here because of my headaches. I mean, I'm not having a headache right now. You see, I had this term paper due today. I've had a couple of really bad headaches this week—made me feel like dying. I just didn't get it done. I told my professor about that, and he said I needed a note from you before he would give me an extension.

Questions

1. Would you provide Shannon with a doctor's note?
2. How would you obtain a thorough headache history from the patient? (See "The Rest of the Story" in Part I)
3. How would you perform a focused physical examination? (See the suggested examinations at the end of "The Rest of the Story" in Part I.)
4. After reading "The Rest of the Story," would you order any special imaging studies?

Discussion

1. This is a fairly common request in a university clinic. Many discussion participants may argue, quite justifiably, that it is too early to answer this question. A successful patient encounter in this situation would not involve simply providing Shannon with a note but engaging the patient in a discussion of her headaches. This may be accomplished in several ways. The physician may, for example, tell Shannon, "I can provide you with a note. That is not a problem. But I'd really like to find out more about these headaches so that I can help you in any way I can."

2. Headache is the seventh most common presenting complaint in ambulatory encounters in the United States (Linet, Stewart, Celentano, Ziegler, & Sprecher, 1989). Unfortunately, many headaches are poorly evaluated by primary care physicians (Lipton, Stewart, Calentano, & Reed, 1991). A detailed history, obtained while keeping the differential diagnosis of headache in mind, is the clinician's most valuable tool in making an accurate diagnosis (Dalessio, 1994).

It is essential during the course of an evaluation of headache to determine whether Shannon has a **primary headache disorder** or headaches **secondary** to some serious organic disease such as meningitis or tumor. This is often an extremely difficult task. The vast majority of headaches are benign in origin. On the other hand, missing a subarachnoid hemorrhage or meningitis could have devastating consequences.

The likelihood that a serious cause of headache is present is much greater in the patient presenting with a first, severe episode rather than with a chronic history of headaches (Raskin, 1995). This point should be clarified first. In addition, Edmeads (1990) describes a set of clinical signs and symptoms that make the possibility of a secondary headache more likely. The "danger signals" include the following:

1. Headache of extraordinary severity (usually patient's worst headache ever).
2. Onset of headache with exertion, suggestive of subarachnoid hemorrhage or increased intracranial pressure.
3. Any abnormality on neurologic examination or abnormality in vital signs, including fever.
4. Nuchal rigidity, suggesting pus or blood in the spinal fluid.
5. Decreased level of consciousness.
6. Worsening headache while under observation.

Presence of any of these should be followed by further investigations, including imaging procedures and/or lumbar puncture.

Edmeads (1990) admits that these criteria are based on his own personal experience and what he perceives as the consensus among fellow neurologists. He identifies a need for consensus-based guidelines that can be tested for validity and then recommended to a wide variety of clinicians. In the interim, his "danger signals" can be applied as a useful tool while obtaining a thorough history and performing a physical examination, as described later, of the patient with headache.

The comprehensive approach to history taking from a patient presenting with headache is not unlike that for other complaints. A number of simplified approaches have been described (Dalessio, 1994; Edmeads, 1990).

The **age at onset** is extremely important. Headaches that first appear later in life are more likely to be associated with organic pathology. By contrast, migraine headaches typically begin in childhood, adolescence, or young adulthood. One should also ask about the **location** of the pain. Pain on one side of the head, which may alternate sides with different episodes, is characteristic of migraine. Unilateral orbital pain is often *cluster headache. Tension-type headaches* may occur anywhere in the head but may also involve the neck or shoulders.

Knowing the **quality** or **characteristics** of the pain sometimes helps in the diagnosis. Migraine headaches are usually throbbing or pounding. In acute subarachnoid hemorrhage, an extremely serious, life-threatening condition, the pain is intense and explosive, often described as the patient's "worst headache ever." In general,

however, the intensity of pain is rarely helpful in distinguishing between a serious and benign cause of headache. Many brain tumors, for example, cause only mild pain (Raskin, 1995).

The **chronology** of the pain is crucial. Headaches that get progressively worse may be a sign of serious pathology. Headaches caused by brain tumors are usually worst before noon and usually of short duration. Migraine headaches may begin upon awakening, often occur on weekends and around holidays, and usually last less than a day. Headaches due to meningeal causes are usually of very acute onset. **Associated signs and symptoms** should be elicited. Cluster headaches, for example, are often associated with rhinorrhea and ipsilateral lacrimation. Migraine headaches may or may not be accompanied by auras, consisting of visual disturbance or unilateral paresthesias. In addition, migraines are often associated with nausea, vomiting, and photo- or phonophobia. Headaches with infectious causes have characteristic symptoms. Meningitis, for example, is associated with fever and nuchal rigidity. Sinusitis is often accompanied by purulent nasal discharge. One should inquire about **precipitating and aggravating** factors. Migraine headaches, for example, may be triggered or made worse by alcohol, fatigue, and food additives. Headaches resulting from intraventricular and posterior fossa tumors may be aggravated by coughing and the Valsalva maneuver.

Dalessio (1994) emphasizes the relationship of headache to **sleep** in obtaining a history. Brain-tumor-related headaches, for example, do not usually disrupt sleep. As noted, migraine headaches may begin upon awakening; they may actually be triggered by very deep sleep.

Family history of headaches is very important, particularly in identifying migraine, which usually has a strong inherited component. In the patient profile, there is no family history of headaches, but participants may wish to question Shannon further in this area.

It is important to keep in mind that a history must be obtained in light of what is immediately known about the patient and what diagnoses are most likely. A diagnosis of migraine or tension-type headaches is common in a young woman like Shannon. Brain tumors are much less common.

3. The history of episodic headaches of 3 months' duration in a young woman is consistent with a **primary headache disorder.** The goal of the physical examination is to find evidence that either does or does not support this conclusion. One should continue to apply Edmeads's danger-signal criteria to whatever extent is possible. In addition, a brief screening, rather than a complete neurological examination, is all that is needed (Edmeads & Pryse-Phillips, 1994). Simply obtaining a history from the patient gives one an idea of his or her **mental state** and **level of consciousness.** While the patient speaks, a brief assessment of **facial muscle power** and **symmetry** can be made. An assessment of the **cranial nerves,** though not comprehensive, can be made by examining the fundi, pupils, eye movements, and corneal reflexes. The **visual fields** should also be assessed.

The **deep tendon reflexes** and **plantar responses** should be tested, as should **proximal and distal muscle power.** Distal power in the upper extremities can be evaluated through grip strength, proximal power by forced flexion of the shoulder that tests the deltoid muscle. Similarly, in the lower extremities, the hip flexors can be tested by asking the patient to bring his or her knees up to the stomach against resistance. Forced dorsiflexion of the toes tests distal power.

A screening test of **sensation** can be accomplished by evaluating light touch on the toes. **Proprioception** can be evaluated by gripping each of the great toes: Grip the toe on its side and move it up or down while asking the patient to determine the direction of movement. A screening test of **cerebellar function** can be accomplished by doing a finger-to-nose test. A **Romberg** test completes the screening neurological examination. See the suggested examinations at the end of "The Rest of the Story" in Part I.

3. Neuroimaging, using CT or MRI, is sometimes performed to rule out the presence of brain tumors and other structural abnormalities. The routine use of such tests in patients with headache and normal neurologic examination is discouraged by the Quality Standards Subcommittee of the American Academy of Neurology (1994). The yield from such investigations is extremely low. In a retrospective case series in which 89 patients with *isolated* headache underwent cerebral computed tomographic scans, the imaging tests added no new information in *any* of the patients (Weingarten, Kleinman, Elperin, & Larson, 1992). Furthermore, in the same study, among 40 patients in whom imaging studies did identify a brain tumor, *none* presented with headache *alone* at the time of diagnosis. A decision to obtain imaging studies in Shannon's case, therefore, cannot be justified.

The Rest of the Story

You tell Shannon that if she has indeed been feeling unwell over the past few days, you will be able to provide her with an appropriate doctor's note. You tell her that you are concerned about her headaches and that you would like to hear more about this problem. You ask her specifically if her headaches began only in the past few days, or some time ago.

"Well, doctor, I guess they started about 3 or 4 months ago. I'm not a complainer, but these headaches are really bad. Sometimes I wake up with a headache, and I'm miserable the rest of the whole day." Shannon tells you that she did not have headaches until 3 months ago, when they began to occur at a frequency of roughly once per week. They last from 4 to 8 hr, and the patient gets only slight relief from regular doses of extra-strength acetaminophen tablets. The headaches have not increased in frequency, duration, or severity over the past 3 months, but she has had two particularly bad headaches over the past week that have, as she first indicated, interfered with her schoolwork. Shannon has noticed that her headaches usually occur on weekends and have had a tendency to interfere more with her social rather than with her academic activities.

Shannon tells you the headaches consist of a throbbing unilateral pain, usually on the left temporal area but sometimes on the right. The patient has noticed no associated change with exertion, no rhinorrhea, tearing, neck stiffness, or any auras of any kind. She has had no fever, nasal discharge or congestion, or any cough. She has noticed no change in the intensity of headache when she changes her position. Shannon has felt very nauseated during her headaches but states that she has only vomited once. She also tells you, "Bright lights and loud noises really bother me when I have headaches. I like to crawl into a cozy dark spot and lie still until it's over."

The patient has not noticed any association with her menstrual cycle, alcohol use, or particular foods. Indeed, she is unable to identify any specific headache trigger. Shannon tells you that her headaches are unrelated to her sleep patterns and that she has been sleeping quite well over the past 3 months.

The patient is unaware of any family history of headache disorders but admits that she has only sporadic contact with her older sisters and that she is not familiar with their particular health concerns.

Suggested Physical Examination: (Corresponding results summarized)

Gen: Alert, very pleasant, slim, articulate young woman
VS: BP = 100/65mmHg; P = 72/min; RR = 18/min; T = 37.2°C
HEENT: No nuchal rigidity

Screening Neurological Examination
    No facial asymmetry; normal speech
    Fundi-normal bilat.; Pupils-PERLA; Normal extraocular movements bilaterally; Corneal reflexes
       normal bilaterally
    Visual fields normal to confrontation
    Deep tendon reflexes normal bilaterally
    Normal bilateral proximal and distal muscle power in upper and lower extremities

Normal sensation to light touch over left and right toes
Normal bilateral proprioception
Normal finger-to-nose test
Romberg test negative

PART II

The Problem

You conclude that Shannon has a *primary* headache disorder, and tell her that it is extremely unlikely that she has any serious underlying disease. She responds, "Well, I'm happy to hear that, Doctor. A friend of mine gets migraines. I was talking to her about my headaches, and they sound pretty similar. Do you think I have migraines?"

Questions

1. What sorts of patients get migraine headaches?
2. How would you respond to Shannon's question?

Discussion

1. The prevalence of migraine headache in relation to age, income, race, and other factors has been studied in a large questionnaire survey of more than 20,000 subjects (Stewart, Lipton, Celentano, & Reed, 1992). Migraine headaches occur more commonly in women. Indeed, in the study, 17.6% of females surveyed reported symptoms consistent with migraine headache. The prevalence of migraines in women rises rapidly after age 20, peaks around age 40, and drops off gradually thereafter. Migraines are somewhat more common in whites than blacks. Interestingly, the prevalence of migraine headache increases with decreasing income, which is inconsistent with the commonly held perception that migraine is more common in the higher socioeconomic classes. Shannon is a young white female. Her background could be described as "middle class." From an epidemiologic point of view, Shannon is not an atypical migraine sufferer.

2. In 1988, the International Headache Society (IHS) issued a new, specific classification system for different types of headache (Headache Classification Committee of the International Headache Society, 1988). In addition, specific definitions of each type of headache based on particular diagnostic criteria were developed, including migraine with and without aura and tension-type headache (see Appendix). This system has been the subject of a great deal of criticism (Becker, Green, Beaufait, Kirk, & Froom, 1993; Smith, 1993). Though a useful tool for research and epidemiologic purposes, the IHS definitions are considered to be too detailed and too difficult to apply in the context of ambulatory care visits to primary care physicians. According to Rapaport (1992), an

"acceptable description" of migraine headaches without aura is the following: "a moderate-to-severe, throbbing, unilateral headache in the temple or around the eye of a woman with a family history of migraine who has developed headaches between the ages of 10 and 25 years . . . usually associated with nausea, vomiting, anorexia, phonophobia, and photophobia, occurring one to four times per month, lasting most of the day and usually improving with sleep." It is hard to understand how this definition represents a significant simplification of the IHS criteria. Solomon and Lipton (1991) have proposed a much simpler scheme, which allows a diagnosis of migraine without aura to be made when any two of the following symptoms are present: unilateral side, throbbing quality, nausea, photo- or phonophobia. Tension headache is usually not accompanied by nausea or photo-/phonophobia. By the Lipton criteria, a diagnosis of migraine without aura can be made in the case of Shannon Stapleton.

If the IHS criteria are strictly applied, the diagnosis of migraine without aura is still supported. Shannon has had more than five attacks of headache, which are unilateral, pulsating or "throbbing," severe enough to interfere with daily activities, and accompanied by nausea and photo- and phonophobia. Furthermore, there is no evidence of a serious neurological disorder. It is unclear in the history that the patient has so far provided whether her headaches are aggravated by physical activity. She did indicate a desire to "crawl into a cozy dark spot and lie still," suggesting that rest is associated with less headache intensity. Aggravation by physical activity has been found to be a particularly useful criterion in distinguishing between migraine and tension headache (Rapaport, 1992), the two most likely diagnoses to consider in an otherwise healthy young woman like Shannon. In any case, when the IHS criteria are strictly applied, a diagnosis of migraine without aura can be made, and one of tension-type headache can be excluded. Shannon should be told this.

PART III

The Problem

You tell Shannon that a diagnosis of migraine without aura is the most likely explanation for her headaches. She responds, "Yeah, I figured that's what it was. I guess I need more than just a doctor's note. These headaches are disrupting my life. That extra-strength Tylenol doesn't do very much for me. I guess there are better medications out there."

Questions

1. In broad terms, how would you classify the approaches to management of migraine headaches?
2. Are you concerned about Shannon's use of the birth control pill?
3. Discuss nonpharmacologic treatments for migraine.

4. What are the indications for pharmacologic, prophylactic therapy?
5. What medications are available for the treatment of migraines?
6. What medication regimen, if any, should Shannon receive?

Discussion

1. The approaches to management of migraines can be broadly classified as **nonpharmacologic** and **pharmacologic.** Both categories can be divided into **prophylactic therapies,** used to prevent attacks of migraine headache, or **abortive and symptomatic therapies,** used during an acute attack of migraine to rid the patient or lessen the severity of the headache.

2. For many years, the presence of migraine headaches in a young woman was considered to be a *relative* contraindication to the use of oral contraceptives (OCPs). This was based on the belief that the incidence of stroke is greater in women who have migraines and use OCPs. It is now believed that migraine headache itself is an independent risk factor for cerebral thromboembolism, and that the use of oral contraceptives in migraine patients does not confer added risk (Collaborative Group for the Study of Stroke in Young Women, 1975; Lidegaard, 1995).

There is considerable evidence that female hormones play a significant role in the pathophysiology of migraine headaches in some women (Silberstein & Merriam, 1991). It follows that oral contraceptives should have some impact on migraine headaches. The effect, however, is highly variable. Oral contraceptives can trigger a first attack of migraine (Kudrow, 1975). Existing migraine headaches may worsen in severity or frequency (Ryan, 1978). Alternatively, migraine headaches may improve with oral contraceptives (Whitty, Hockaday, & Whitty, 1966). Many patients on OCPs experience no change in the pattern of migraine headaches (Silberstein & Merriam, 1991). In summary, the effect of oral contraceptives is unpredictable. Shannon has been using her birth control pills for 3 years. Her headaches are of relatively recent onset. It is extremely unlikely that the pill is a migraine trigger. Furthermore, it is hard to say what effect, if any, stopping the birth control pill would have on Shannon's migraines.

All things considered, Shannon's use of oral contraceptive pills should not raise too much concern. There is no good reason to discontinue the pill or switch to another variety at this time.

3. Nonpharmacologic therapies will be discussed first. These are mostly prophylactic approaches, but they also include some symptomatic/abortive treatments. **Trigger identification and avoidance** is emphasized as part of a comprehensive management plan (Sheftell, 1993), although only 10% to 15% of migraine sufferers are able to identify a specific trigger (Edmeads & Pryse-Phillips, 1994). The likelihood of identifying one or more triggers is increased by keeping a *headache calendar* (Schulman & Silberstein, 1992; see Appendix) on which the onset, duration, and severity of headaches is recorded, together with the patient's activities, emotional state, medications taken (if any), and recently consumed foods and drinks. Sheftell divides triggers into **hormones, diet, changes, sensory stimuli,** and **stress.**

The hormonal influence on migraine headaches has already been mentioned. Female migraine sufferers often experience onset of headache during the first three days of menstruation (Johannes et al., 1995). Furthermore, 14% of women with migraines experience headaches exclusively during menses (Nattero, 1982). This is the disorder known as **menstrual migraine.** Shannon has given no indication that any phase of her menstrual cycle is associated with headaches, but a well-kept headache calendar may reveal otherwise.

Foods and drinks that can trigger migraines include alcohol, chocolate, aged cheeses, monosodium glutamate (a preservative found in many Chinese foods), nuts, and coffee and other caffeinated beverages. At the very least, Shannon should be asked to record the consumption of such products in relation to her headaches. Some advocate complete avoidance of all such products, or *dietary modification* as an immediate management strategy for migraine headaches (Sheftell, 1993).

Among *changes* that can trigger migraine are weather conditions, seasons, and modification of sleep patterns. **Sensory stimuli** include flickering lights and particular odors. Stress can take many forms in a young woman like Shannon, including exams or assignments or difficulties in her relationships with friends, family, or her boyfriend Todd. All these potential triggers should be explained to Shannon so that her success in identifying one or several related to her headaches will be maximized. Just as dietary modification can be immediately recommended to a patient presenting with migraines, other recommendations to avoid *potential* triggers can be made, such as good sleep hygiene and ways to relieve stress (such as exercise). Such recommendations are consistent with "healthy living" in general.

A number of other prophylactic non-pharmacologic approaches to migraines have been used, including biofeedback therapy, meditation, and acupuncture. The effectiveness of such therapies needs further evaluation before they can be universally recommended to migraine sufferers. In any case, these methods have been advocated as an adjunct to, rather than a replacement for, other nonpharmacologic and pharmacologic treatments (Schulman & Silberstein, 1992).

Of interest: In a randomized, double-blind, placebo-controlled crossover study, the aromatic plant **feverfew** was found to decrease the frequency of migraine attacks by 24% in patients belonging to a migraine self-help group (Murphy, Heptinsall, & Mitchell, 1988). Feverfew is widely used as an herbal prophylactic remedy in the United Kingdom.

During an acute migraine attack, the pain of headache can be somewhat lessened by applying cold compresses to the head or tying a tight band around it to decrease throbbing. Vigorous massage of the scalp muscles can actually abort an attack (Edmeads & Pryse-Phillips, 1994).

3. Baumel (1994) recommends prophylactic pharmacologic therapy for patients who have more than two migraine attacks per month, those with a lesser frequency of attacks but more severe headaches that are refractory to acute therapy, and those with a predictable pattern of headaches (e.g., women with menstrual migraines). By these criteria, Shannon should benefit from prophylactic medications.

4. As noted, there are both prophylactic and abortive, or symptomatic, medications. As the precise etiology of migraine is uncertain, the mechanism of action of many of these medications has yet to be determined. **Methysergide,** an ergot alka-

loid, is generally only used in severe cases of migraine as a prophylactic agent. It has serious side effects, including vascular constriction and retroperitoneal fibrosis, with prolonged use. **Calcium-channel blockers,** especially *verapamil,* have been used successfully in prophylaxis. *Flunarizine,* a relatively new calcium-channel blocker available in Canada but not currently in the United States, is among the most effective prophylactic agents.

Nonsteroidal anti-inflammatory drugs (NSAIDs), when used on a regular basis, are able to decrease the frequency of migraine headaches (Buring, Peto, & Hennekens, 1990). Other medications used in migraine prophylaxis include *antidepressants* (especially *amitryptilline*) and the anticonvulsant *valproate.*

The most commonly used prophylactic medications are the beta-adrenergic blockers. Indeed, a beta-blocker is considered the best established choice ("Drugs for Migraine," 1995). Commonly used preparations include *propanolol,* 80 to 240 mg/day, and *timolol,* 20 mg/day. Prophylactic therapy need not be continued indefinitely. After a trial of 3 to 6 months with one prophylactic agent, the medication can be withdrawn. The decrease in frequency of migraines usually continues, and medication may not need to be restarted (Edmeads & Pryse-Phillips, 1994).

There is a large number of medications used in abortive (symptomatic) therapy. Commonly used analgesics such as NSAIDs, either alone (e.g., *Naproxen*) or in combination (e.g., *Fiorinal—a combination of aspirin, caffeine, and butalbital*) may be effective in controlling the symptoms of mild to moderate migraine headaches. *Acetaminophen* preparations can also be used (e.g., *Tylenol, Midrin*). More powerful analgesic agents, such as the narcotics, **meperidine,** and **butorphanol** nasal spray, are also an option for treatment of migraine but are, obviously, prone to dependence and abuse.

The serotonin agonists **ergotamine** and **dihydroergotamine** have been used for many years to treat migraine headaches. Ergotamine is more effective if used early during an attack. It should be used only for short periods, as it can cause dependence and consequent rebound headache upon discontinuation. Its adverse effects include nausea and vomiting, which can be minimized by simultaneous administration of an anti-emetic. Ergotamine is available in oral and suppository forms. Dihydroergotamine, which has fewer side effects, is available in an injectable form as well as a newly available nasal spray.

Sumatriptan (Imitrex) has received a great deal of publicity in recent years. A short-acting serotonin agonist, it is effective in relieving migraine symptoms or aborting migraine completely. It is available in oral and a self-injectable subcutaneous form. Sumatriptan is considerably more expensive than other migraine treatments. It is slightly more effective than dihydroergotamine (DHE) in relieving migraine symptoms in the first 2 hr after administration. At 4 hr, both medications are equally effective. At 24 hr, DHE is more effective. Moreover, DHE is associated with a much lower rate of headache recurrence after 24 hr ("Drugs for Migraine," 1995).

A number of other drugs are used to abort acute, severe migraine, including the antiemetics *promethazine* and *chlorpromazine* and corticosteroids, such as parenteral *dexamethasone.* These agents are often used in the emergency room setting.

5. There is no precise answer to this question. Exclusively oral treatment may

be a good, simple starting point. Shannon could benefit from both prophylactic and symptomatic (abortive) therapy. One effective regimen could be *timolol, 20mg/ day,* and oral *sumatriptan, 100mg* (maximum dose of 300mg/day), during an acute attack. Timolol, like other beta-blockers, is known to cause fatigue, depression, and orthostatic hypotension. Sumatriptan has a favorable side-effect profile but can cause chest pressure, particularly in patients with coronary heart disease. See "The Rest of the Story," which follows.

The Rest of the Story

You engage Shannon in a detailed discussion on the treatment of migraine headaches. You start with nonpharmacological approaches and tell her about identification and avoidance of migraine triggers. You also tell Shannon about the importance of good sleep hygiene, exercise, and ways to relieve stress in promoting good health in general, as well as a potential way to prevent migraine headaches. The patient is grateful for this advice and tells you,

> Well, I know what you're saying. Those things are important. I do sleep regular hours. I guess I could get some exercise. I really should do something. Jane takes an aerobics class. I've thought about joining in. It seems like it may be a lot of fun.

You tell Shannon that the aerobics class is a good idea. She denies a great deal of stress or any symptoms of depression or anxiety. In her words, "I guess I'm a pretty happy person."

Shannon agrees to keep a headache diary or calendar for the next couple of months to help identify triggers. You discuss preventive and abortive or symptomatic medication treatments. You recommend timolol, 20mg/day, and sumatriptan, 100mg po during acute attacks. Shannon seems receptive to your recommendations and agrees to take the medications as prescribed. You complete a note for her professor as requested and ask her to return in 1 month's time.

PART IV

The Problem

Shannon returns as scheduled. She has had three attacks of migraine over the past month but none during the last 10 days. Early during each of the attacks, she took sumatriptan as prescribed and experienced nearly complete relief with one tablet within 3 to 4 hours. The headaches have not interfered with her social or academic activities.

Shannon has maintained a headache calendar. Each of her three headaches began in the morning, two on a Sunday and one on a Tuesday. Shannon could identify no food, drink, weather change, emotional state, or other factor as a trigger in any of the headaches. Each headache occurred at a different phase in her menstrual cycle.

The patient seems quite pleased with the results of treatment, especially with the sumatriptan she has found to be so effective. She reports no fatigue, depressive symptoms, dizziness, lightheadedness, or chest pressure.

On physical examination:

Gen: Healthy-looking, pleasant young woman
BP = 110/60—no orthostatic change

Questions

1. How would you gauge the success of your migraine treatment?
2. Describe how you would manage the case from this point.

Discussion

1. There is little question that treatment of Shannon's headaches has been very successful. She appears to respond very well to the sumatriptan. Successful prophylaxis with beta-blockers usually takes several weeks of treatment to become apparent (Edmeads & Pryse-Phillips, 1994). In this respect, it is a good sign that Shannon has had no headaches for the past 10 days. Preventive therapy for migraines is considered successful if it reduces the frequency, duration, and intensity of attacks by 50% or more (Baumel, 1994). As noted earlier, like Shannon, most migraine sufferers are unable to identify one or more triggers.

2. The present medication regimen is working well. No immediate changes are needed. The timolol could be discontinued after 6 months. Shannon could be encouraged to continue keeping a headache diary, although, with successful treatment, the frequency of her headaches should continue to decrease, and there should be fewer headaches to record. She could be seen in 3 to 6 months' time to monitor her progress.

Conclusion

You ask Shannon to continue the present medication regimen and refill her prescriptions accordingly. You also ask her to continue to keep a record of her headaches. She returns to see you in 4 months and tells you immediately that she has been doing extremely well. She has had two headaches since her last visit, both of much less severity than those of several months ago and both responding quickly to one dose of sumatriptan. She continues to experience no side effects of either medication. Shannon's headache diary has revealed no triggers.

You ask Shannon to continue the timolol for 2 more months only and to return should she begin to experience headaches at an increased frequency. She tells you,

Oh yes, I'll definitely come back if I get bad headaches again. I want to thank you for all your help. And Doctor, I need a complete checkup some time, including a Pap smear. I'd like to come back and see you for that. By the way, I did join that aerobics class!

You tell Shannon you would be happy to look after her other health care needs and congratulate her for starting a program of regular exercise.

References

Baumel, B. (1994). Migraine: A pharmacologic review with newer options and delivery modalities. *Neurology, 44*(Suppl. 3), S13-S17.

Becker, L. A., Green, L. A., Beaufait, D., Kirk, J., & Froom, J. (1993). Use of CT scans for the investigation of headache: A report from ASPN, Part 1. *Journal of Family Practice, 37*, 129-134.

Buring, J. E., Peto, R., & Hennekens, C. H. (1990). Low-dose aspirin for migraine prophylaxis. *Journal of the American Medical Association, 264*, 1711-1713.

Collaborative Group for the Study of Stroke in Young Women. (1975). Oral contraceptives and stroke in young women. *Journal of the American Medical Association, 231*, 718-722.

Dalessio, D. J. (1994). Diagnosing the severe headache. *Neurology, 44*(Suppl. 3), S6-S12.

Drugs for migraine. (1995). *Medical Letter, 37*, 17-20.

Edmeads, J. (1990). Challenges in the diagnosis of acute headache. *Headache, 30*(Suppl.), 537-540.

Edmeads, J., & Pryse-Phillips, W. (1994, August). A painless approach to migraine headache. *Patient Care*, pp. 13-21.

Headache Classification Committee of the International Headache Society. (1988). Classification and diagnostic criteria for all headache disorders, cranial neuralgias and facial pain. *Cephalalgia, 8*(Suppl. 7), 1-96.

Johannes, C. B., Linet, M. S., Stewart, W. F., Celentano, D. D., Lipton, R. B., & Szklo, M. (1995). Relationship of headache to phase of the menstrual cycle among young women: A daily diary study. *Neurology, 45*, 1076-1082.

Kudrow, L. (1975). The relationship of headache frequency to hormone use in migraine. *Headache, 15*, 36-49.

Lidegaard, O. (1995). Oral contraceptives, pregnancy and the risk of cerebral thromboembolism: The influence of diabetes, hypertension, migraine and previous thrombotic disease. *British Journal of Obstetrics and Gynaecology, 102*, 153-159.

Linet, M. S., Stewart, W. F., Celentano, D. D., Ziegler, D., & Sprecher, M. (1989). An epidemiologic study of headache among adolescents and young adults. *Journal of the American Medical Association, 261*, 2211-2216.

Lipton, R. D., Stewart, W. F., Calentano, D. D., & Reed, M. L. (1991). Undiagnosed migraine headaches: A comparison of symptom-based and reported physician diagnosis. *Cephalalgia, 11*(Suppl.), 89-90.

Murphy, J. J., Heptinsall, S., & Mitchell, J.R.A. (1988, July). Randomised double blind placebo-controlled trial of feverfew in migraine prevention. *Lancet, 2*(8604), 189-192.

Nattero, G. (1982). Menstrual headache. In M. Critchley (Ed.), *Advances in neurology* (Vol. 33; pp. 215-216). New York: Raven.

Quality Standards Subcommittee of the American Academy of Neurology. (1994). Practice parameter: The utility of neuroimaging in the evaluation of headache in patients with normal neurologic examinations. *Neurology, 44*, 1353-1354.

Rapaport, A. M. (1992). The diagnosis of migraine and tension-type headache, then and now. *Neurology, 42*(Suppl. 2), 11-15.

Raskin, N. H. (1995). Headache. In L. P. Rowland (Ed.), *Merritt's textbook of neurology* (9th ed.; pp. 42-45). Media, PA: Williams and Wilkins.

Ryan, R. E. (1978). A controlled study of the effect of oral contraceptives on migraine. *Headache, 17*, 250-252.

Schulman, E. A., & Silberstein, S. D. (1992). Symptomatic and prophylactic treatment of migraine and tension-type headache. *Neurology, 42*(Suppl. 2), 16-21.

Sheftell, F. D. (1993). Pharmacologic therapy, non-drug therapy, and counseling are keys to effective migraine management. *Archives of Family Medicine, 2*, 874-879.

Silberstein, S. D., & Merriam, G. R. (1991). Estrogens, progestins, and headache. *Neurology, 41*, 786-793.

Smith, R. (1993). Headaches: An area of special responsibility for family practice. *Journal of Family Practice, 37*(2), 126-127.

Solomon, S., & Lipton, R. (1991). Criteria for the diagnosis of migraine in clinical practice. *Headache, 31*, 384-387.

Stewart, W. F., Lipton, R. B., Celentano, D. D., & Reed, M. L. (1992). Prevalence of migraine headache in the United States: Relation to age, income, race, and other sociodemographic factors. *Journal of the American Medical Association, 267*, 64-69.

Weingarten, S., Kleinman, M., Elperin, L., & Larson, E. B. (1992). The effectiveness of cerebral imaging in the diagnosis of chronic headache. *Archives of Internal Medicine, 152*, 2457-2462.

Whitty, C.W.M., Hockaday, J. M., & Whitty, M. M. (1966). The effect of oral contraceptives on migraine. *Lancet, 1*, 856-859.

Appendix
International Headache Society Definition of Migraine

1.1 Migraine without aura (previously used terms: common migraine, hemicrania simplex)

Diagnostic criteria
A. At least five attacks fulfilling B through D
B. Headache lasting 4 to 72 hr (untreated or unsuccessfully treated)
C. Headache has at least two of the following characteristics:
   1. Unilateral location
   2. Pulsating quality
   3. Moderate or severe intensity (inhibits or prohibits daily activities)
   4. Aggravation by walking stairs or similar routine physical activity
D. During headache, at least one of the following:
   1. Nausea and/or vomiting
   2. Photophobia and phonophobia
E. At least one of the following:
   1. History, physical, and neurologic examinations do not suggest one of the disorders listed in groups 5 through 11
   2. History and/or physical and/or neurologic examinations do suggest such disorder, but it is ruled out by appropriate investigations
   3. Such disorder is present, but migraine attacks do not occur for the first time in close temporal relation to the disorder

1.2 Migraine with aura (previously used terms: classic migraine; classical migraine; ophthalmic, hemiparesthetic, hemiplegic, or aphasic migraine)

Diagnostic criteria
A. At least two attacks fulfilling B
B. At least three of the following four characteristics:

1. One or more fully reversible aura symptoms indicating focal cerebral cortical and/or brainstem dysfunction
2. At least one aura symptom develops gradually over more than 4 min or two or more symptoms occur in succession
3. No aura symptom lasts more than 60 min; if more than one aura symptom is present, accepted duration is proportionally increased
4. Headache follows aura with a free interval of less than 60 min (it may also begin before or simultaneously with the aura)
C. At least one of the following:
   1. History, physical, and neurologic examinations do not suggest one of the disorders listed in groups 5 through 11
   2. History and/or physical and/or neurologic examinations do suggest such disorder, but it is ruled out by appropriate investigations
   3. Such disorder is present, but migraine attacks do not occur for the first time in close temporal relation to the disorder

Migraine with Typical Aura

Diagnostic criteria
A. Fulfills criteria for 1.2 including all four criteria under B
B. One or more aura symptoms of the following types:
   1. Homonymous visual disturbance
   2. Unilateral paresthesias and/or numbness
   3. Unilateral weakness
   4. Aphasia or unclassifiable speech difficulty

SOURCE: Rapoport (1992). Reproduced with permission from *Neurology*, Vol. 42, Supplement 2, p. 14. Copyright by Advanstar Communications Inc. Advanstar Communications Inc. retains all rights to this article.

Tension-Type Headache

2.1 Episodic tension-type headache (previously used terms: tension headache, muscle contraction headache, psychomyogenic headache, essential headache, idiopathic headache, and psychogenic headache)

Diagnostic criteria

A. At least 10 previous headache episodes fulfilling criteria B through D listed below; number of days with such headache < 180/year (< 15/month)
B. Headache lasting from 30 min to 7 days
C. At least two of the following pain characteristics:
   1. Pressing/tightening (nonpulsating) quality
   2. Mild or moderate intensity (may inhibit, but does not prohibit, activities)
   3. Bilateral location
   4. No aggravation by walking stairs or similar routine physical activity
D. Both of the following:
   1. No nausea or vomiting (anorexia may occur)
   2. Photophobia and phonophobia are absent, or one but not the other is present

2.1.1 Episodic tension-type headache associated with disorder of pericranial muscles (previously used terms: muscle contraction headache)

Diagnostic criteria

A. Fulfills criteria for episodic tension-type headache
B. At least one of the following:
   1. Increased tenderness of pericranial muscles demonstrated by manual palpation of pressure algometer
   2. Increased EMG level of pericranial muscles at rest during physiologic tests

2.1.2 Episodic tension-type headache not associated with disorder of pericranial muscles (previously used terms: idiopathic headache, essential headache, psychogenic headache)

Diagnostic criteria

A. Fulfills criteria for episodic tension-type headache
B. No increased tenderness of pericranial muscles. If studied, EMG of pericranial muscles shows normal levels of activity

2.2 Chronic tension-type headache (previously used terms: chronic daily headache)

Diagnostic criteria

A. Average headache frequency 15 days/month (180 days/year) for 6 months, fulfilling criteria B through D
B. At least two of following pain characteristics:
   1. Pressing or tightening quality
   2. Mild or moderate severity (may inhibit or prohibit activities)
   3. Bilateral location
   4. No aggravation by walking stairs or similar routine physical activity
C. Both of the following:
   1. No vomiting
   2. No more than one of the following: Nausea, photophobia, or phonophobia
D. At least one of the following:
   1. History, physical, and neurologic examinations do not suggest one of the disorders listed in groups 5 through 11
   2. History and/or physical and/or neurologic examinations do suggest such disorder, but it is ruled out by appropriate investigations
   3. Such disorder is present, but tension-type headache does not occur for the first time in close temporal relation to the disorder

2.2.1 Chronic tension-type headache associated with disorder of pericranial muscles

2.2.2 Chronic tension-type headache not associated with disorder of pericranial muscles

SOURCE: Rapoport (1992). Reproduced with permission from *Neurology*, Vol. 42, Supplement 2, pp. 12-13. Copyright by Advanstar Communications Inc. Advanstar Communications Inc. retains all rights to this article.

Headache Calendar

#1 Mild headache

#2 Moderate headache

Name _____ Month _____ Year _____   #3 Incapacitating headache

	01 02 03 04 05 06 07 08 09 10 11 12 13 14 15 16 17 18 19 20 21 22 23 24 25 26 27 28 29 30 31
Morning	
Afternoon	
Evening	
Sleeptime	

Medication

Relief 0-1-2-3   (0)-None   (1)-Slight relief   (2)-Moderate relief   (3)-Complete relief

Triggers:

Periods:

SOURCE: Sheftell (1993, p. 875). Used by permission.

5. TYPE II DIABETES

Mr. William Hodge

*Goal: The goal of this group discussion exercise is
to develop and evaluate the participants' understanding
of the diagnosis and management of Type II diabetes.*

Specific Objectives: Upon completion of the exercise, participants should be able to accomplish the following:

1. List the risk factors for development of Type II diabetes and screen appropriate patients.
2. Recall the rationale for treatment of Type II diabetes.
3. Counsel a patient recently diagnosed with Type II diabetes about nonpharmacologic approaches to management.
4. List the four classes of medications presently available for the treatment of Type II diabetes and explain the advantages and drawbacks of each.
5. Administer appropriate pharmacotherapy in a timely fashion.
6. Design a program of ongoing care for the Type II diabetic that incorporates regular medical evaluation, counseling, appropriate referrals according to present guidelines, and, what is most important, takes into consideration the special individual needs of the patient.

PART I

The Patient

Social History

Mr. William Hodge is a 54-year-old African American man who lives and works in the city of Beaumont, Texas. The son of Lucy and Harold Hodge, William was born and raised in Galveston, where he attended school until age 15. He held a number of different jobs throughout his youth, finally landing one with a Catholic high school in Beaumont, where he was employed as a custodian and later a groundskeeper. He presently works as an "all-purpose" repairman, responsible for maintenance of heating and cooling systems as well as minor adjustments to plumbing and electricity. A beloved figure among the school's students and teachers, Mr. Hodge is affectionately known as "Big Willie."

William met Carla Hayes in 1973. Carla was just 18 years old at the time. The two pursued a relationship for several years and were finally married in 1979. Carla and William had two children: Reggie, now 16, and Dwayne, 15. The marriage fell apart in 1984. According to the patient, "I was a lousy husband and was no father at all." William spent little time with his wife and children, and under the circumstances, Carla left, taking her two young sons with her. She remarried in 1986 and presently lives with her husband, Drew, her two sons, and Tyla, her daughter from her second marriage. The patient maintains a cordial relationship with his ex-wife and does occasionally spend time with his children. The patient himself has not remarried and is not presently involved in an intimate relationship. He rents the upstairs of a small home in Beaumont and has lived alone since separation from his wife.

William is a devout Catholic and attends church on a regular basis. He has a number of close friends. He enjoys playing cards and watching television. He volunteers for a number of charities organized through his church. A passionate fan of professional football, William has attended a number of Houston Oilers games.

William's ex-wife and two sons live in Galveston. He has six brothers and sisters scattered throughout the United States. He remains in contact with his older brother, Walter, 65, a retired factory worker who lives in St. Louis, Missouri, and his older sister, Myra, 55, who lives in Galveston. The patient's mother, Lucy, 86, lives in a nursing home in St. Louis.

Past Personal and Family Medical History

The patient had an eventful childhood from a medical point of view. In his words, "I was a kid with really bad asthma. Every time I got a cold I got the asthma real bad." He recalls several admissions to the hospital with asthma attacks, which gradually disappeared by the time he was 14 years old.

While playing on the beach when he was 11, William accidentally stepped on a piece of cut glass, lacerating his left foot. His mother had warned him just that morning to wear sandals, as the beach was full of such hazards. To avoid what he foresaw as a severe scolding, William covered his foot in petroleum jelly "to ease the pain" and slid a wool sock over it. Unfortunately, the pain increased steadily, and 3 days passed before young William came sobbing to his mother with the whole story. He cried in agony as she pulled the dirty sock off to find a foot covered in blood and pus. She rushed him to hospital, where part of his foot was eventually amputated.

William says, "I have been overweight as long as I can remember." As he puts it, "When I was born, the nurse didn't need to wrap me in a blanket 'cause I came with plenty of insulation." At age 13, William weighed 100kg, and a concerned family physician recommended a strict diet. Unfortunately, this effort was completely unsuccessful, and the patient remains morbidly obese to this day.

William has had episodic back pain since he was around 35. This has always resolved within a few days, but he does miss several days of work a year as a result. He has seen a family physician for this problem, who has told him it is due to "lumbar strain."

The patient has never smoked. His consumption of alcohol is minimal, limited to one or two beers while playing cards with friends. He has a voracious appetite, catered to by virtually every fast-food enterprise in Beaumont. He presently uses ibuprofen from time to time for back pain. He takes no other medications.

William's mother Lucy suffers from senile dementia, incontinence, Type II diabetes, and chronic atrial fibrillation. She has been in a nursing home for 12 years and has frequent bouts of pneumonia that require hospitalization. The patient's father passed away in 1978 at the age of 69 as a result of metastatic prostate cancer.

The patient's brother, Walter Hodge, has Type II diabetes and, like William, suffers from obesity. His sister Myra is in comparatively good health, with no history of major illnesses or surgery. William's two children are in perfect health. Unfortunately, William is not in contact with his other siblings, and their health status is unknown to him.

William Hodge belongs to a health maintenance organization that covers 100% of the cost of doctor's visits, medical supplies, and hospitalizations, as well as 90% of the cost of all prescription medications.

The Problem

You are a family physician in a small city with easy access to all diagnostic facilities and specialists. William Hodge, a 54-year-old African American man, comes to you for a periodic health examination. Upon completion, your main concern is Willliam's weight, which is presently 128.5kg. You ask him to return in 1 week's time to discuss dietary strategies and exercise as a means of weight loss. William agrees. Neither you nor William have any other major concerns.

As part of the periodic health evaluation, you draw a serum random glucose level and total blood cholesterol. You also administer a tetanus-diphtheria booster immunization.

Two days later, the results of his blood tests are available to you. His total serum cholesterol is 4.8mmol/l (185.3 mg/dL). His random glucose was 14.5mmol/l (261mg/dL).

Questions

1. Was it reasonable to include a random serum glucose as part of the periodic health examination? Based on this result, is William diabetic?

Discussion

1. Neither the Canadian Task Force on the Periodic Health Examination (1994) nor the U.S. Preventive Services Task Force (1996) recommends universal routine screening for non-insulin-dependent diabetes mellitus (NIDDM), as the yield from such testing would be very low. Both organizations, however, encourage individualized screening for diabetes on the basis of the presence of risk factors. Risk factors include obesity; a family history of diabetes; and certain ethnic origins, in- cluding Native American, Hispanic, and African American. This is also consistent with the recommendations of the American Diabetes Association (ADA, 1996b), the World Health Organization, and the British Diabetic Association (Engelgau, Aubert, Thompson, & Herman, 1995). As William is at increased risk, screening for diabetes is not unreasonable. The preferred test for screening, however, is a *fasting* serum glucose level in an asymptomatic patient like William. The criteria estab-

lished by the National Diabetes Data Group (1979) require a fasting blood glucose of 7.8mmol/l (140mg/dL) or greater for a diagnosis of diabetes to be made. This should be confirmed on a repeat test. In other words, William Hodge cannot be diagnosed with diabetes on the basis of an elevated random serum glucose. A random glucose level of 11.1mmol/l (200mg/dL) or greater is diagnostic only in patients who present with classic symptoms of diabetes mellitus such as polyuria and polydipsia. The patient should be told to return for two fasting serum glucose levels.

PART II

The Problem

You call William and tell him to return on two separate days after fasting overnight for blood glucose testing. He agrees, and 5 days later, his results return as 11.5mmol/l (207mg/dL) and 13.2mmol/l (237.6mg/dL), respectively. You call the patient again and tell him his results are abnormal and that he needs to return for a complete evaluation. He sounds a bit anxious on the phone. "Doc, so I have diabetes?" he asks. You tell him that his results indicate that he does have diabetes but that he requires further evaluation to determine how bad his illness is at present. He arranges for follow-up in 3 days and returns as scheduled.

Questions

1. What should be the agenda for William's next visit?

Discussion

1. William is obese, over 30 years old, and, according to his last visit, has no symptoms of diabetes. There is little doubt that he has *NIDDM*, or *Type II*, diabetes. Reactions to the news of this diagnosis are variable. William should certainly be asked about how he feels about the diagnosis, as well as what he knows about the disease. He should be made aware that with a sound management plan, in which he plays an active role, life can be as normal as possible. The American Diabetes Association (1994) has superb guidelines for the initial office evaluation of such patients. The goal is to determine the patient's present disease status and to assess the risk of diabetic complications. The history includes a more specific inquiry into diabetic symptoms, as they may have been overlooked by doctor or patient in a periodic health examination. Also important is information about eating patterns and exercise, as well as prior or current skin, foot, dental, and urinary tract infections. Past medical history, cardiac risk factors, family history, and lifestyle information are needed as well. Much of this information has been provided in the patient profile. The American Association of Clinical Endocrinologists (AACE, 1995) has published a useful inventory of questions to be included in an initial visit.

The physical examination should include height, weight, and blood pressure determinations with orthostatic measurements. (Of course, this information would have been gathered in William's periodic health examination.) Ophthalmoscopic, oral, thyroid, cardiac, abdominal, skin, and extremity examination are also recommended by the ADA (1994). Laboratory evaluation should include a glycated hemoglobin, serum creatinine, and urinalysis. A fasting plasma glucose and fasting lipid profile is recommended as well. William has already had serial fasting blood glucose determinations. A complete lipid profile screening is not recommended as part of the periodic health examination (U.S. Preventive Services Task Force,

1996). Despite William's normal total blood cholesterol level, strict adherence to the guidelines issued by the ADA (1994), AACE (1995), or Canadian Diabetes Advisory Board (CDAB) (Expert Committee of the CDAB, 1992) mandates obtaining a lipid profile at present. The need for other tests, such as a TSH, should be individualized. All three organizations above recommend an EKG, which may detect evidence of past asymptomatic myocardial damage.

A recommended initial evaluation of Mr. Hodge, together with corresponding summarized results, is presented in "The Rest of the Story" (Part II).

The Rest of the Story

You tell William once again that the results of his blood sugar tests indicate that he has diabetes, and you ask him how he feels about that. He responds, "Yeah, my whole family's got it pretty much. I guess I'm not surprised. I want to keep things under control. I don't want to wind up on insulin."

William already has a surprisingly good understanding of the nature of diabetes, which he says he acquired from family members. You briefly review, however, the pathophysiology of diabetes as well as complications. You tell him that there are a number of approaches to control of blood sugar that should be tried before resorting to insulin and that a comprehensive team approach to management, in which William is the key player, should allow him to lead a fairly normal life.

William reports no recent increased appetite or change in weight. In his words, "I'm heavy as hell as usual." He reports no polydipsia, polyuria, or fatigue. He reports no visual disturbances. He has had no recent infections. The patient reports no numbness or tingling in his hands or feet. He reports no difficulty in obtaining an erection.

The patient does not exercise at all. He has four large meals a day: Usually breakfast consists of bacon, fried eggs, and cereal. He buys lunch at the high school cafeteria and dinner at one of many fast-food restaurants along a busy commercial strip in Beaumont. He normally has a "snack" before bed—usually a "hoagie" or a "sloppy joe." A bag of potato chips is usually at his side. He has a number of friends who love to barbecue on weekends, and he rarely passes up their hospitality.

Suggested Physical Examination (with corresponding summarized results)

Gen: Pleasant, obese, African American male. Looks stated age
  height = 1.75m; wt. = 129kg; BP = 135/90—no significant orthostatic change

HEENT:

    Eyes: fundi (visualized reasonable well; mydriatics not given)

    No hemorrhages; no dilated veins; no cotton-wool spots or hard exudates

    Otherwise normal appearance

    Oral: poor dentition with many fillings; no caries; no infections

    Thyroid: normal

CVS: normal

Abdomen: significant truncal obesity; otherwise normal

Skin: normal

Extremities: amputation at mid-metatarsal level of left foot; otherwise normal

Screening neurologic examination: normal sensation over hands and feet; no muscle wasting noted; normal deep tendon reflexes.

Suggested Laboratory Results (with corresponding summarized results)

Glycosylated hemoglobin: 9.5% (< 6% is regarded as normal, < 8% acceptable, < 10% fair, > 10% poor)

Serum creatinine: normal

Urinalysis: normal

Lipid profile: normal

EKG: unremarkable

PART III

The Problem

You review William's laboratory results, and he arranges for a follow-up appointment in 5 days, at which you plan to work with William to derive a management plan.

The patient returns as scheduled. He tells you he continues to feel well, and that he has "stopped trying to eat sugar." By this William indicates that he has completely avoided sweets and has begun using artificial sweeteners in coffee and cereal. You tell him that this is a respectable effort but that complete dietary management of his diabetes is more complicated and includes a number of different strategies. You review the laboratory results with the patient.

Questions

    1. How would you begin to manage William's diabetes?

Discussion

1. William's laboratory results reveal no evidence of diabetic complications. His glycosylated hemoglobin level indicates he has "fair" glycemic control.

Family physicians play an important role, not only in the diagnosis of diabetes but in its initial management. Indeed, familiarity with a comprehensive and rational approach to the management of Type II diabetes is essential knowledge for the practicing family physician. The physician and patient rarely work alone in this context, however. Most guidelines advocate the involvement of other health professionals and their integration into a *Diabetes Health Care* Team (DHC). Their roles are discussed below. How does one begin to examine the question of management?

Understanding the management of diabetes begins with a review of the goals of diabetic care. According to the ADA (1994), the two major goals of management of Type II diabetes are to achieve normal metabolic control and to prevent microvascular and macrovascular complications. Furthermore, specific objectives include the elimination of symptoms if present, helping the patient achieve a normal weight, and improvement of cardiovascular risk factors. Achievement of normal metabolic control and prevention of complications are not mutually exclusive goals. Though the value of their results is still controversial, two major studies have demonstrated that good glycemic control in both Type I (Diabetes Control and Complications Trial Research Group, 1993) and Type II (Ohkubo et al., 1995) diabetics delays the onset and slows the progression of diabetic nephropathy, retinopathy, and neuropathy.

Therapeutic modalities used to achieve the goals specified above include diet, exercise, pharmacologic intervention, and patient education. For newly diagnosed asymptomatic patients with NIDDM, diet and exercise are the principal components of initial management. William's present diet, even ignoring his diabetes, is certainly not compatible with good health. He has a huge caloric intake and appears to make food choices with little discretion. A healthy diet designed to optimize glucose control would likely be a drastic change for William, and it requires a great deal of motivation and encouragement. This is one area in which the DHC team can be expanded from doctor and patient to include a qualified dietician with experience in the field of diabetes. Alternatively, the primary care physician can provide William with a suitable diet, but in most parts of North America, the help of an experienced dietician is usually available and should be exploited. Below is a brief review of general dietary goals that, when applicable, can be explained to William prior to and in between his visits to a dietician. Dietary modification is not easy, and reinforcement by different members of the DHC team may encourage the patient to comply with recommendations.

The position statement of the ADA provides a good overview of nutrition therapy in diabetic care (ADA, 1996c). There are five main goals: (a) maintenance of as near-normal blood glucose as possible, (b) achievement of optimal serum lipid levels, (c) adjustment of caloric intake to maintain reasonable weight, (d) prevention and treatment of acute complications of insulin-treated disease, and (e) improvement of general health apart from diabetes. William's lipid profile is normal, and for the time being he is not on insulin therapy. The remaining goals are applicable. The current philosophy of dietary intervention is to recommend a diet based on individual goals and a nutrition assessment. During an assessment, a dietician should determine what William is able and willing to do to meet the goals. In other words, there is no longer a standard "diabetic diet" in which the intake of particular nutrients is well defined.

Exercise has many beneficial effects in patients with Type II diabetes. It increases insulin sensitivity and may reduce the need for insulin and other hypoglycemic agents. It is an adjunct to diet as a means of weight reduction. Exercise has a favorable impact on cardiovascular risk factors other than diabetes (e.g., lipids, blood pressure). Finally, quality of life is enhanced through improved strength, increased flexibility, improved mood, and stress reduction. How does one approach the issue of exercise with William? This will probably not be an easy matter. Many patients with Type II diabetes are sedentary, and any form of exercise represents a major change in lifestyle.

The ADA (1994) recommends a thorough evaluation prior to beginning most forms of exercise. This includes a cardiovascular examination and exercise stress test, as well as neurologic and ophthalmologic examinations and precise determination of glycemic control. Patients are advised to obtain suitable equipment (e.g., proper athletic footwear). This seems overly cautious. After all, it is unlikely that William would be willing or able to engage in any intense aerobic activity such as jogging. Indeed, the ADA identifies a walking program as the minimum form of exercise that should be considered. This is likely a good starting point for William. Aerobic activity should ideally be carried out at a heart rate of 60% to 80% of maximum, but even 50% may be of some benefit. William could probably achieve this through vigorous walking. The ADA (1994) makes it clear that a stress test is not needed prior to beginning this sort of less-intense aerobic activity, during which the heart rate rarely exceeds 110/min. Other forms of activity, such as lifting weights (not recommended for patients with hypertension or diabetic retinopathy), can be considered, depending on William's interest.

It is recommended (ADA, 1994) that exercise sessions take place in the evening (after 4:00 p.m.), as this reduces hepatic glucose output and decreases fasting glycemia, or after meals, to reduce postprandial hyperglycemia. Exercise should be carried out a minimum of three times a week, for a duration of 30 to 40 min per session. The guiding principle should be that an exercise prescription should be highly individualized and that any activity is better than none. The issue should be discussed with William from this standpoint.

As noted, nutrition therapy and exercise are "first-line" strategies to achieve glucose control in patients with Type II diabetes. Pharmacologic therapy is used when these strategies fail. At the present time, therefore, medications should not be part of the management plan.

William is a partner in the DHC team, and patient education is therefore an extremely important component of the initial management plan. This, of course, is provided to some extent in every encounter with Mr. Hodge's family physician. There is a great deal that William needs to know to play a major role in the control of his illness. Throughout North America, there is widespread access to diabetes education centers staffed by professional diabetes educators, social workers, podiatrists, psychologists, nutritionists, and others. Discussion participants should know that although family physicians play an extremely important role in the management of patients with Type II diabetes, the resources of diabetes centers are still invaluable and should be routinely used. At the very least, a qualified diabetes educator can be integrated into the DHC team. Patient education is effective in reducing diabetic complications, in decreasing foot problems, in diminishing hospitalizations, and in improving long-term glycemic control (AACE, 1995). The goals of education are to help patients adhere to the management plan and acquire new skills and behaviors.

Diabetes educators provide patients with a wide variety of valuable information and skills. These will not be discussed in detail here, but one skill in particular deserves further comment. Self-monitoring of blood glucose (SMBG), though most useful for Type I diabetics and Type II diabetics on pharmacologic therapy, nevertheless serves to remind William of his diabetes and can make him aware of the impact of diet and exercise on his blood glucose (Expert Committee of the CDAB, 1992). In this context, periodic self-monitoring helps to increase compliance with the therapeutic plan. Home glucose monitors and test strips are presently affordable and widely available. The technique of self-monitoring is easily taught to the majority of patients. Recommendations for the frequency of self-monitoring vary. The AACE (1995) recommends a frequency of at least twice daily for all diabetic patients.

Obviously, patients taking insulin need to monitor their glucose quite often. A good place to start is to encourage William to test his fasting blood sugar daily or perhaps three times a week. He may wish to increase this frequency depending on his comfort with the procedure. Self-monitoring should be accompanied by accurate record keeping, consisting of a log of blood glucose that should be brought to every encounter with the DHC team.

There are clearly many issues to discuss with William at an encounter dealing with initial management of his diabetes. It is best to limit the agenda to a few straightforward items and to make it clear that diabetic care is an ongoing process that will require multiple follow-up visits. For this visit, it would be reasonable to expand the DHC team by referring the patient to a nutritionist and a diabetes educator as described and to discuss exercise as a strategy to improve glycemic control. The goals of therapy and the complications of diabetes should be reviewed. A discussion of foot care can be included. As always, William should be encouraged to express any concerns and to ask questions about his condition.

PART IV

The Problem

You engage William in a thorough discussion of management of diabetes. You tell him that you will both be part of a diabetic health care team that will also include a nutritionist and a diabetes educator, both available through a local diabetes center. You discuss exercise and its benefits. William indicates that he is not interested in any vigorous activity at this point: "I can't run or nothing. I mean, I only got half a left foot. I sort of hobble along as it is."

William agrees to begin a regular program of evening walking—daily for half an hour. He has a special pair of shoes, designed to accommodate his amputated anterior left foot and to correct for gait imbalance, that are suitable for the purpose. You briefly review the goals of dietary therapy. You explain to the patient the importance of wearing good footwear, keeping feet clean, avoiding foot injury, and inspecting the feet frequently for signs of damage or infection. You ask William if he has any concerns at this time.

> Well, Doctor, I mean I ain't happy with having diabetes, but everything you said about diet and exercise is good stuff—common sense. I should have been doing that all along. I'm definitely going to follow through with it. I don't want to wind up on insulin like my brother. And you know that I know all about foot problems. I take better care of my feet—well, what's left of them—than anyone else alive. But I think it would be good to go to the diabetes center to get as much information as I can.

You tell William that you are impressed that he is so motivated to tackle his diabetes. He is scheduled for an appointment at the diabetes center in 2 days, at which time he will have comprehensive sessions with a nutritionist and a nurse educator.

Questions

1. When would you like William to return for a follow-up visit, and what will be your agenda?

Discussion

1. There is no correct answer to this question, and fellow discussion participants will likely come up with a variety of responses depending on their perception of the patient and his illness. It is important to remember that the family physician is part of a DHC team and that the other professional members are valuable sources of information. A phone call to the diabetes center to see how successful William is in learning and following dietary advice, self-monitoring, record keeping, foot care, and so on is a simple and effective way of keeping track of comprehensive diabetic care. William can be contacted often to find out how he is feeling and how his exercise program is going. Furthermore, his impression of the care provided by the diabetes center is very important. This informal contact with the patient and other members of the team can take place frequently after William's last office visit.

The CDAB (Expert Committee of the CDAB, 1992) recommends office visits at intervals of 4 and 8 weeks after the initial management visit. An interim history should be obtained at each visit that includes symptoms, if any; results of self-monitoring; problems with adherence with the therapeutic plan; and psychosocial issues. Weight and blood pressure are valuable parameters. Other components of the physical examination may be performed if needed based on the presence of symptoms or abnormalities at the initial assessment. Elements of continuing diabetic care such as glycohemoglobin determination and ophthalmologic referral are provided at regular, specified intervals but are not needed at the 4- and 8-week visits. See "The Rest of the Story," which follows, for a description of William's progress during the first 8 weeks of comprehensive, coordinated diabetic care.

The Rest of the Story

You decide to call Sharon, the diabetes educator involved in William's care, and Maxine, his nutritionist, 10 days after William's office visit. Sharon tells you that William is a very motivated patient who was able to learn the technique of self-monitoring very easily. He was also eager to learn about foot care (especially as he had such a terrible experience with his left foot as a child) and about record keeping. Sharon also tells you that she reviewed the goals of diabetic care with William and reinforced the importance of continuing the walking program. William has told her that he has been walking daily for 30 min, although not always in the evening.

Maxine tells you that the patient was eager to learn about a "proper diet" but told her he has had a great deal of difficulty in curbing his consumption to reasonable levels. She prescribed for him a balanced diet of approximately 2,000 calories/day that included some of his favorite foods, such as those he would purchase from fast-food restaurants. Adherence to the diet, she tells you, will require that William become accustomed to smaller portions and be willing to introduce a number of healthy foods to his daily intake. Maxine was impressed with William's level of motivation, and she looks forward to working with him on a regular basis. William is to see both Sharon and Maxine in 1 month's time.

You call William shortly after speaking with the diabetes center staff. He tells you that he is very pleased with the care he is receiving from you and the other members of the team. You tell him that you spoke to both the nutritionist and educator and that you will continue to keep in touch with them. William tells you he has been walking regularly, sometimes in the evening, but usually very early in the morning, just before work, when "it's cool." The high temperature in Beaumont has been running in the range of 36°C for several days. He walks around his neighborhood for about 30 min each day.

At his 4-week visit, William continues to report no symptoms of diabetes. He tells you he feels quite well in general and that the walking has improved his energy level. You review his blood glucose log book. William has been taking daily fasting measurements for the past 3 weeks. The range of values is 8.2mmol-l (148mg/dL) to 15.5mmol-l (279mg/dL), with a mean of 10.8mmol-l (194mg/dL). William's weight is 131.5kg. His blood pressure is 130/75.

William is not surprised by the increase in weight. "I'm really having trouble with that diet. I get so damn hungry." He is also aware that his blood glucose has been above the normal range on a regular basis. You tell William that you are impressed with William's adherence to the exercise program and his self-monitoring but that he needs to work on the dietary management aspect. You review the importance of diet and make some suggestions on how to limit intake, such as substituting water or low-calorie drinks for soda pop and buying smaller portions of food. You tell him that Maxine will likely have more detailed suggestions on how to improve his diet. William is looking forward to returning to the diabetes center next week.

Prior to his 8-week visit, you review the patient's progress with the staff at the diabetes center. Maxine tells you William continues to have difficulty restricting his caloric intake. However, he has no trouble in making healthy food choices. Indeed, the patient now eats a variety of foods and has curbed his consumption of high-fat fast foods. This, Maxine insists, is a very positive development. Sharon tells you it is a pleasure to work with William because of his level of motivation; he has a great deal of interest in self-monitoring and remaining as healthy as possible.

PART V

The Problem

At his 8-week visit, William continues to have no symptoms of diabetes. He remains in good spirits. His logbook shows that he has missed only 1 day of blood glucose monitoring, when he spent a weekend at a friend's place and forgot his glucometer. The range of values is 7.5mmol-l (135mg/dL) to 15.0mmol-l (270mg/dL), with a mean of 11.3mmol-l (203mg/dL). On the positive side, William now weighs 125kg, a loss of 6.5kg. His blood pressure remains normal.

Questions

1. How would you assess the success of nonpharmacologic therapy, and how would you proceed from this point?

Discussion

1. There is little question that diet and exercise have had a positive impact on William. He reports an increased energy level. He has learned to make healthy food choices. He is improving his level of fitness by walking daily. He has lost weight. Unfortunately, his glycemic control has not improved. Improvement in control is often evident with a weight loss of 5% to 10% of original body weight. William has lost roughly 5%.

The lack of success so far in controlling blood glucose through diet and exercise alone is not unexpected. In a recent British study, 95% of newly diagnosed patients with Type II diabetes failed to achieve reasonable control of blood glucose after a 3-month trial of nonpharmacologic therapy (United Kingdom Prospective Diabetes Study Group, 1995). According to the ADA (1996a), fewer than 10% of diabetic patients are able to achieve long-term control through diet and exercise. Despite this abysmal success rate, nonpharmacologic therapy remains the first choice for the newly diagnosed asymptomatic Type II diabetic. It is important to remember that following a good diet and exercising are behaviors that should be pursued by all diabetic patients. If and when pharmacologic therapy is warranted, diet and exercise remain important adjuncts. In this context, starting with nonpharmacologic therapy seems to be a reasonable strategy. When does one add medications to the management scheme? This is not an easy question to answer. The ADA (1996a) recommends a trial of 3 months of diet and exercise before considering pharmacologic therapy. The CDAB (AACE, 1995) recommends a trial of only 8 weeks before proceeding to pharmacologic therapy. As William remains asymptomatic and continues to lose weight, it is not unreasonable

to allow him to continue dietary and exercise therapy for 1 more month before considering medications.

PART VI

The Problem

You decide to continue to recommend diet and exercise as therapy for William's diabetes for another month, and you tell the patient that medication will probably be needed if there is no improvement in glucose control in 1 month's time.

William seems a little disappointed by this. "Now, I'm doing everything right. I eat right. I walk every day. Just can't get that sugar down."

You tell William that his efforts to improve his diet and level of activity are admirable, but that in the majority of patients, such behavior change is not enough to achieve control of blood sugar.

William returns in 1 month's time. He continues to feel very well. He has been keeping excellent records of his fasting blood glucose. The range of values and mean are virtually identical to those recorded prior to his last visit. His weight is 123.6kg. His blood pressure remains normal.

Questions

1. Describe your management of the case from this point.

Discussion

1. It is clear that diet and exercise are not enough to control the patient's diabetes. It is time to consider pharmacologic therapy. There are four classes of medications presently available in North America for control of blood glucose. These include the sulfonylureas, which have been in use for over 40 years and are known to increase insulin secretion. Metformin, a biguanide, has been available in Canada for a number of years but has only recently become available in the United States. It acts by decreasing glucose production in the liver and stimulating hepatic glucose uptake. The third class of medications is that of the alpha glucosidase inhibitors, including the recently available acarbose, which inhibit enzymes that break down starches and therefore delay carbohydrate absorption and serum glucose elevation. Finally, there is insulin, discovered in Canada more than 70 years ago and widely available in a number of injectable preparations. It remains the most effective agent for blood glucose control. The choice of initial agent should be individualized. In a patient presenting with typical symptoms of diabetes such as significant polyuria and polydipsia, it is inappropriate to begin therapy with a sulfonylurea. Insulin is the preferred

treatment. In patients like William who are asymptomatic, according to the ADA (1996a), any of the other three classes of medications can be used as first-line therapy. Experience with acarbose in North America is limited. The sulfonylureas, like insulin, are known to cause weight gain in patients with Type II diabetes. This is a side effect William can certainly do without. Sulfonylureas are also associated with episodic hypoglycemia, and their use requires cautious monitoring.

There is no ideal first-line agent for control of diabetes. There are a number of experts, however, who presently advocate the use of metformin as initial pharmacologic therapy in obese Type II diabetics (Bailey, 1992; Gearhart & Forbes, 1995; Tan & Nelson, 1996). Metformin does not cause significant hypoglycemia. Furthermore, it is not associated with weight gain. The major disadvantage is cost. A month's supply costs approximately three times as much as a comparable dose of glyburide, the most commonly used sulfonylurea ("Metformin for Non-Insulin," 1995). Metformin also produces a number of unpleasant gastrointestinal side effects in a significant number of patients, including a metallic taste, diarrhea, vomiting, and anorexia. Indeed, it has been postulated that these side effects are actually responsible for the favorable impact of metformin on body weight ("Metformin for Non-Insulin," 1995).

The usual starting dose of metformin is 500mg bid, taken with the morning and evening meal. The typical maintenance dose is 850mg bid. The maximum is 850mg tid.

It may be wise, although metformin is not associated with significant hypoglycemia, to encourage the patient at some point to monitor his blood glucose more frequently to gather more information about his glycemic control.

It has been approximately 3 months since the diagnosis of diabetes was made. William requires specific elements of ongoing care at this time (ADA, 1996c). His feet should be examined for vascular status, damage to skin, and sensation. He requires a funduscopic examination, preferably with dilatation. A glycosylated hemoglobin level should be obtained.

PART VII

The Problem

You examine William's feet and find no evidence of recent damage, loss of sensation, or vascular compromise. Funduscopic examination with dilatation reveals no evidence of retinopathy. You obtain serum for determination of glycosylated hemoglobin.

You decide to start William on metformin, at a dose of 500mg bid. You warn him about the side effects. You inform him about the cost, as he is required to pay 10%. He tells you that he is prepared to do this and that it does not constitute an intolerable financial burden.

William returns in 2 weeks. He continues to feel very well. He reports no dysgeusia, nausea, vomiting, abdominal pain, or diarrhea. He has been taking his medication regularly, and continues to eat well and exercise. He has been keeping excellent records of his blood glucose. The range of fasting values is 8.5mmol/l (153mg/dL) to 12.5mmol/l (225mg/dL), with a mean of 10.0mmol-l (180mg/dl). His glycosylated hemoglobin level returns as 8.8%. You decide to increase his dose of metformin to 850mg bid. You ask William if he is interested in monitoring his blood glucose more frequently, as this may provide a more accurate picture of his glycemic control. He indicates that he has no difficulty increasing the frequency of checks. You ask him to take an additional reading approximately 2 hr after supper each day.

The patient returns once again. He remains asymptomatic and has been very compliant with the management plan. His logbook reveals fasting glucose values ranging from 4.5mmol-l (81mg/dL) to 9.0mmol-l (162mg/dL), with a mean value of 7.5mmol-l (135mg/dL). His postprandial values range from 6.0mmol-l (108mg/dL) to 13.5mmol-l (243mg/dL), with a mean of 10.8mmol-l (194mg/dL).

Questions

1. Are you satisfied with the degree of glucose control?
2. When would you like to see William again, and what elements of continuing care would you incorporate into the management plan?

Discussion

1. With a mean fasting glucose of 7.5mmol-l (135mg/dL) and a mean postprandial glucose of 10.8mmol-l (194mg/dL), it is likely that William presently has "acceptable" metabolic control of diabetes (Gearhart & Forbes, 1995). His previous glycosylated hemoglobin value of 8.8% falls in the fair-to-acceptable range, but this will be likely to improve on the present dose of metformin. One can conclude that William appears to be comfortable with the management plan and that it has produced satisfactory results. At the present time there is no great need to make significant changes in an effort to have better control over his diabetes.

2. Ongoing diabetic care is extremely important. The ADA (1996c) recommends quarterly or semiannual regular visits for reassessment of diabetes. As noted previously, a medical history that includes symptoms, a review of self-monitoring, other illnesses, and social and psychological concerns is necessary at each regular visit. Furthermore, the physical examination should include weight and blood pressure as well as inspection of the fundi and feet. A glycohemoglobin level is recommended quarterly in all insulin-treated patients. The ADA (1996c) makes no strict recommendations as to the frequency in non-insulin-treated patients but does recommend regular testing until glycemic control goals are met. Alternatively, a fasting laboratory plasma glucose can be obtained periodically as a measure of control and as a gauge of the accuracy of the patient's self-monitoring.

Although the fundi should be examined regularly by the physician providing comprehensive diabetic care, an annual complete visual examination performed by an experienced optometrist or opthalmalogist is recommended. Finally, a routine urinalysis is recommended annually for the detection of proteinuria, a sign of diabetic nephropathy. Of course, other elements of the periodic health examination should be incorporated into regular visits for monitoring diabetes.

PART VIII

The Problem

You decide to follow William every 3 months for a year. He continues to report no symptoms. He takes his medication regularly. His physical examination is unchanged, except that he is slowly losing weight, at a rate of approximately 1kg/month. He remains in good spirits and has been following a healthy diet as well as a regular routine of daily walking. He has visited the diabetes center on a couple of occasions, mainly to ask questions about the nutritive value of certain foods but also to inform Sharon and Maxine of his progress. The results of self-monitoring, fasting blood glucose, and glycosylated hemoglobin indicate that William has acceptable control. At the end of the 1-year period, you decide that William is doing very well. He visits an opthalmologist, who finds no evidence of retinopathy. You obtain a urinalysis that is normal. You decide to follow William at a less frequent interval of every 6 months.

Three weeks prior to his scheduled 6-month follow-up appointment, William calls your office and asks to see you as soon as possible. You ask him to come in the next day. When asked how he has been feeling, the patient responds, "Well, pretty lousy, Doctor. I mean, I didn't think I should wait another 3 weeks. My sugars are going out of control, too."

When asked to qualify his feeling "lousy," William tells you that he has been increasingly fatigued for the past 3 or 4 months. He reports a very low energy level. As a consequence, over the past month he has discontinued his exercise program. He complains of decreased appetite, but otherwise he continues to pursue a healthy diet. William has been taking his medications regularly. He has called in sick to work on four occasions over the past 2 months. He reports increased thirst and frequent urination, especially at night. He reports no visual disturbances or other symptoms.

Upon inspection of his logbook, you notice that William has been monitoring his fasting glucose regularly but taking 2-hr postprandial readings only roughly once a week. His fasting values have been gradually climbing. The average over the past month is 15.0mmol/l (170mg/dL). The mean postprandial reading is 17.0mmol/l (306mg/dL). His blood pressure is normal. His fundi and feet are normal. A urinalysis obtained shows no evidence of ketones or protein. His weight is 107kg. His weight at his previous visit was 116kg.

Questions

1. How would you explain William's lack of glycemic control?
2. How would you change the management plan?

Discussion

1. William has poor glycemic control. Furthermore, his diabetes is manifested by fatigue, polydipsia, and polyuria. He has lost considerable weight, but whether this is due to diabetes or to the positive lifestyle changes he has made is unclear. What is certain is that the present management plan is inadequate. The metformin William

takes is no longer able to control his diabetes. This situation, in which control was originally achieved with an oral agent and then lost, is called a secondary drug failure and occurs in approximately 5% to 10% of patients per year (ADA, 1994). There are multiple possible causes. First, one should consider lack of compliance with the management plan. Failure to comply with diet or to take medications on a regular basis can lead to deterioration of metabolic control. There is no evidence of this in William's case. Second, the occurrence of a stressor such as an infectious disease or cardiovascular event raises the amount of insulin required for adequate control. William should be asked specifically about such a stressor, and, if needed, appropriate testing and treatment should be carried out. See "The Rest of the Story," which follows. Finally, it is important to remember that diabetes is a progressive disease and that what was adequate therapy at one time may no longer be enough because of deterioration of pancreatic beta-cell function. For this reason, William's poorly controlled diabetes should not come as a surprise.

2. There are several different pharmacologic options at this point. One could maximize the dose of metformin, but given that William is quite symptomatic and has control that is not nearly adequate, this is unlikely to have a major impact. One could add a second oral agent, either acarbose or a sulfonylurea. Alternatively, one could add insulin to the regimen. There is evidence of benefit of combined insulin and biguanide therapy (Guigliano et al., 1993), but experience with this combination is limited in North America. The most effective and prudent way to achieve glycemic control is likely to be monotherapy with insulin (Expert Committee of the CDAB,

1992; Gearhart & Forbes, 1995; Tan & Nelson, 1996). Other options put forth by fellow discussion participants should not be discounted, however. William has expressed concerns about insulin therapy before, and these should certainly be re-explored. As his present deterioration probably represents a natural progression of his diabetes, he will most likely need insulin as long-term therapy. He will need to visit the diabetes center on a regular basis for education on insulin storage, dosage adjustment, and self-administration. During the period in which insulin is first administered, frequent glucose self-monitoring is needed so that any adjustments in dosage and scheduling can be made. The majority of Type II diabetics can be controlled with a single dose of intermediate-acting insulin (e.g., *NPH* or *Lente*) each morning before breakfast (Nussbaum, 1995; Tan & Nelson, 1996). A starting dose of 10 to 15 units is recommended by some, and this can gradually be increased by 2 units a day by the patient, depending on the results of self-monitoring (Nussbaum, 1995). Rosenzweig (1994) recommends a starting morning dose of 0.2 to 0.5 U/kg of body weight, which in William corresponds to a much higher 21 to 54 units of insulin. Insulin requirements are unpredictable and vary widely, from 5 to 10 to hundreds of units per day. The goal should be fasting glucose values of no greater than 7.8mmol-1 (140mg/dL) and postprandial (2-hr) values of no more than 11.1mmol-1 (200mg/dL) (Gearhart & Forbes, 1995).

Insulin therapy is not without its hazards. The most common side effect is hypoglycemia. Hypoglycemia is defined as a blood glucose of less than 3.3mmol-1 (60mg/dL) and can be confirmed by the patient through self-monitoring. It is acutely manifested by increased sympathomimetic activity in the form of sweating, palpitations, tremor, and weakness. Neuroglycopenic symptoms, including fatigue and changes in mental status, occur when blood sugar declines slowly. William needs to be informed about these symptoms and take adequate measures to correct hypoglycemia if present. He should have a convenient source of sugar available, such as fruit juice, sugar cubes, or glucose tablets, which he should consume if he starts to experience symptoms of hypoglycemia. Some advocate that insulin-treated diabetics carry a syringe with glucagon for intramuscular self-administration, should a hypoglycemic reaction occur (Nussbaum, 1995). Some patients, especially those who have had diabetes for a number of years or have been on intensive insulin programs, develop hypoglycemic "unawareness" in which the warning signs of hypoglycemia are not perceived. This is another reason for William to perform frequent self-monitoring early in the course of insulin therapy, as it permits him to assess his own reaction to varying levels of blood glucose.

The Rest of the Story

William denies any recent cough, fever, cold symptoms, myalgias, nausea, vomiting, diarrhea, dysuria, or skin infections. He denies any history of chest pain, shortness of breath, or diaphoresis. He denies any change in his duties at work. He remains in good spirits, although he feels "very run down" and is disappointed that he doesn't have his usual level of energy.

To detect asymptomatic myocardial damage, you obtain an EKG, which is completely normal.

PART IX

The Problem

You tell William that his diabetes has progressed and that insulin therapy is the best way to achieve control at this point. You remind him that he was concerned about insulin therapy in the past, and you ask him to now express these concerns.

William tells you,

Well, back then I was really worried. I didn't think I could poke myself all the time for blood. I don't think I would have any trouble injecting insulin. I guess I'm worried that taking insulin means I'm going downhill as far as the diabetes. I don't want to go blind or nothing like that.

You tell William that diabetes is a progressive disease and that many patients eventually require insulin therapy for adequate control. You inform him that there is evidence that good control can prevent unfortunate effects such as blindness and that you will continue to monitor him for this and other complications. You recommend that William monitor his blood sugar four times a day for the next several weeks, as insulin therapy is titrated. You refer him once again to the diabetes center for education on insulin therapy.

William agrees with this plan. He visits the diabetes center for education on how to store, administer, and adjust the dose of insulin and is immediately started by you on 20 units of NPH each day before breakfast. He agrees to monitor his sugar before breakfast, 2 hr after lunch, 2 hr after dinner, and just before bedtime. You tell him that he may require much more than 20 units of insulin per day and ask him, if he feels comfortable, to increase the dose by 2 units per day if his fasting values are greater than 7.8mmol-1 (140mg/dL) or if his post-prandial values are greater than 11.1mmol-1 (200mg/dL).

William tells you, "Well, I'll try to play around with the dose, but I'm a bit scared of it. Can I call you if I have any questions or run into problems?"

You inform the patient that you welcome any questions or concerns he may have, particularly about self-adjustment of insulin dosage, and remind him that it may take some time to achieve good control with insulin. You draw a serum sample for glycosylated hemoglobin and ask him to return in 10 days.

On his return, William tells you that he feels a little better. He has been keeping excellent records and has been performing self-monitoring as recommended. He has not increased his dose of insulin. He complains of being very fatigued and sleepy in the afternoon. He no longer reports any polyuria or polydipsia. He has no visual complaints. He states that his appetite has improved considerably over the past week and that he is worried he may have gained some weight. He has had increased energy late in the day and has resumed his walking program in the evening. He has not missed work for the past 8 days. He reports no other symptoms. The most recent glycosylated hemoglobin level returns as 9.2%. A summary of his self-monitoring log for the past 10 days is found in "The Rest of the Story" at the end of Part 9. His blood pressure remains normal. He presently weighs 107kg.

Questions

1. After reviewing William's glucose log in "The Rest of the Story" (Fig. 5.1), what conclusions can you draw?
2. What changes, if any, would you make to the insulin regimen?

Discussion

1. One general observation from William's logbook data is that he does appear to respond to relatively small amounts of intermediate-acting insulin, and it is probably wise that he did not attempt to increase his dose. The chronology of this response, however, is a wholly different matter. Type II diabetics respond in different ways to intermediate-acting insulin, and these responses can be classified in particular patterns. One third of patients are so-called *early* or *type A* responders, who experience their peak insulin effect shortly after noon and often develop afternoon hypoglycemia. This is William's pattern. Others respond with a normal peak effect of insulin 6 to 12 hours after administration. These *late* or *type C*

responders often develop hypoglycemia overnight.

2. Type A patients often benefit by modifying the insulin regimen so that two thirds of the total daily dose is given before breakfast and one third before dinner. William should be instructed to do this, to continue self-monitoring frequently, and to return in a relatively short period of time (1 to 2 weeks). Incidentally, the most recent glycosylated hemoglobin level of 9.2%, which reflects glucose regulation over the preceding 3 months, corresponds to *fair* metabolic control.

The Rest of the Story

Hour/Day	1	2	3	4	5	6	7	8	9	10
AC (breakfast)	8.4	9.3	6.5	7.0	7.6	7.2	7.0	8.0	7.8	7.1
Postprandial/afternoon	4.2	3.8	5.0	4.0	3.5	6.0	4.3	3.6	3.8	4.5
Postprandial/supper	9.0	9.8	12.2	11.5	11.8	11.8	14.2	12.5	9.8	10.5
HS	8.5	9.0	6.5	5.5	5.5	7.0	6.8	8.0	7.5	7.5

NOTE: mmol-l are Système International units used in most parts of the world. In the United States, however, the conventional units are mg/dL. To convert mmol-l to mg/dL, simply multiply by 18.

Figure 5.1   Summary of William's Self-Monitoring Logbook for the Past 10 Days (Capillary blood glucose in mmol-l)

Conclusion

You ask William to take 14 units of NPH before breakfast and 7 before supper. You also ask him to return in 10 days.

Upon return he states that he feels very well. He no longer feels fatigued in the afternoon. He has no obvious symptoms of diabetes. As always, he has been keeping excellent records and has had no difficulty with the frequency of self-monitoring nor with the new insulin regimen. He continues to exercise and eat well.

His logbook (see Fig. 5.2) results for the past 10 days are found in "The Rest of the Story" at the end of this section. You and William are both satisfied with the degree of glucose control. You tell William that he need monitor his blood glucose only twice daily from this point, once before breakfast and once before supper. You review the signs and symptoms of hypoglycemia. You re-emphasize that diabetic care is an ongoing process. As he has recently started insulin therapy, you recommend regular visits at 3- rather than 6-month intervals for the following year. You assure William that you are available to answer questions and concerns and that he should not hesitate to contact you for that purpose. You make it clear that he need not wait until his regular appointment, should he feel it is necessary to see you. You remind him that the resources of the diabetes center remain available.

He thanks you for your help and tells you he looks forward to seeing you again.

The Rest of the Story

Hour/Day	1	2	3	4	5	6	7	8	9	10
AC (breakfast)	8.0	6.5	6.8	7.5	7.8	5.8	6.6	6.5	7.0	6.8
Postprandial/afternoon	7.0	8.2	8.0	7.5	7.5	7.8	8.4	8.2	7.3	8.0
Postprandial/supper	9.2	8.4	8.6	6.0	9.0	7.4	7.6	7.4	7.2	7.0
HS	6.5	6.2	5.4	4.8	5.0	6.0	5.8	5.0	6.1	6.5

Figure 5.2   Summary of William's Self-Monitoring Logbook for the Past 10 Days (Capillary blood glucose in mmol-l)

References

American Association of Clinical Endocrinologists. (1995). Guidelines for the management of diabetes mellitus. *AACE On-Line.* Retrieved November 9, 1996 from the World Wide Web: http://www.aace.com/clin/guides/diabetes_guide.html

American Diabetes Association. (1994). *Medical management of non-insulin-dependent (Type II) diabetes* (3rd ed.). Alexandria, VA: Author.

American Diabetes Association. (1996a). Consensus statement: The pharmacological treatment of hyperglycemia in NIDDM. *Diabetes Care, 19,* S54-S61.

American Diabetes Association. (1996b). Position statement: Screening for diabetes. *Diabetes Care, 19,* S5-S7.

American Diabetes Association. (1996c). Position statement: Standards of medical care for patients with diabetes mellitus. *Diabetes Care, 19,* S8-S15.

Bailey, C. J. (1992). Biguanides and NIDDM. *Diabetes Care, 15,* 755-772.

Canadian Task Force on the Periodic Health Examination. (1994). *The Canadian guide to clinical preventive health care.* Ottawa: Minister of Supply and Services Canada.

Diabetes Control and Complications Trial Research Group. (1993). The effect of intensive treatment of diabetes on the development and progression of long-term complications in insulin dependent diabetes mellitus. *New England Journal of Medicine, 329,* 977-986.

Engelgau, M. M., Aubert, R. E., Thompson, T. J., & Herman, W. H. (1995). Screening for NIDDM in nonpregnant adults: A review of principles, screening tests, and recommendations. *Diabetes Care, 18,* 1606-1618.

Expert Committee of the Canadian Diabetes Advisory Board. (1992). Clinical practice guidelines for the treatment of diabetes mellitus. *Canadian Medical Association Journal, 147,* 697-712.

Gearhart, J. G., & Forbes, R. C. (1995). Initial management of the patient with newly diagnosed diabetes. *American Family Physician, 51,* 1953-1962.

Giugliano, D., Quatraro, A., Consoli, G., Minei, A., Ceriello, A., De Rosa, N., & D'Onofrio, F. (1993). Metformin for obese, insulin-treated diabetic patients: Improvement in glycaemic control and reduction of metabolic risk factors. *European Journal of Clinical Pharmacology, 44,* 107-112.

Metformin for non-insulin dependent diabetes mellitus. *Medical Letter, 37,* 41-42.

National Diabetes Data Group. (1979). Classification and diagnosis of diabetes mellitus and other categories of glucose intolerance. *Diabetes, 28,* 1039-1057.

Nussbaum, S. R. (1995). Approach to the patient with diabetes mellitus. In A. H. Goroll, L. A. May, & A. G. Mulley (Eds.), *Primary care medicine* (3rd ed.; pp. 554-564). Philadelphia, PA: J. B. Lippincott.

Ohkubo, Y., Kishikawa, H., Araki, E., Miyata, T., Isami, S., Motoyoshi, S., Kojima, Y., Furuyoshi, N., & Shichiri, M. (1995). Intensive insulin therapy prevents the progression of diabetic microvascular complications in Japanese patients with non-insulin-dependent diabetes mellitus: A randomized prospective 6-year study. *Diabetes Research and Clinical Practice, 28,* 103-117.

Rosenzweig, J. L. (1994). Principles of insulin therapy. In C. R. Kahn & G. C. Weir (Eds.), *Joslin's diabetes mellitus* (13th ed.; pp. 461-484). Malvern, PA: Lea & Febiger.

Tan, G. H., & Nelson, R. L. (1996). Pharmacologic treatment options for non-insulin-dependent diabetes mellitus. *Mayo Clinic Proceedings, 71,* 763-768.

United Kingdom Prospective Diabetes Study Group. (1995). United Kingdom Prospective Diabetes Study (UKPDS) 13: Relative efficacy of randomly allocated diet, sulphonylurea, insulin, or metformin in patients with newly diagnosed non-insulin dependent diabetes followed for three years. *British Medical Journal, 310*, 83-88.

U.S. Preventive Services Task Force. (1996). *Guide to clinical preventive services*. Baltimore, MD: Williams and Wilkins.

6. HYPERLIPIDEMIA

Mr. Nigel Waugh

> *Goal: The goal of this exercise is to evaluate and develop
> the participants' understanding of the detection, assessment,
> and management of lipid disorders in an adult patient.*

Specific Objectives: Upon completion of this group discussion exercise, each participant should be able to accomplish the following:

1. Describe which populations to screen for hypercholesterolemia.
2. List the major risk factors for cardiovascular disease.
3. Define the goals of therapy for lipid disorders on the basis of the number of cardiovascular risk factors present.
4. Describe a stepwise approach to dietary therapy in the adult patient with high cholesterol.
5. Describe the various classes of lipid-lowering medications and the advantages and disadvantages of each.

PART I

The Patient

Social History

Nigel Waugh is a 45-year-old co-owner of a software company who lives just outside Santa Cruz, California, and works in Sunnyvale, California. Born and raised in Southampton, United Kingdom, Nigel is the second of four children of the late Matthew Waugh and his wife Cybill. The patient attended private school in England and completed a bachelor's degree in mathematics at the University of Manchester. It was there that Mr. Waugh cultivated a fascination with computers. In his words,

> There wasn't much back then in terms of computers. I was getting tired of *real analysis* and other aspects of pure mathematics. I wandered into a computer lab one day and the people were doing really interesting things. I learned one thing pretty quickly—I was in the wrong place.

Nigel applied successfully for graduate studies in computer science at the University of California at Berkeley in 1973.

The patient remembers his time at Berkeley as perhaps the best years of his life. In his words, "It was an absolutely wonderful place. So many people from so many places with so many different ideas." It was at Berkeley that Nigel met his wife, Sharifa Haddad, then an undergraduate student from Egypt. It was also back then that the patient met Frank Dermott, an ambitious fellow computer science student who convinced Nigel to quit graduate school and join him in starting a company. "It was a risky business," according to Nigel. "After all, I had come to America to study. Frank was a bit of a renegade. His father was a cowboy in New Mexico. He had guts, and it paid off for both of us." Frank and Nigel started a small company in 1975 that designed custom-made software for large industries. *Valley Horizons* was an almost instant success and has flourished ever since.

Nigel and Sharifa were married in 1976. Sharifa, who has an MBA, has been a vital part of the software company since its inception. She, her husband, and Frank Dermott are three of the company's executives. The Waughs have three children: Jeremy, 18 years old; Courtenay, 16; and Sarah, 13. The family has a net worth of approximately $100 million and lives on a 40-acre ranch outside Santa Cruz.

Most who meet Nigel describe him as an incredibly energetic, charming, and likable person. His interests are extremely varied. He enjoys golfing and riding horses. He is an avid collector of vintage automobiles. This hobby itself has grown into a business of considerable value. He describes himself as a "soccer fanatic" and has encouraged his children to become involved in the sport. In fact, Jeremy, a freshman at Stanford University, plays for its varsity soccer team.

Nigel and Sharifa Waugh are involved in a number of philanthropic activities. The couple has established a foundation that buys used, outdated computers, refurbishes them, and supplies them to poor rural schools in South Africa, the native country of Nigel's parents. The Waughs also sponsor a number of foster children throughout the developing world.

The patient describes his background as "Anglo-Saxon." When asked about his religious affiliation, he responds, "I've never been a religious person. I guess I'm an Anglican. Sharifa is a Copt. That makes us pretty different, I guess. Of course, we both celebrate Christmas!"

Past Personal and Family Medical History

The patient had a healthy childhood and adolescence. He became myopic in his late teens and has needed visual correction ever since. To date, Nigel has never been hospitalized with any acute illnesses or surgery. The patient has never smoked. He describes his alcohol consumption as "minimal"—roughly one or two glasses of wine on an average of once a month. The patient presently uses no medications.

Nigel's father Matthew, a professor of African history, died in 1980 at the age of 58 after suffering a heart attack. According to Nigel, "My father was pretty much healthy until then. Just collapsed one day and died in hospital a day later." The patient's mother, Cybill, 70, lives in Southampton, England, and is in good health. She had a hysterectomy in 1979 for heavy menstrual bleeding.

The patient's older brother, Randolph, 47, a businessman in Cape Town, South Africa, has had two heart attacks, the first at age 36 and the second 1 year ago. He has no other health problems. The patient's younger brother, Daniel, 41, of Southampton, and his younger sister, Felicity, 40, of Glasgow, Scotland, are both in excellent health. Nigel's children are also perfectly healthy.

Nigel and his family have extensive medical, dental, and life insurance.

The Problem

You are a family physician in a prosperous suburban area with complete access to all diagnostic facilities and a full spectrum of specialists. Nigel Waugh, a 45-year-old man, comes to you for a periodic health examination. He feels perfectly well. Two concerns arise after your initial evaluation. First, the patient is 177cm tall and weighs 98kg, with a body mass index (BMI) of 31.3 kg/metres squared. Second, the patient, who is a golf enthusiast and who travels frequently to tropical countries for business or pleasure, has a habit of exposing his bare skin to intense sunlight. You provide general advice on how to limit his fat and cholesterol intake and follow a balanced diet. You also advise Nigel to avoid extreme midday sun as much as possible and otherwise to wear protective clothing and sunscreen in intense sunshine. The patient agrees to follow your advice. Upon conclusion of the encounter, you decide it would be best to screen the patient for hypercholesterolemia by obtaining a blood test.

Questions

1. What are Nigel Waugh's risk factors for cardiovascular disease?
2. Is the decision to screen for hypercholesterolemia justifiable?
3. What specific serum values would you obtain?

Discussion

The recommendations in this Discussion section are largely based on those of the second Adult Treatment Panel (ATP II) of the National Cholesterol Education Program (NCEP, 1993).

1. ATP II (NCEP, 1993) identified six important risk factors for cardiovascular disease: age 45 years or more in men and 55 or more in women without premature menopause, cigarette smoking, diabetes mellitus, history of myocardial infarction or sudden cardiac death before age 55 in first-degree male relatives and before age 65 in first-degree female relatives, high-density lipoprotein (HDL) cholesterol level < 0.9mM (35mg/dL), and hypertension. Furthermore, as a high HDL cholesterol level (> 1.6mM, or 60mg/dl) is protective against cardiovascular disease, it is considered to be a *negative* risk factor that can cancel the presence of another positive risk factor. A high triglyceride level is not considered to be an independent risk factor for cardiovascular disease. Its presence is usually accompanied by other lipid disturbances or other risk factors, such as diabetes and obesity. Extremely high triglyceride levels may, however, cause pancreatitis. Nigel, therefore, is at increased cardiovascular risk because of

his age and family history. His HDL cholesterol is not yet known.

2. There is considerable evidence that a low HDL, rather than a high total cholesterol (most of which is derived from a high low-density lipoprotein [LDL] cholesterol), is a major risk factor for cardiovascular disease. The LDL cholesterol, however, has been the target of therapy, and lowering the LDL and, consequently, the total cholesterol level has been shown to reduce morbidity and mortality. By contrast, there is less available evidence at present to support raising the HDL to prevent cardiovascular incidents. Three large, multicenter placebo-controlled trials have shown that treating high cholesterol in asymptomatic men aged 30 to 59 years can reduce the risk of future cardiovascular events (Committee of Principal Investigators, 1978; Frick et al., 1987; Lipid Research Clinics, 1984). For this reason, screening for hypercholesterolemia in this population is recommended by the National Cholesterol Education Program (1993), the U.S. Preventive Services Task Force (1996), the Canadian Consensus Conference (1988), and the American College of Physicians (1996). The decision to screen for hypercholesterolemia, therefore, is supported by considerable evidence and a number of very prominent authorities.

3. A serum total blood cholesterol level and, if possible, a serum HDL level are the preferred initial screening tests for hypercholesterolemia (NCEP, 1993). Fasting specimens are not needed. Laboratory error and biological variation within the same individual is, for a number of reasons, quite common (Cooper, Myers, Smith, & Schlant, 1992). The U.S. Preventive Services Task Force therefore recommends at least two measurements, and a third if the two differ by more than 16%. The Canadian Task Force on the Periodic Health Examination (1994) recommends a minimum of three separate measurements.

PART II

The Problem

You decide to obtain nonfasting total cholesterol and HDL levels on two separate occasions and ask Mr. Waugh to return in 1 week's time. The results are shown below:

1. Total blood cholesterol 7.3mM (284.7mg/dL); HDL 0.80mM (31.2mg/dL)
2. Total blood cholesterol 7.2mM (280.8mg/dL); HDL 0.82mM (32.0mg/dL)

Questions

1. How would you interpret Nigel's results?
2. How would you proceed with management of this case?

Discussion

1. The ATP II has designated a value above 6.2mmol/l (240mg/dL) as *high* total cholesterol. This level corresponds roughly to the 80th percentile of cholesterol values in the American population, above which the risk for cardiovascular disease rises very steeply. *Borderline-high* cholesterol is 5.2 to 6.2mmol/l (200-239mg/dL), and a *desir-*able level is below 5.2mmol/l (200mg/dL). As noted in Part 1, an HDL level below 0.9mmol/l is abnormal. Nigel, therefore, has high total cholesterol and low HDL.

2. The next step is to further characterize Nigel's lipid abnormalities by obtaining a fasting lipoprotein analysis that will allow calculation of serum LDL.

PART III

The Problem

You obtain two fasting lipoprotein analyses. The results are shown below. Nigel is available to return to your office within a few days.

	First Analysis	Second Analysis
Total cholesterol	7.2mmol/l (280.8mg/dL)	7.1mmol/l (276.9mg/dL)
HDL cholesterol	0.8mmol/l (31.2mg/dL)	0.8mmol/l (31.2mg/dL)
Total triglycerides	6.0mmol/l (273.0mg/dL)	5.8mmol/l (226.2mg/dL)

Questions

1. From the data above, determine Nigel's LDL cholesterol level.
2. How would you characterize Nigel's LDL cholesterol level?
3. How would you proceed with management of this case?

Discussion

1. Direct determination of LDL is difficult and expensive. The LDL level can be estimated using the following formula:

LDL cholesterol = (Total cholesterol – HDL Cholesterol) – (Triglycerides/5)

In Nigel's case,

LDL = (7.2mmol/l – 0.8mmol/l) – (6.0mmol/l/5) = 5.2mmol/l, or 202.8mg/dL, and

LDL = (7.1mmol/l – 0.8mmol/l) – (5.8mmol/l/5) = 5.1mmol/l, or 198.9mg/dL.

2. An LDL cholesterol level greater than 4.1mmol/l or 160mg/dL is considered *high risk*.

3. Nigel should now undergo a thorough clinical evaluation, the purpose of which is to determine whether a familial lipoprotein disorder is present or whether the high LDL is secondary to another dis-

ease process. The three most common secondary causes of hypercholesterolemia are diabetes, hypothyroidism, and nephrotic syndrome. Screening for these conditions can be easily accomplished with a fasting serum glucose, sTSH level, and urine dipstick for protein (Freeman, 1995). The ATP II recommends such tests only *if indicated.* There is no reason to suspect that Nigel has nephrotic syndrome. He feels "perfectly well" and presumably has no symptoms of hypothyroidism. As obesity is an independent risk factor for the development of diabetes, and the patient is significantly overweight, it would not have been unreasonable to screen for diabetes as part of the periodic health examination. In addition, the patient's lipid profile, characterized by high LDL, low HDL, and elevated triglycerides, is common in patients with poorly controlled non-insulin-dependent diabetes. Furthermore, as diabetes often presents without any signs or symptoms, a patient who feels "perfectly well" may indeed be diabetic. For these reasons, screening for diabetes as a secondary cause of lipid disturbance is a reasonable intervention.

There are many inherited forms of hyperlipidemia, several of which are extremely rare disorders. A discussion of all of these is certainly beyond the scope of this exercise. Among common inherited forms is the heterozygous form of *familial hypercholesterolemia,* which affects roughly 1 in 500 persons. Its clinical features include premature atheroscle-rosis, often presenting in the form of myocardial infarction in men in the fourth and fifth decades. Other features include the presence of **xanthomas,** yellowish nodules or plaques composed of lipid-laden histiocytes. These occur on the tendons of the hand, knee, elbow, and ankle and are found in roughly 75% of patients with this lipid

disorder (Brown & Goldstein, 1991). Cholesterol deposits are also often found on the eyelids, in a form called **xanthelasma,** and on the cornea, as **arcus corneae,** an opaque, grayish ring within the junction of the sclera and cornea.

Multiple lipoprotein-type hyperlipidemia is a common inherited lipid disorder with three characteristic patterns of abnormalities: hypercholesterolemia alone (type 2a), hypertriglyceridemia alone (type 4), and both hypercholesterolemia and hypertriglyceridemia (type 2b). Affected individuals often have a strong family history of heart disease. Xanthomas are not present. It is difficult to distinguish this disorder from the more common **polygenic hypercholesterolemia,** which is simply the diagnosis in the majority of those with hypercholesterolemia and probably results from both genetic and environmental factors. Nigel's lipid profile is consistent with both multiple lipoprotein-type hyperlipidemia, type 2b, and with polygenic hypercholesterolemia. As the approach to management is identical, there is no practical reason to distinguish between the two.

As both familial hypercholesterolemia and more rare forms of lipid disorders commonly present with xanthomas and other superficial lipid deposits, physical examination to rule out the presence of such findings is a suitable way to exclude the possibility of an inherited lipid disorder. Most rare inherited disorders actually present early in life, with very high cholesterol levels and with severe consequences. They are unlikely to be present in Nigel. The patient has a strong family history of heart disease, and it may be prudent to ask him if he is aware of any familial history of lipid disorders.

The remaining components of a clinical evaluation, upon diagnosis of hyperlipidemia, include a thorough examination of the cardiovascular system and an examination for hepatosplenomegaly, which may occur with excessive lipid deposition in some disorders (Roederer, 1995). See "The Rest of the Story" at the end of this section for a suggested clinical evaluation upon diagnosing hyperlipidemia, and Nigel's corresponding results. Note that some components would probably have already been included in his periodic health examination.

The Rest of the Story

Nigel is unaware of any family history of lipid disorders. The results of your physical examination are summarized below.

wt. = 98.2kg
BP = 125/80mmHg
Skin: no xanthomas in tendons of hands, around knees, elbows, or on Achilles tendons
HEENT: no arcus cornea; no xanthelasmae on eyelids
CVS: normal heart sounds
normal peripheral pulses
no carotid, abdominal, or femoral bruits
Abdomen: no hepatosplenomegaly

You ask Nigel to return the next day for a fasting blood glucose specimen, which returns as 5.5mmol/l (99mg/dL).

PART IV

The Problem

After reviewing Nigel's clinical evaluation, you ask him to return to your office to discuss therapy for hypercholesterolemia. He agrees and comes back 2 weeks later.

Questions

1. What sort of therapy would you initiate?
2. What are the goals of therapy?
3. Are there natural dietary supplements that can help reduce lipid levels?

Discussion

1. There is sound evidence to support dietary measures, specifically the restriction of intake of saturated fat and cholesterol, as a means of lowering LDL cholesterol, which, as noted, is the primary target of therapy. Indeed, diet is the first-line

therapy recommended for hypercholesterolemia by the ATP II. It follows a two-step approach. The American Heart Association's (1986) Step 1 Diet recommends an intake of no more than 8% to 10% of calories from saturated fat, no more than 30% of calories from fat overall, and a daily cholesterol intake of less than 300mg/day. Such a diet is consistent with healthy living in general and is recommended for and followed by a number of people without high cholesterol. For this reason, it is best to get an idea of what Nigel's diet is presently like and to see how close his intake is to the recommendations in the Step 1 program. The Step 2 diet is more restrictive and can be employed should the Step 1 diet fail to achieve the desired effect on lipids.

2. The goals of dietary therapy can be defined precisely in terms of LDL cholesterol levels. As outlined by the ATP II, goals are dependent on the number of cardiovascular risk factors present. Dietary therapy is initiated at an LDL level of 3.4mmol-l (130mg/dL) when two or more risk factors are present (such as in Nigel's situation). The goal is to reduce LDL below this level. With fewer than two risk factors, the threshold LDL level at which dietary therapy is initiated rises to 4.1mmol-l (160mg/dL). When coronary heart disease is already present, it drops to 2.6mmol-l (100mg/dL).

Beyond specific LDL target levels, another goal of dietary therapy is to promote weight loss through caloric restriction. Weight loss serves to reduce LDL levels independently beyond those that can be achieved through reduction in cholesterol and saturated fat intake alone. Weight loss and exercise together also help to reduce

triglycerides, raise HDL cholesterol, and reduce the risk of diabetes. The effect, therefore, is to reduce the overall risk of cardiovascular disease.

In summary, the initial approach to hypercholesterolemia in this patient involves significant lifestyle modification, including exercise and a diet that restricts saturated fat, cholesterol, and calories. These recommendations should be carefully explained to Nigel, who can then incorporate them in a way that suits his lifestyle.

3. The general public is bombarded with a great deal of often conflicting information about the value of many common foods, vitamins, and supplements. Among these is no shortage of products promoted as having a positive effect on serum lipids.

The addition of fiber to cholesterol-lowering diets has been studied extensively. Some water-soluble high fiber supplements, such as psyllium, are known to have a beneficial effect on serum lipids (Bell, Hectorne, Reynolds, Balm, & Hunninghake, 1989). There is controversy as to whether oat bran has a cholesterol-lowering effect. It has been recently postulated that any beneficial effect of oat bran on serum lipids is due to displacement of other foods high in cholesterol and saturated fat from the diet. In a randomized double-blind trial in which a diet supplemented with foods high in oat bran was compared to a placebo diet in which the supplement was a low-fiber wheat, both products had a similar favorable impact on serum cholesterol (Swain, Rouse, Curley, & Sacks, 1990). In other words, oat bran was found to have no intrinsic hypolipidemic effect.

Garlic supplements have been used in Germany for many years to reduce lipid levels. The presumed active ingredient is *allicin,* formed enzymatically from the precursor, *alliin,* when garlic cloves are crushed. In a 12-week double-blind randomized study of garlic tablets given at a dose of 900mg/day, supplementation was found to produce a modest but significant decrease in total cholesterol and LDL cholesterol, compared to a placebo (Jain, Vargas, Gotzkowsky, & McMahon, 1993). This is one part of a fairly large body of evidence from similar trials that supports the use of supplemental garlic as a lipid-lowering agent (Mader, 1990; Vorberg & Schneider, 1990). Garlic is available in a variety of preparations with varying degrees of acceptability in terms of taste and odor.

The use of water-soluble fiber products, such as psyllium, and supplementing one's diet with garlic can be discussed with Nigel.

See "The Rest of the Story," which follows.

The Rest of the Story

At his return appointment, you review Nigel's laboratory results and tell him that he requires therapy to reduce his cholesterol level to a point that reduces his risk of cardiovascular disease. Nigel does not seem at all surprised by his high cholesterol level. "Oh, yes," he says. "Well, I eat poorly, you know. I guess I have to be careful from now on."

You tell Nigel that dietary management of his lipid disorder is first-line therapy. You explain the recommendations of the AHA Step 1 Diet and ask the patient to give you an idea of what his dietary intake is like on a typical day.

Well, first of all, at our house there are two people who prepare meals: Gracie in the morning and Franco at supper. Gracie pampers me. She makes anything I want for breakfast. My wife and the kids are much more careful about what they eat. Sharifa really keeps the rest of the family in line. For my part, if I want Belgian waffles, I get Belgian waffles—and lots of them!

Several catering companies and restaurants supply lunch to the executive offices at our company. It's usually a pigfest around noon—and I'm the King Pig! It's usually something new every day. My secretary takes care of it. I love Indian and Thai food for lunch.

For supper, Franco cooks up a storm. It's all very rich, and his desserts are amazing. This is all when I'm *in* town. I do much of my eating in airplanes, in New York, London, or Cape Town, and then it's often rich Indian or Middle-Eastern snacks and meals. I can assure you, I'm not following any special "heart" diet!

You tell Nigel that he is correct in that his diet is far from the AHA Step 1. You ask him if he is willing to make dietary changes and to incorporate exercise into his lifestyle. He responds,

Oh yes, definitely. I've been meaning to make some serious changes for a while. I know how bad my family history is. I definitely want to get in shape. What I can do is ask Gracie and Franco to prepare only Heart Association-approved meals. I will make sure that I get proper meals at work, in restaurants, hotels, etc. It won't be hard to arrange. My wife hired a personal trainer a couple of years ago. Anyway, she gave up after a couple of months, but the guy was great. He told me he could help me too. I'll give him a call and get started on a routine. I've been meaning to do that for a long time. I mean, I do golf, but that is just not enough.

PART V

The Problem

You tell Nigel that it is very fortunate that he has such great resources at his disposal to help him make lifestyle changes. He agrees to follow a Step 1 diet and to begin a program of regular exercise. You mention the benefits of weight loss on lipids but decide that changes in dietary content and exercise should lead to gradual decrease in weight, and you decide to delay any further deliberate caloric restriction. You review the effects of high-fiber, water-soluble supplements and garlic on serum lipids. Nigel tells you, "Oh, that gritty Metamucil stuff. I guess I could try it. Garlic is no problem—I love it! That gritty stuff looks very unappetizing, though."

Questions

1. When would you like to see Nigel again? What will be your agenda for the next visit?

Discussion

1. The ATP II recommends that those beginning a Step 1 diet be seen in 4 to 6 weeks and 3 months later as well, to assess compliance with diet and any change in serum lipids. As total cholesterol levels generally closely parallel LDL levels, a nonfasting total cholesterol is adequate to monitor progress. A substantial decrease in total cholesterol can be followed by a fasting lipid profile to confirm a corresponding decrease in LDL. Serial total cholesterol measurements can be obtained and averaged because, as noted previously, significant variation is common.

PART VI

The Problem

Nigel returns 5 weeks later. Two total cholesterol measurements taken within the past few days average **7.1mmol/l (276.9mg/dL)**. You review these results with him. He seems a little disappointed, especially as he has been "sticking to his diet to the letter." You tell him that treatment of hypercholesterolemia often requires a long-term commitment for measurable success. His personal trainer has involved him in a program of graded aerobic exercise. Nigel tells you he feels better and has more energy. You congratulate him on his work in changing his lifestyle. You advise Nigel to continue with his lifestyle modification program and to return in 2 months.

Nigel returns as scheduled. Two recently drawn total cholesterol levels average **7.1mmol/l (276.9mg/dL)**. Nigel has established a rigorous routine of diet and exercise and now weighs 91kg.

Questions

1. Where would you go from here?

Discussion

1. A minimum of 6 months of dietary therapy is recommended as initial management of hypercholesterolemia. At this point, one can consider the more restrictive AHA Step II diet, in which less than 7% of calories are consumed as saturated fat and cholesterol intake is limited to 200mg/day. Despite Nigel's access to carefully pre- pared food, he may benefit from the assistance of a dietician, who can further explain the Step II diet and how to maintain it. Once again, the patient should be seen 4 to 6 weeks and 3 months later, and his total cholesterol should be measured at similar intervals to monitor progress.

PART VII

The Problem

You briefly review Nigel's blood tests and tell him that a more restrictive diet can be pursued to help achieve the desired lipid levels. He seems a little bit discouraged but tells you, "Oh well. At least I feel better and I'm losing weight." You tell Nigel that his success in lifestyle modification itself is likely to have a long-term beneficial impact on his health. You discuss the Step II diet, in which the patient appears to be very interested. You refer him to a qualified dietician and ask him to return as previously for follow-up and cholesterol measurements.

At his follow-up visit 4 weeks later, Nigel tells you he finds the Step II diet rather bland, although his dietician has made some excellent suggestions on how to "eat well" within its limitations. He has followed the diet carefully, with the exception of one indiscretion 1 week ago that consisted of several "greasy kebabs" in London, England. The average of two total cholesterol measurements drawn in the past few days is **6.8mmol/l (265.2mg/dL).**

Two months later, Nigel returns and tells you he continues to feel fit and well. He now jogs for 20 min roughly four times a week. His weight is now 86.9kg. Two recently obtained total serum cholesterol levels return as **6.7mmol/l (261.3mg/dL)** and **6.3mmol/l (245.7mg/dL).** You decide to obtain two fasting lipid profiles, the results of which are shown below:

1. Total cholesterol 6.3mmol/l (245.7mg/dL)
   HDL 0.84mmol/l (32.8mg/dL)
   Triglycerides 5.5mmol/l (214.5mg/dL)
   Calculated LDL 4.4mmol/l (170.0mg/dL)

2. Total cholesterol 6.3mmol/l (245.7mg/dL)
   HDL 0.89mmol/l (34.7mg/dL)

Triglycerides 5.2mmol/l (202.8mg/dL)
Calculated LDL 4.4mmol/l (170.0mg/dL)

Questions

1. What management options are available at this point?
2. Describe the various types of pharmacotherapy for hypercholesterolemia and their corresponding effects on different lipid components.
3. What pharmacotherapy, if any, would you consider?

Discussion

1. The goal is to reduce Nigel's LDL level to 3.4mmol/l (130mg/dL) or below. One can draw two important conclusions at this point. First, it is evident that Nigel has been following his diet carefully. Second, dietary intervention and exercise are having a modest, but definitely significant, positive impact on his lipid profile and a profound impact on his overall health, fitness, and sense of well-being. Unfortunately, Nigel has not met his target level for LDL cholesterol after 6 months. One option is to recommend an even more restrictive diet, with further reductions in intake of cholesterol and saturated fat. Nigel, however, already finds the Step II diet quite unpalatable and may find it difficult to adjust to further restrictions.

Another option is drug therapy. The ATP II specifies an LDL of 4.1mmol/l or greater in patients with two or more other risk factors as the level at which drug therapy should be considered after an adequate trial of diet. The decision to initiate medication should not be taken lightly, as some lipid-lowering drugs are associated with unpleasant side effects and may be needed indefinitely. In a patient unaccustomed to taking medication regularly, this would represent a major commitment. It is important to note that lipid-lowering medications are an adjunct to, and not a substitute for, continued dietary therapy.

2. Lipid-lowering drugs include three *major* categories, namely the **bile acid sequestrants, nicotinic acid** (niacin), and the **HMG-CoA reductase inhibitors.** In addition, there is **probucol** and, also, the **fibric acid derivatives** such as gemfibrozil.

The **bile acid sequestrants,** such as cholestyramine and colestipol, can lower LDL cholesterol by approximately 20% ("Choice of Lipid," 1996) and are known to be an effective primary preventive measure for coronary heart disease (Lipid Research Clinics, 1984). They have a relatively insignificant impact on HDL and may actually raise triglyceride levels. The bile acid sequestrants are associated with a variety of adverse gastrointestinal symptoms, including nausea, heartburn, and bloating. The gritty texture of most preparations is also unpalatable to many patients. Side effects can be minimized by using these medications in modest doses of 8 to 10 gms prior to meals and adding a water-soluble high fiber supplement such as psyllium, which, as discussed previously, itself has intrinsic lipid-lowering value.

Nicotinic acid decreases LDL cholesterol by 15% to 30% and triglycerides by

20% to 50%, and it is the most effective medication in raising HDL, with levels rising 20% to 30%. Its use is limited by its side effects, which include flushing, pruritus, fatigue, and a variety of gastrointestinal symptoms. Flushing can be minimized by increasing the dose gradually and taking 80 to 325 mg aspirin 30 min prior to administration (Fortmann & Maron, 1997). Niacin is available in both immediate (IR) and sustained (SR) release forms. The latter is associated with significant hepatotoxicity and is not recommended (Etchason et al., 1991; Henkin, Johnson, & Segrest, 1990).

The well-studied **HMG-CoA reductase inhibitors** (lovastatin, pravastatin, simvastatin, and fluvastatin) inhibit the rate-limiting step in cholesterol synthesis. They are the most effective LDL-lowering drugs, decreasing levels by 20% to 30%. They also modestly decrease triglyceride levels, but they have a relatively insignificant impact on HDL. The HMG-CoA reductase inhibitors have a favorable side-effect profile, but at present it is unknown whether very long-term use is associated with any adverse effects.

The effect of pravastatin on the incidence of myocardial infarction and death from cardiovascular disease in asymptomatic men with hypercholesterolemia has been studied in a large randomized double-blind placebo-controlled trial in Scotland (Shepherd et al., 1995). The medication was associated with a 31% decrease in relative risk of adverse coronary events over a follow-up period of 4.9 years.

The fibric acid derivatives and probucol, although effective in reducing triglycerides, have only a slight beneficial effect on LDL and no proven impact on cardiovascular mortality.

3. As noted, the HMG-CoA reductase inhibitors, bile acid sequestrants, and niacin will all lower LDL, which has been shown to reduce morbidity and mortality. Nigel, however, also has low HDL, a major risk factor for cardiovascular disease. Though compelling evidence for the benefit of raising HDL is still pending, the ATP II (NCEP, 1993) recommends that agents that raise HDL be given strong consideration in patients with low HDL. Niacin, therefore, is a good choice for Nigel.

PART VIII

The Problem

Nigel returns to discuss his results and further management. You tell him that dietary management and exercise have had a significant impact on his lipid profile, but that to meet his LDL target, more aggressive therapy will most probably be needed. You review the options of further dietary restrictions, bile acid sequestrants, HMG-CoA reductase, and niacin. Nigel tells you he feels his diet is already very restrictive and that he is not too interested in making further restrictions.

You and Nigel both agree on therapy with niacin. You warn the patient about the common side effects and begin with a low dose of 100mg tid with meals, gradually increasing it to

500mg po tid over the course of 3 weeks. He is to take 80mg aspirin 30 min prior to each niacin dose to minimize flushing.

Questions

1. When would you like to see Nigel again?

Discussion

1. After starting pharmacologic therapy, a lipid profile should be obtained 4 to 6 weeks and 3 months later. Nigel's compliance with diet and medications can be assessed on each of these occasions. If the target LDL is met, repeat levels can be drawn every four months (NCEP, 1993). It is recommended that liver function tests, glucose, and uric acid be checked once a dose of 1.5gm/day of niacin is reached and three times a year thereafter.

Conclusion

Nigel returns 4 weeks later. He feels well. He has been taking niacin as instructed and did initially experience considerable flushing, which has since abated. A calculated LDL obtained the previous day returns as **3.7mmol/l (144.3mg/dL)**. His HDL is **0.89mmol/l (34.7mg/dL)**. There is no evidence of hepatotoxicity and no abnormalities of glucose or uric acid. Though Nigel's HDL is essentially unchanged, he is pleased with the decrease in LDL. You decide to continue with the same dose of niacin.

Prior to his 3-month visit, his calculated LDL level is measured as **3.2mmol/l (124.8mg/dL)** and HDL as **1.1mmol/l (42.9mg/dL)**. His other serum chemistries remain normal. He is following his diet and medication regimen carefully and continues to feel well. You congratulate Nigel once again on his overall lifestyle modification program, and you ask him to return every 4 months for a year for continued monitoring. He agrees and thanks you for all your help.

References

American College of Physicians. (1996). Clinical guidelines. Part I: Guidelines for using serum cholesterol, high-density lipoprotein cholesterol, and triglyceride levels as screening tests for preventing coronary heart disease in adults. *Annals of Internal Medicine, 124*, 515-517.

American Heart Association. (1986). Dietary guidelines for healthy American adults: A statement for physicians and health professionals by the nutrition committee, American Heart Association. *Circulation, 74*, 1465A-1468A.

Bell, L. P., Hectorne, K., Reynolds, H., Balm, T. K., & Hunninghake, D. B. (1989). Cholesterol-lowering effects of psyllium hydrophilic mucilloid. *Journal of the American Medical Association, 261*, 3419-3423.

Brown, M. S., & Goldstein, J. L. (1991). The hyperlipoproteinemias and other disorders of lipid metabolism. In J. D. Wilson, E. Braunwald, K. J. Isselbacher, R. G. Petersdorf, J. B. Martin, A. S. Fauci, & R. K. Root (Eds.), *Harrison's prin-*

ciples of internal medicine (12th ed.). New York: McGraw-Hill.

Canadian Consensus Conference on the Prevention of Heart and Vascular Disease by Altering Serum Cholesterol and Lipoprotein Risk Factors. (1988). Canadian Consensus Conference on Cholesterol: Final report. *Canadian Medical Association Journal, 139*(11 Suppl.), 1-8.

Canadian Task Force on the Periodic Health Examination. (1994). *The Canadian guide to clinical preventive health care.* Ottawa: Minister of Supply and Services Canada.

Choice of lipid-lowering drugs. (1996). *Medical Letter, 38,* 67-70.

Committee of Principal Investigators. (1978). A cooperative trial in the primary prevention of ischemic heart disease using clofibrate (Report). *British Heart Journal, 40,* 1068-1118.

Cooper, G. R., Myers, G. L., Smith, S. J., & Schlant, R. C. (1992). Blood lipid measurements: Variations and practical utility. *Journal of the American Medical Association, 267,* 1652-1660.

Etchason, J. A., Miller, T. D., Squires, R. W., Allison, T. G., Gau, G. T., Marttila, J. K., & Kottke, B. A. (1991). Niacin-induced hepatitis: A potential side effect with low-dose time-release niacin. *Mayo Clinic Proceedings, 66*(1), 112-113.

Fortmann, S. P., & Maron, D. T. (1997). Diagnosis and treatment of lipid disorders [CD-ROM, Chap. 2]. *Scientific American Medicine, 9,* 3.

Freeman, M. W. (1995). Approach to the patient with hypercholesterolemia. In A. H. Goroll, L. A. May, & A. G. Mulley (Eds.), *Primary care medicine* (pp. 139-151). Philadelphia, PA: J. B. Lippincott.

Frick, M. H., Elo, O., Haapa, K., Heinonen, O. P., Heinsalmi, P., Helo, P., Huttunen, J. K., Kaitaniemi, P., Koskinen, P., & Manninnen, V. (1987). Helsinki Heart Study: Primary prevention trial with gemfibrozil in middle-aged men with dyslipidemia. Safety of treatment, changes in risk factors, and incidence of coronary heart disease. *New England Journal of Medicine, 317,* 1237-1245.

Henkin, Y., Johnson, K. C., & Segrest, J. P. (1990). Rechallenge with crystalline niacin after drug-induced hepatitis from sustained-release niacin. *Journal of the American Medical Association, 264*(2), 241-243.

Jain, A. K., Vargas, R., Gotzkowsky, S., & McMahon, F. G. (1993). Can garlic reduce levels of serum lipids? A controlled clinical study. *American Journal of Medicine, 94,* 632-635.

Lipid Research Clinics. (1984). Coronary primary prevention trial results, I: Reduction in incidence of coronary heart disease. *Journal of the American Medical Association, 251,* 351-364.

Mader, F. H. (1990). Treatment of hyperlipidemia with garlic-powder tablets: Evidence from the German Association of General Practitioners' multicenter placebo-controlled double-blind study. *Arzneimittelforschung, 40,* 1111-1116.

National Cholesterol Education Program (NCEP) Expert Panel on Detection, Evaluation, and Treatment of High Blood Cholesterol in Adults (Adult Treatment Panel II). (1993). Summary of the second report. *Journal of the American Medical Association, 269,* 3015-3023.

Roederer, G. O. (1995). Dyslipidemias. In J. Gray (Ed.), *Therapeutic choices.* Ottawa: Canadian Pharmaceutical Association.

Shepherd, J., Cobbe, S. M., Ford, I., Isles, C. G., Lorimer, A. R., MacFarlane, P. W., McKillop, J. H., & Packard, C. J. (1995). Prevention of coronary heart disease with pravastatin in men with hypercholesterolemia. *New England Journal of Medicine, 333*(20), 1301-1307.

Swain, J. F., Rouse, I. L., Curley, C. B., & Sacks, F. M. (1990). Comparison of the effects of oat bran and low-fiber wheat on serum lipoprotein levels and blood pressure. *New England Journal of Medicine, 322,* 147-152.

U.S. Preventive Services Task Force. (1996). *Guide to clinical preventive services* (2nd ed.). Baltimore, MD: Williams and Wilkins.

Vorberg, G., & Schneider, B. (1990). Therapy with garlic: Results of a placebo-controlled, double-blind study. *British Journal of Clinical Practice, 44*(Suppl. 69), 7-11.

7. OUTPATIENT MANAGEMENT
OF HEART FAILURE

Mr. Stewart Ross

Goal: The goal of this group discussion exercise is
to evaluate and develop the participants' understanding
of the management of heart failure in an outpatient setting.

Specific Objectives: Upon completion of this group discussion exercise, each participant should be able to accomplish the following:

1. Recognize the signs and symptoms of heart failure.
2. Order appropriate investigations upon initial presentation of a patient with heart failure.
3. Counsel a patient recently diagnosed with heart failure about nonpharmacologic approaches to management.
4. Administer pharmacologic therapy in an appropriate and timely fashion.
5. Recognize the important psychological impact of heart failure as a multifaceted illness and assess a patient's coping abilities in this respect.

PART I

The Patient

Social History

Mr. Stewart Ross is a married 68-year-old Scottish-Canadian man who lives in Berwick, Nova Scotia. Born in Annapolis Royal, NS, the patient is the second child of the late Mr. Angus Ross and the late Eileen Ross. Stewart grew up in the Annapolis Valley region of Nova Scotia, where he attended school until age 14. Never a keen or successful student, he left to work in a small corner store owned by his uncle, all the while dreaming of fighting the war in Europe. The war passed young Stewart by, but, looking for adventure, he enlisted with the Canadian armed forces in 1946, with whom he spent 2 years. His military posting took him no further from home than St. Jean, Province of Quèbec. Frustrated by the military's insistence on discipline and protocol, a homesick Stewart returned to the Valley in 1948 and worked on the family farm outside Annapolis Royal with his parents and brothers.

Stewart met Charlotte McNeil, a slim, shy 19-year-old at a church picnic in 1952. In his words, "I hate to use a cliché, but it really was love at first sight." The two were married in 1953. Stewart quickly found a job with a shipyard in Saint John, New Brunswick, where the couple lived from 1953 to 1962.

While in Saint John, the Ross's children, Brian, now 42 years old; Joan, 41; and Alan, 36, were born. Stewart worked long, difficult hours while his wife worked equally hard looking after the children. Sadly, a wave of layoffs hit the shipyard in 1962, and Stewart lost his job. No longer able to make ends meet in Saint John, the Rosses returned to Nova Scotia, to the old farmhouse in which Stewart grew up, which his older brother had inherited. Stewart's experience at the shipyard served him well. He was a skilled welder and sheetmetal worker, and he started his own business in the Valley, repairing agricultural machinery.

The 1960s were a very happy time for the Ross family. The repair shop did very well. Stewart and Charlotte enjoyed raising their three children immensely. The Rosses' extended family was a very close-knit clan. Stewart's brothers and their families were never more than a short distance away. Stewart and Charlotte were always a happy couple. Stewart's older brother, Alexander, once remarked about them, "Even as they get older, they're still like two school kids falling in love for the first time."

As changes in technology hit the agricultural machinery industry, Stewart's repair shop gradually became obsolete through the late 1960s and early 1970s. With four full-time employees, he diversified the business in 1974 and became a general contractor. Ross General Contracting took on jobs as diverse as landscaping, roofing, and even plumbing. By 1980, Stewart Ross was one of the most successful general contractors in the region. In 1989, he sold the business and retired to the community of Berwick.

Today, Stewart and Charlotte Ross live in a beautiful Victorian brick home in Berwick, Nova Scotia. Their three children have long since moved away and started families of their own. The Rosses are an inseparable couple who enjoy fishing, taking long walks, shopping for antiques, and visiting their children and grandchildren. As Stewart puts it, "We like to get outdoors and be active. We've never owned a television set."

The Rosses are devout Presbyterians and rarely miss Sunday service at their local church. Stewart Ross is a card-carrying member of the provincial Liberal party and has helped with several local campaigns in previous election years.

Past Personal and Family Medical History

The patient had, in his words, "a pretty healthy childhood." He does recall his mother mentioning that he was struck by scarlet fever at age 5. At age 15, a large scale, used to weigh vegetables, fell on Stewart's right foot, fracturing his first proximal phalanx. The remainder of the patient's childhood and adolescence were unremarkable from a medical perspective.

In 1956, Stewart spent 5 days in the hospital with what he describes as a "nasty pneumonia." This was his only hospitalization until 1985, when the patient suffered an anterolateral myocardial infarction. Stewart describes that experience this way:

I was out trying to fix one of the trucks. It was bloody hot outside and I was sweating bullets. Suddenly I felt this tightening across my chest, and my jaw and ears started to hurt. I knew I was in trouble. I called for Charlotte. I was in agony when the ambulance brought me into hospital.

Stewart has not experienced any chest pain of any kind since his discharge from the hospital in 1985. To date, there are no other significant events in the patient's medical history.

The patient smoked approximately one pack of cigarettes a day from 1947 to 1985, when his family physician helped him to quit after his heart attack. Stewart drinks about 12 shots of whisky or brandy a week, usually with dinner. His only medication at the present time is enteric-coated aspirin, at a dose of 325mg/day.

The patient's father, Angus Ross, died in 1956 of a heart attack. He was 60 years old. Eileen Ross died in 1972 of metastatic cancer of the colon. She was 71 years old.

Stewart has an older and a younger brother. Alexander Ross, 70, of Halifax, NS is a married father of four and grandfather of nine. He has insulin-dependent Type II diabetes and has also had symptomatic benign prostatic hyperplasia, which required surgery last year. Charles Ross, 65, of Kentville, NS is a married, retired father and grandfather who, according to Stewart, is "as healthy as a horse." He has had no serious illnesses, surgery, or hospitalizations.

Stewart and Charlotte's three children are in generally good health. Joan had a hysterectomy in 1992 for heavy menstrual bleeding and fibroids. The Rosses' four grandchildren are in perfect health.

The Problem

You are one of three family physicians in a small town. There is a community hospital approximately 50 km away with a nearly full complement of specialists and diagnostic facilities. Mr. Stewart Ross, a married 68-year-old man, comes to your office and tells you he "has been out of breath recently." He reports that he has always tried to keep active but that that has been impossible over the past couple of months because even mild exertion makes him short of breath.

Stewart tells you, "Gosh, I used to be able to go out and work in the yard for hours. Now I start to feel winded on the way to the backyard." Stewart tells you he usually has no difficulty climbing the stairs in his house, but now occasionally he does feel slightly short of breath after climbing the two flights to the top floor. The Ross home is located on top of a small hill up from the road, and it is there that Stewart has noticed the greatest difficulty. "I actually have to stop two or three times on my way up the hill. It's crazy." The patient is unable to tell you when exactly he started to become "winded" easily, but he has been developing gradually poorer activity tolerance over the past 2 to 3 months. Over the past 3 weeks, something even more distressing has taken place. "I've actually woke up in the middle of the night a few times feeling out of breath. It's awful. It wakes Charlotte up too. I have to stand up and get some fresh air before I start to feel better again."

Stewart also reports feeling generally fatigued and lacking energy recently. In his words, "Charlotte has all these ideas for traveling, shopping, gardening, and other things. I just don't feel up to it." He reports no change in weight, no fever, and no other constitutional symptoms.

Stewart reports no chest pain or pressure, no orthopnea, no palpitations, and no swelling of his extremities. He reports no recent cough, sputum, or wheezing. He has been otherwise well. The results of his physical examination upon initial evaluation are summarized below:

Gen: Very pleasant male in no apparent distress. Looks stated age

VS: Ht. = 1.83m; Wt. = 87.2kg; BP = 120/80 (no pulsus alternans) (no significant orthostatic changes); P = 80/min; RR = 22/min; T = 37.3°C

Thorax and lungs: Symmetrical thorax. Normal expansion. Normal breath sounds. Fine crepitations heard bilaterally in both lung bases

Cardiovascular: JVP = 4.5cm above sternal angle at 30deg elevation of head

   Carotid pulses normal

   Apical impulse palpable in 5th left interspace, 8cm from midsternal line

   Normal S1, S2. No S3 or S4

   No murmurs

Peripheral vascular: Normal pulses in lower extremities

   No peripheral edema

Questions

1. How would you proceed with an evaluation of Mr. Ross's problem?

Discussion

1. Stewart Ross's clinical picture is certainly consistent with a diagnosis of heart failure. Heart failure is a very prevalent disease associated with considerable morbidity and mortality. Family physicians can play an important role in its diagnosis and management. For these reasons, there is no shortage of excellent diagnostic and treatment guidelines available from Canada (Canadian Cardiovascular Society, 1996), the United Kingdom (Dargie & McMurray, 1994), Europe (Task Force on Heart Failure of the European Society of Cardiology, 1995), and the United States (American College of Cardiology/American Heart Association Task Force on Practice Guidelines, 1995; Konstam et al., 1994). Recommendations for how to proceed with an initial evaluation in a patient suspected of having heart failure, like

Stewart Ross, are quite similar in most countries. In continuing to evaluate Mr. Ross, one must try to put together a strategy for ordering blood tests and other investigations. What must be known is the rationale for ordering tests. In this context, tests have three main purposes. First, they may find evidence supporting the diagnosis of heart failure. Second, they may help rule out other disease entities (e.g., pulmonary pathology) as a cause of the patient's symptoms. Finally, they may help identify conditions that can cause or aggravate heart failure, precipitating the patient's visit. During the group discussion, any suggestion for initial diagnostic evaluation should be rationalized using this three-part strategy.

In patients presenting with typical signs of heart failure such as exertional and paroxysmal nocturnal dyspnea, like Mr. Ross, an electrocardiogram is universally recommended as a means of identifying a precipitant. Acute ST-T wave changes may indicate acute myocardial ischemia, a common cause of heart failure. Rhythm disturbances that can also cause failure, such as atrial fibrillation, can be identified. Previous infarction, which reduces left ventricular performance, may manifest itself in the form of Q waves. This is a finding one would expect in the case of Stewart Ross. Low-voltage waves on the EKG are a sign of pericardial effusion that can also impair cardiac performance. Left ventricular hypertrophy identified on an EKG is a sign of diastolic dysfunction, a cause of heart failure in which systolic function is often unimpaired.

A CBC can rule out anemia, which can cause heart failure by decreasing oxygen-carrying capacity. A urinalysis can serve a useful purpose (Konstam et al., 1994). It detects proteinuria, a sign of nephrotic syndrome, and red cell casts, a sign of glomerulonephritis, both of which can mimic heart failure, as patients with these conditions often present with peripheral edema (Mair, 1996). Mr. Ross does not have edema, so in his case, a urinalysis would not be useful in this respect. A urinalysis is not part of the routine, recommended, initial evaluative procedures in the guidelines of the Canadian Cardiovascular Society (1996) nor those suggested by Dargie and McMurray (1994).

A serum creatinine and/or urea level is indicated to identify renal failure and consequent volume overload as a cause of heart failure. A decreased serum albumin level is also consistent with an increased extravascular volume and should be identified (ACC/AHA Task Force, 1995; Konstam et al., 1994). Serum electrolytes, as well as glucose, phosphorus, magnesium, and calcium levels, are recommended tests, according to the American College of Cardiology/American Heart Association (ACC/AHA Task Force, 1995). Identifying disturbances in these values would be useful prior to starting any pharmacologic therapy. Tests of thyroid function (i.e., T_4 and TSH) are recommended to rule out heart failure provoked by hypo- or hyperthyroidism.

A chest radiograph is helpful in identifying pulmonary disease, which may explain Stewart's symptoms. Furthermore, signs of heart failure such as cardiomegaly and redistribution of pulmonary vasculature can be readily identified.

The most important element of diagnosis in a suspected case of heart failure is some measure of cardiac performance. This can be achieved through an echocardiogram or radionuclide ventriculography. Echocardiography is much more widely available, but a radionuclide ventriculogram provides a more precise estimate of systolic ejection fraction, the component of cardiac performance, which is impaired in the majority of cases of heart failure.

Coronary artery disease is the most common cause of heart failure (Rahimtoola, 1989). Roughly half of all patients presently free of angina but with a history of myocardial infarction have significant areas of ischemic myocardium (Konstam et al., 1994). There is a great deal of controversy about how to approach such patients, like Stewart Ross, from the perspective of evaluation of ischemia and revascularization. Should Stewart undergo noninvasive or invasive evaluation to detect stenotic coronary arteries and areas of myocardial ischemia even though he is free of chest pain? Revascularization procedures have not been found to increase the quality or length of life in patients like Mr. Ross (Baker, Jones, et al., 1994). At the present time, the Agency for Health Care Policy and Research (AHCPR; Konstam et al., 1994) recommends noninvasive evaluation for myocardial ischemia in patients who present with symptoms of heart failure and a previous history of myocardial infarction but who presently have no angina. The ACC/AHA (ACC/AHA Task Force, 1995) recommends either noninvasive evaluation or cardiac catheterization (coronary arteriography) under the same circumstances. A number of noninvasive tests for ischemia are available, including treadmill exercise testing and thallium perfusion scintigraphy. As the benefit of re-vascularization is questionable in patients like Stewart Ross, any discussion participant who elects not to evaluate him for myocardial ischemia either through noninvasive or invasive means can do so justifiably. In any case, in the AHCPR guidelines (Konstam et al., 1994), noninvasive testing is not part of the initial evaluation but is recommended after the patient has received pharmacologic therapy and advice about nonpharmacologic strategies to reduce symptoms, and also after he or she has been counseled adequately about the benefits and risks of revascularization. At that time, a decision to undergo noninvasive testing can be made.

The results of the wide variety of investigations based on the guidelines mentioned above are available in "The Rest of the Story," which follows.

The Rest of the Story

Suggested initial evaluation (with accompanying summarized results; all values are in SI units if not otherwise specified)

EKG: rate 72/min. Normal voltage. Normal sinus rhythm. Normal axis. No evidence of LVH. No acute ST-T changes. Significant Q waves in leads I, aVL, V1-V5

CBC: hematocrit = 44.5

    hemoglobin = 14.2 g/dl

    leukocytes = 7.2

    platelets 245

    All other parameters normal

Urinalysis: No proteinuria. No RBC or other casts. Otherwise normal

Electrolytes: sodium = 142

    potassium = 3.8

    plasma CO_2 = 24

    chloride = 100

Creatinine = 58

Albumin = 40

Phosphate = 1.15

Magnesium = 0.83
Calcium (total) = 1.88
TSH = 3.40
Thyroxine (T$_4$, total) = 50

For the benefit of discussion participants, they should be told that all serum values above are within normal limits.

> Chest Radiograph: Radiologist's reports reads: "There is increased prominence of the pulmonary vasculature. The cardiothoracic ratio is slightly increased to just above 0.5. There is no present evidence of clinically significant pulmonary edema nor of any intrapulmonary disease."
> Echocardiogram: Summary of report (2D Echo): No valvular abnormalities. Moderate left and right ventricular hypertrophy. Impaired left ventricular contractions. Systolic ejection fraction, approximately 30%

Radionuclide ventriculography is not readily available at the community hospital to which Stewart Ross has been sent for many of his tests.

PART II

The Problem

You send Mr. Ross for an initial evaluation the same day he comes to your office. He is sent to a community hospital for blood tests and other investigations, the results of which are available to you within 24 hr. He returns the next day and tells you, "Had a rough night. Woke up a couple of times out of breath. Opened the window to get some fresh air. Charlotte complained that it was freezing. It's just awful, Doctor. Have you got any answers?"

Questions

1. After reviewing the results of Mr. Ross's initial evaluation in "The Rest of the Story," above, are you convinced that his symptoms are the result of heart failure? If so, how would you describe the severity of his illness at present?
2. Describe how you would counsel the patient about his illness and ways in which he can monitor and control its severity.
3. What sort of pharmacotherapy would you administer at this point?

Discussion

1. There is little question, especially given Mr. Ross's echocardiogram result, that his symptoms are due to heart failure and, more specifically, to left ventricular systolic dysfunction. Grading the severity of the disease according to ability to func-

tion rather than according to technical parameters such as systolic ejection fraction and cardiac output is highly practical. The functional classification of heart failure developed by the New York Heart Association (Barnett, Pouleur, & Francis, 1993) is widely used to describe the severity of disease based on activity limitation. Stewart has symptoms of heart failure with mild to moderate exercise. At present, therefore, he has NYHA Class II to Class III heart failure.

2. Heart failure is a very serious illness with a dismal prognosis. The psychological impact of heart failure is profound. Among the most important roles of family physicians in the management of this disease is the provision of adequate counseling and education. In this regard, Dracup et al. (1994) provide a superb review of appropriate counseling for patients newly diagnosed with heart failure.

First, patients newly diagnosed with heart failure should have some understanding of their illness. Stewart could be told, for example, that his symptoms are the result of the inability of his heart to pump blood adequately, leading to a backing up of fluid, congesting his lungs. He should know that shortness of breath and fatigue are common and expected symptoms of heart failure.

Many of Dracup et al.'s (1994) counseling recommendations involve self-monitoring of symptoms and signs, as well as lifestyle modifications. Stewart should be told that any sudden worsening of dyspnea or onset of orthopnea or increased frequency of PND is a marker for worsening heart failure and warrants immediate medical attention. He should monitor his weight daily, bringing to the attention of

his family physician any changes of more than 2.25kg since his last visit. This, he should know, represents a significant alteration in fluid balance that requires immediate medical care.

Dietary recommendations for patients with heart failure are controversial. To discourage fluid overload, a low-sodium diet has been a long-standing recommendation. The degree to which sodium should be restricted is uncertain. Limiting sodium intake to 3g/day, which can be achieved by avoiding salty foods (e.g., potato chips) and not adding salt to foods represents a reasonable degree of sodium restriction (Dracup et al., 1994) that Stewart can maintain. The role of alcohol restriction in the health of patients with heart failure is uncertain. Alcohol is known to depress ventricular performance (Gould, Zahir, DeMartino, & Gomprecht, 1971). Stewart's intake of brandy and whisky is quite heavy. He could benefit from limiting his consumption to one drink per day.

Bed rest is no longer regarded as conventional therapy for heart failure. Indeed, in some studies, exercise capacity has been shown to improve in heart failure patients involved in an exercise program (Conn, Williams, & Wallace, 1982; Lee, Ice, Blessey, & Sanmarco, 1979). Dracup et al. (1994), however, state that there is insufficient evidence to recommend a formal exercise or rehabilitation program. Stewart should continue to remain as active as possible, participating in his usual vigorous recreational activities to a reasonable degree of tolerance.

As noted previously, heart failure has a very poor prognosis. Stewart should be informed of this. The annual mortality rate for NYHA Class II patients is 5% to 10%

(Kannel, 1989). Stewart's wishes with regard to cardiopulmonary resuscitation are a matter that should be discussed in the collaborative environment of his physician's office rather than only in the event of a catastrophic downturn in his condition. Charlotte should be part of this discussion. Stewart's reaction to the news of the serious nature of his illness must be assessed. He may be interested in a support group if available. Of equal importance, his family physician should be available to answer any questions or address any concerns he may have, in a supportive fashion.

It is recommended that all patients with heart failure be vaccinated against influenza and pneumococcus (Konstam et al., 1994). The current visit is an opportunity to provide an initial reminder to Stewart to obtain these vaccinations in the near future.

3. Pharmacologic therapy in mild to moderate heart failure has two main purposes. First, it serves to relieve symptoms, such as dyspnea. Second, it serves to preserve left ventricular function and improve the quality and length of life. In reference to this second purpose, there is now abundant evidence that angiotensin-converting-enzyme (ACE) inhibitors reduce both morbidity and mortality in patients with all degrees of heart failure (Braunwald, 1991; CONSENSUS Trial Study Group, 1987; SOLVD Investigators, 1991). It is recommended that all patients with left ventricular dysfunction, whether symptomatic or asymptomatic, be started on ACE inhibitors. In patients without evidence of significant volume depletion (e.g., orthostatic hypotension), 12.5mg tid of *captopril* (or 2.5mg tid of *enalapril*) can be started (Baker, Konstam, Botorff, & Pitt, 1994). Side effects of ACE inhibitors include symptomatic hypotension and cough. About 2.2% to 5.5% of patients receiving enalapril will develop symptomatic hypotension. Cough is a commonly reported side effect of ACE inhibitors, but it is less prevalent than many physicians realize. In the SOLVD (1991) trial, 37% of patients receiving enalapril complained of cough, compared to 31% of those in the placebo group. As many patients with heart failure develop cough, it should not immediately be attributed to ACE inhibitors. Stewart should be told about these side effects and their incidences. He should also know that ACE inhibitors prolong survival as well as improve functional status. In the SOLVD (1991) trial, enalapril reduced the 4-year mortality of patients with Class II heart failure from 40% to 35%. Functional status, measured in terms of improvement in NYHA class, increased in 40% to 80% of patients by an average of 0.5 to 1.0 functional classes.

Diuretics are an important component of therapy in symptomatic heart failure. Whereas some advocate treatment with ACE inhibitors alone in patients with mild symptoms (Baker, Konstam, et al., 1994), others promote an individualized approach to diuretics in which they are started at the same time as ACE inhibitors (ACC/AHA Task Force, 1995) in symptomatic patients. As Stewart has mild to moderate (Class II to III) heart failure, initiating therapy with diuretics, together with an ACE inhibitor, is a reasonable approach. Therapy is usually begun with thiazide diuretics (Baker, Konstam, et al., 1994). An adequate starting dose is 25 to 50 mg of *hydrochlorothiazide* (HCTZ) per day. Stewart should be told that diuretics work by promoting loss of excess fluid and that they should therefore improve his symptoms.

PART III

The Problem

You provide Stewart with the results of the investigations performed. You tell him he has mild to moderate heart failure and explain to him what that means in plain terms. You counsel him about lifestyle modifications, self-monitoring, and drug treatments. You also discuss the prognosis of patients with his condition and the need at some point to discuss issues such as advance directives and cardiopulmonary resuscitation. At that point, Stewart appears noticeably dismayed.

> Well, I knew you didn't have good news, Doctor. You know, when I had my heart attack, I though I was a goner for sure. I thanked God I pulled through that. I guess I was hoping that Charlotte and I would still have many good years left together.

You tell Mr. Ross that you realize that the diagnosis of heart failure is a difficult one to absorb. You also tell him that with lifestyle modifications, self-monitoring, and medication, he can expect to improve the quality and length of his life. He says, "Well, I've got to go home and tell Charlotte. It won't be easy. She worries about me so much."

You tell Stewart that Charlotte should be as involved in the treatment plan as possible, as her life will certainly be profoundly affected by his illness, and she can be of a great deal of help in assisting with changes in lifestyle and so on. Stewart agrees to begin therapy with captopril (12.5mg tid) and HCTZ (50mg qday). He agrees to monitor his weight daily, make changes to his diet and alcohol intake, and receive the appropriate vaccinations. You tell him it is beneficial for him to remain as physically active as possible. He tells you that he and Charlotte will make decisions together about advance directives in a careful, unhurried fashion.

You briefly discuss the role of revascularization in patients with heart failure and its questionable benefit. Stewart indicates that he does not wish to undergo testing for myocardial ischemia in the near future. He thanks you for all your help.

Questions

1. When would you like to see Stewart again? What would you do at his next appointment?

Discussion

1. Mr. Ross requires close follow-up for a number of reasons. First, his shortness of breath needs reevaluation after a reasonable therapeutic period. Second, you need to know how he is coping with his illness from a psychological standpoint. The diagnosis of heart failure can have a major impact on mood and even on sexual functioning. These issues should be explored. Furthermore, Baker, Konstam, et al. (1994) note that all patients started on ACE inhibitors need to be examined in approxi-

mately 1 week (or sooner) to monitor renal function, potassium, and symptoms of hy-potension. One week is probably a reasonable interval prior to overall reassessment.

PART IV

The Problem

Stewart returns 1 week later accompanied by his wife. He had blood drawn for serum potassium and creatinine a day prior to his return. You have received the results, which are within normal limits. He tells you he has noticed no significant improvement in his condition.

> Things have stayed pretty much the same, Doctor. Still have to stop a couple of times on the way to the house. I've been doing everything we talked about. Weigh myself every morning—no real change there. Charlotte makes sure I take my medications. I don't touch the salt shaker. I haven't had a sip of whisky. It's frustrating, you know. I was hoping to be a bit better.

Stewart reports no chest pain or orthopnea. He has had one episode of PND during the past week. He reports no cough. He complains of no dizziness or lightheadedness. He remains generally quite fatigued.

When asked to describe his mood, Stewart tells you that he feels frustrated but not depressed. He has been sleeping fairly well except for the night he awoke short of breath. His appetite has been very good. You mention to both Charlotte and Stewart that in conditions like these, sexual function can often be affected, and you ask Stewart if he has had any difficulties in this respect. To this, he smiles and turns to his wife, "I guess we're still doing OK in that department, right, sweetheart?"

Charlotte tells you,

> I suppose we're doing as well as we always have. We're as active in that as we have been. It's just that Stewart is such an active person in so many ways. I think that he's gotten a little down by sitting around the house.

His physical examination is unchanged.

Questions

1. Describe how you would proceed with management of this case.

Discussion

1. One can draw certain conclusions from Mr. Ross's repeat visit. Unfortunately, he has had little improvement in his symptoms using HCTZ and low-dose cap-

topril. There is every indication that this patient has been compliant with the treatment plan. He appears to be able to tolerate the ACE inhibitor without the side effects of cough or hypotension. His ability to cope with his illness has been somewhat thwarted by a lack of improvement in his symptoms. The fact that Charlotte has accompanied him and is obviously involved in the treatment plan is a very positive development.

According to Baker, Konstam, et al. (1994), under the preceding circumstances, it is time to make some changes in pharmacologic management. The dose of ACE inhibitor should gradually be increased over the next 2 weeks to 50mg tid, which is the dose used in large-scale clini-

cal trials. Stewart's main concern at the present time, his dyspnea, requires a different approach to diuresis. Once a patient has been unresponsive to 50mg/day of HCTZ, a loop diuretic should be tried, usually furosemide at a dose of 20 to 40 mg/day. Stewart should be commended for his adherence to the overall treatment plan and told that often it is hard to find a good medication regimen to relieve symptoms. Once again, close follow-up (1 to 2 weeks) is needed at this stage of management to monitor symptoms, side effects of medications, and coping abilities. Serum potassium should be monitored closely, as often as each 3 days during titration of diuretic and ACE inhibitor therapy.

PART V

The Problem

You tell Mr. Ross and his wife that they are pursuing all the right strategies to minimize the impact of Stewart's heart failure. You also tell them that unfortunately, it is often hard to find the right combination of medications to provide the greatest relief of symptoms. You ask Stewart to discontinue the HCTZ, and you start him on 40mg/day of *furosemide*. You also increase his dose of captopril to 25mg tid for 1 week and 50mg tid thereafter, as he appears to be tolerating this medication well. You ask that he return in 2 weeks for reassessment. Stewart and Charlotte agree to this plan and tell you they are hopeful for some improvement in the interim.

Stewart and his wife return as scheduled. He has had serum potassium levels drawn every 4 days, all of which are normal. Stewart tells you,

Well, I guess things are a little better. I haven't woke up in the middle of the night out of breath at all. Everything else is a bit better. Same weight. Same damn hill I used to put to shame ten times a day that I wind up staring at for five minutes before I start climbing, 'cause I know I'm not going to make it to the top in one go. At least now I only have to stop once on the way up.

Charlotte, feeling the need to corroborate Stewart's sentiments, says, "Doctor, I think those medicines are helping Stew. He is starting to improve."

Stewart continues to report no cough, dizziness, or lightheadedness. He has been in fairly good spirits, especially as he has noticed some improvement. His physical examination remains unchanged.

Questions

1. Would you consider starting Mr. Ross on digoxin?

Discussion

1. Digoxin has been widely used to treat heart failure for many years. It should not, however, be indiscriminately prescribed to all patients with left ventricular dysfunction. Baker, Konstam, et al. (1994) note that digoxin provides the most benefit to patients with severe heart failure and to those who remain symptomatic after optimal treatment with ACE inhibitors and diuretics. At this point, Stewart is not receiving nearly the maximum recommended dose of furosemide (Mair, 1996). Doubling the dose is a good starting point in optimizing pharmacologic managment (Brater, Day, Burdette, & Anderson, 1984) and further improving his symptoms. Digoxin can be considered if Stewart continues to fail to respond to increasing doses of diuretic.

Conclusion

You double Mr. Ross's dose of furosemide, making it 80mg per day. You administer both influenza and pneumococcal vaccinations and ask Stewart to return in 2 weeks. You tell him, however, that if he notices any deterioration he should return sooner.

Stewart Ross and his wife return 2 weeks later. His potassium levels have been normal. The patient tells you he has been doing quite well.

> Well, Doctor, I've finally noticed a big improvement. I haven't been short of breath much at all—only when I'm out working in the yard for a fairly long time. I mean, I don't feel 16 years old, but I think I'm doing OK. I can get up to my house. I huff and puff a bit, but it's no big deal. I've been sleeping very well—no more waking up out of breath.

On physical examination, Stewart has lost 1.5kg since his last visit. You are unable to hear any crepitations in his chest, and his JVP has decreased to 3cm above the sternal angle at 30 degrees of elevation of the head. The rest of his physical examination is unchanged.

You tell Mr. Ross that you are delighted with his progress. You re-emphasize the importance of dietary restrictions, physical activity, and self-monitoring. You arrange for follow-up in 1 month's time, prior to which Stewart should have another serum potassium level drawn. You tell Stewart and Charlotte that, should they have any questions or concerns, or if Stewart's condition deteriorates in any way, they should contact you as soon as possible.

Once again, a cordial Mr. and Mrs. Ross thank you for your help and tell you they look forward to seeing you again. They tell you they will consider the issue of advance directives in the interim and will return prepared to discuss this matter with you.

References

American College of Cardiology/American Heart Association Task Force on Practice Guidelines (Committee on Evaluation and Management of Heart Failure). (1995). Guidelines for the evaluation and management of heart failure (Report). *Journal of the American College of Cardiology, 26,* 1376-1398.

Baker, D. W., Konstam, M. A., Botorff, M., & Pitt, B. (1994). Management of heart failure: I. Pharmacologic treatment. *Journal of the American Medical Association, 272,* 1361-1366.

Baker, D. W., Jones, R., Hodges, J., Massie, B. M., Konstam, M. A., & Rose, E. A. (1994). Management of heart failure: III. The role of revascularization in the treatment of patients with moderate or severe left ventricular systolic dysfunction. *Journal of the American Medical Association, 272,* 1528-1534.

Barnett, D. B., Pouleur, H., & Francis, G. S. (1993). *Congestive heart failure: Pathophysiology and treatment.* New York: Marcel Dekker.

Brater, D. C., Day, B., Burdette, A., & Anderson, S. (1984). Bumetanide and furosemide in heart failure. *Kidney International, 26,* 183-189.

Braunwald, E. (1991). ACE inhibitors: A cornerstone of the treatment of heart failure. *New England Journal of Medicine, 325,* 351-353.

Canadian Cardiovascular Society. (1996). *Canadian Cardiovascular Society Consensus Conference: Guidelines for the management of heart failure.* Toronto: Publications Ontario.

Conn, E. H., Williams, R. S., & Wallace, A. G. (1982). Exercise responses before and after physical conditioning in patients with severely depressed left ventricular function. *American Journal of Cardiology, 49,* 296-300.

CONSENSUS Trial Study Group. (1987). Effects of enalapril on mortality in severe congestive heart failure. *New England Journal of Medicine, 316,* 1429-1435.

Dargie, H. J., & McMurray, J.J.V. (1994). Diagnosis and management of heart failure. *British Medical Journal, 308,* 321-328.

Dracup, K., Baker, D. W., Dunbar, S. B., Dacey, R. A., Brooks, N. H., Johnson, J. C., Oken, C., & Massie, B. M. (1994). Management of heart failure: II. Counseling, education and lifestyle modifications. *Journal of the American Medical Association, 272,* 1442-1446.

Gould, L., Zahir, M., DeMartino, A., & Gomprecht, R. F. (1971). Cardiac effects of a cocktail. *Journal of the American Medical Association, 218,* 1799-1802.

Kannel, W. (1989). Epidemiological aspects of heart failure. *Cardiology Clinic, 7,* 1-9.

Konstam, M. A., Dracup, K., Bottorff, M. B., Brooks, N. H., Dacey, R. A., Dunbar, S. B., Jackson, A. B., Jessup, M., Johnson, J. C., Jones, R. H., Luchi, R. J., Massie, B. M., Pitt, B., Rose, E. A., Rubin, L. J., & Wright, R. F. (Eds.). (1994). Heart failure: Evaluation and care of patients with left-ventricular systolic dysfunction (Clinical Practice Guideline No. 11, AHCPR Publication no. 94-0612). Rockville, MD: Department of Health and Human Services, Public Health Service, Agency for Health Care Policy and Research.

Lee, A. P., Ice, R., Blessey, R., & Sanmarco, M. E. (1979). Longterm effects of physical training on coronary patients with impaired ventricular function. *Circulation, 60,* 1519-1526.

Mair, F. S. (1996). Management of heart failure. *American Family Physician, 54,* 245-254.

Rahimtoola, S. H. (1989). The hibernating myocardium. *American Heart Journal, 117,* 211-221.

SOLVD Investigators. (1991). Effect of enalapril on survival in patients with reduced left-ventricular ejection fractions and congestive heart failure. *New England Journal of Medicine, 325,* 293-302.

Task Force on Heart Failure of the European Society of Cardiology. (1995). Guidelines for the diagnosis of heart failure. *European Heart Journal, 16,* 741-751.

8. GASTROESOPHAGEAL

REFLUX DISEASE

Mr. Roger Edstrom

*Goal: The purpose of this exercise is to evaluate and develop
the participants' understanding of the assessment and treatment
of gastroesophageal reflux disease (GERD).*

Specific Objectives: Upon completion of this exercise, each participant should be able to accomplish the following:

1. List the common and uncommon symptoms of GERD and its complications.
2. Describe the nonpharmacological approach to GERD symptoms.
3. List the major categories of medications used in the treatment of GERD.
4. Describe the special diagnostic procedures used in the assessment of GERD and their indications.
5. Explain the pathophysiology of esophageal reflux.
6. Prescribe effective maintenance therapy for a patient with healed esophagitis.

PART I

The Patient

Social History

Roger Edstrom is a divorced 64-year-old truck driver who lives in Medford, Oregon. Originally from Fort Bragg, California, Roger is the oldest of two children born to a sawmill worker, an immigrant to the United States from Norway, and his American-born wife. The patient was part of a close-knit, hard-working family. Roger left school at the age of 14 to work alongside his father in the sawmill. He is fiercely proud of his "working-class" roots and claims to have "never used a pen and paper and never been afraid to get my hands dirty." That commitment to physically demanding labor has led Roger to a number of different jobs. He has worked in a silver mine; a pulp and paper mill; and, for a short time, as a longshoreman. He has been an independent truck driver for the past 26 years. He transports goods all across the western United States and Canada, completing three and sometimes four deliveries a week, which involve driving up to 10 continuous hours.

Roger was first married in 1955. He was divorced 7 years later. He has two children from this marriage—Jeremy, 39, and Alice, 38, both of whom live in the Los Angeles area and are married, with children of their own. Aside from a Christmas card each year, Mr. Edstrom has little contact with his children or grandchildren. He remarried in 1970 to Corinne, 16 years his junior. The marriage fell apart in 1974. The couple had no children.

Although he spends a lot of time on the road, the patient owns a small house in Medford. He is also an active member of a local Methodist parish. He has a number of close friends with whom he enjoys fishing and hunting.

Past Personal and Family Medical History

Roger's childhood was characterized by a number of "bumps and bruises" acquired through sports and other activities, but he had no serious illnesses or surgeries. The patient had no serious problems until age 47, when he was diagnosed with essential hypertension by a family physician in Medford. He has been treated with various medications and is presently taking diltiazem, 180mg po qday. The patient takes no other medications and reports no other chronic illnesses. He has no known allergies.

Roger has been smoking one pack of cigarettes a day for the past 45 years. He has recently switched to a low-tar brand. The patient drinks quite heavily on weekends, sometimes consuming 10 to 12 beers a night.

The patient has not seen a physician for just over 18 months and presently has no health insurance whatsoever.

Roger's father passed away in 1964 at the age of 58 from a heart attack. His mother died in 1991 at the age of 81. She had been diagnosed with dementia of the Alzheimer's type in 1987. The patient's younger sister, Annette, 63, lives with her husband in Astoria, Oregon. To the best of Roger's knowledge, she is in excellent health, as are Roger's children.

The Problem

You are a family physician in the city of Medford, Oregon. A complete range of diagnostic facilities and specialist services is at your disposal. Roger Edstrom, a 64-year-old man, comes to your office and complains that "my heartburn has been really acting up." Roger describes a burning sensation in his chest that rises into his throat. "I've been popping antacids like crazy," he tells you. "Anyway, it's starting to get real bad."

Questions

1. What is heartburn? How common and how serious is this problem?

2. What further information would you like to obtain as part of the initial history?

3. How would you perform a focused physical examination?

Discussion

1. Roger describes typical heartburn—a burning substernal sensation rising into the neck and sometimes the throat. Heartburn is one among a spectrum of symptoms that comprise **gastroesophageal reflux disease (GERD),** the condition in which the esophagus is exposed to gastric contents. Another less common symptom of GERD is regurgitation. Some patients describe "chest pain" in association with GERD that can sometimes be difficult to distinguish from pain of cardiac origin. Uncommon GERD symptoms include nocturnal cough, wheezing, hoarseness, and sore throat (Beck & Pearson, 1993).

GERD is an extremely common condition. Roughly 10% of the American population reports heartburn daily, and more than 30% report intermittent heartburn (DeVault & Castell, 1994). The vast majority have mild symptoms that they self-treat with over-the-counter antacids and H2-blockers. Perhaps for this reason, GERD is not always viewed as a serious condition by many clinicians (Fennerty et al., 1996). Recently, efforts have been made to evaluate the impact of chronic GERD symptoms on quality of life. The *Psychological General Well-Being Index* (PGWB) is a tool used to measure the subjective well-being of patients suffering from chronic conditions. Patients are asked a series of questions relating to six specific areas: anxiety, depressed mood, positive well-being, self-control, general health, and vitality (Croog et al., 1986). Dimenas (1993) describes the application of the PGWB to a large number of patients suffering from either untreated duodenal ulcer or untreated reflux esophagitis. Such patients had scores on the PGWB comparable to those of patients with severe angina pectoris, and actually worse than those with mild congestive heart failure. Though the PGWB is widely recognized as a valid measure of quality of life, whether the results described by Dimenas are valid or relevant is unclear. In any case, the idea that GERD is an extremely common problem with a profound and often underestimated impact on quality of life is a reasonable one.

2. Roger already gives a convincing history consistent with GERD symptoms. Further details can be elicited to support the diagnosis and determine the severity of symptoms.

Heartburn is the classic symptom of GERD, occurring shortly after meals and usually relieved temporarily with antacids. The chronology of heartburn and the use of antacids and their effect should, therefore, be ascertained. As gastric contents reflux more easily into the esophagus in recumbent or bent-over positions, exacerbation of symptoms in these circumstances also supports the diagnosis. The presence of other manifestations of GERD, such as respiratory symptoms, chest pain, and regurgitation, should be determined. Patients with advanced GERD may present with dys- or odynophagia. An inquiry into other gastrointestinal symptoms may also be of value. Roger is certainly at increased risk of cardiovascular disease, given his smoking, hypertension, and family history. It is reasonable to conduct a brief functional inquiry to rule out coronary artery disease as a source for what Roger describes as heartburn.

An assessment of the severity of symptoms is important. The range of severity of GERD is great, from mild and easily self-treated to severe and debilitating. Knowing the severity of symptoms and the impact on quality of life provides invaluable information about the patient's illness experience and helps the primary care physician gauge the expediency and aggressiveness with which treatment should be instituted. There are many ways to gauge the severity of GERD symptoms. Velanovich, Vallance, Gusz, Tapia, and Harkabus (1996) have developed a "quality of life scale" specifically for patients with gastroesophageal reflux disease (see Appendix). The scale was incorporated into a brief questionnaire easily administered to patients and designed to assess the severity and chronology of symptoms and their impact on daily activities. Discussion participants may wish to incorporate this instrument into the diagnostic interview,

although a less formal evaluation is sufficient at this stage. Simply asking Roger, for example, how bad his heartburn symptoms are and how they disrupt his life is a good strategy.

3. The physical examination in patients with reflux disease is usually unremarkable (Beck & Pearson, 1993). Some rare conditions, however, such as scleroderma, have reflux as a symptom, and findings associated with such diseases may be found on physical examination. In the case of Roger Edstrom, simple examination of the patient's body habitus and vital signs is sufficient in the absence of any abnormalities obtained from the history. Some discussion participants may also wish to perform an abdominal examination.

PART II

The Problem

You ask Roger for more details about his heartburn. He tells you he has had the problem intermittently for several years but that it has been getting steadily worse over the past 4 or 5 months. He tells you, "I'm not a complainer, but this is getting intolerable." Roger tells you he usually has heartburn an hour or two after meals. It is particularly bad when lying down. When asked how his symptoms affect his daily life, Roger tells you that heartburn often wakes him from sleep. "I wake up, have to get out of bed and take some antacids, before I can try getting to bed again. I really haven't been sleeping well because of this problem." The patient is unaware that his heartburn is made worse by bending over.

Roger does not describe his problem as "chest pain" or pressure. He reports no diaphoresis, palpitations, syncope, or dyspnea. The "heartburn" is not aggravated by physical activity and does not radiate to his jaw, arms, or back. The patient reports no regurgitation, cough, wheezing, hoarseness, sore throat, or any dys- or odynophagia. Roger reports no change in appetite, weight, bowel habits, or stool. He reports no abdominal pain, nausea, or vomiting.

The patient has been treating his symptoms with antacid tablets. He gets relief, but only for a short time. He tells you repeatedly that the problem is getting steadily worse and that he is looking for a "quick solution." He describes himself as "addicted to food" and says that he wishes he "didn't have to pay the price of such bad heartburn." Roger has, however, made no changes to his diet and has not noticed that any particular foods make his heartburn worse. In his words, "Doctor, I guess I'm hoping there's a pill I can take to get rid of this problem for good."

The results of your limited physical examination are shown below:

Gen: Obese gentleman who looks his stated age
Ht. = 177cm; Wt. = 118.5kg; BP = 160/100; P = 78, reg.; RR = 18/min; T = 37.1°C
Abdomen: No scars or distension, soft, nontender, no masses or organomegaly, normal bowel sounds

Questions

1. What causes esophageal reflux?
2. Why are GERD symptoms worse at night?
3. What are the complications of GERD?
4. What lifestyle modifications should Roger make to alleviate his symptoms?

Discussion

1. Reflux of gastric contents into the esophagus was once thought to result from a single mechanism in an individual patient. It is now recognized that, in most cases, several factors contribute to reflux and its symptoms (Marshall, 1995). **Dysfunction of the lower esophageal sphincter** (LES), which normally provides a "pressure valve" on gastric contents, is a common contributor to the problem of reflux. Very few patients with GERD have an incompetent or hypotensive LES. The most common abnormality of this defense mechanism is episodic inappropriate relaxation, which allows reflux to take place. Many substances, including fatty foods, chocolate, caffeine, alcohol, cigarettes, and many medications, can cause transient decreases in LES tone and consequent reflux.

A **hiatal hernia,** in which the gastroesophageal junction is "pushed up" from an intra-abdominal position to an intrathoracic one, was once regarded as the principal abnormality in patients with GERD. Although the majority of patients with GERD have hiatal hernias, most patients with hiatal hernias do not have reflux symptoms. Current evidence suggests that a hiatal hernia may play an important, but not exclusive, role in promoting reflux of gastric contents (Weinberg & Kadish, 1996).

All persons have reflux from time to time. The healthy esophagus normally clears acidic fluid quickly. Saliva is able to neutralize any remaining fluid and prevent esophageal injury. **Impaired esophageal clearance** of refluxed gastric contents is thought to contribute to symptoms in roughly half of GERD patients (Weinberg & Kadish, 1996). This can occur because of esophageal peristaltic dysfunction.

Delayed gastric emptying contributes to GERD in some patients. It is aggravated by smoking and high-fat meals. Finally, it should be noted that **impaired mucosal defense** is thought to contribute to esophageal injury in the form of esophagitis, which will be discussed in greater detail.

2. The beneficial and obvious effects of gravity, which prevent acid reflux in the upright position, are lost in the supine position. GERD symptoms are consequently worse at night. Furthermore, most people are unaware that swallowing and salivation, two effective mechanisms to clear and

neutralize refluxed acid, virtually cease at night (Marshall, 1995).

3. In general terms, the major complications of GERD can be classified as **esophagitis, Barrett metaplasia,** and **extraesophageal manifestations.**

Esophagitis refers to the damage that takes place in some patients with prolonged exposure of the esophagus to gastric contents. Such damage is usually only apparent with histopathological examination. Severe damage, in the form of erosions and ulcerations, can, however, be visualized endoscopically (Kahrilas, 1996). **Esophageal strictures** sometimes result following ulcerations. **Barrett metaplasia** is a serious histopathologic consequence of chronic GERD in which the normal squamous epithelium of the esophagus is replaced by columnar epithelium. Patients with Barrett metaplasia have a 30- to 40-fold increased risk of developing adenocarcinoma of the esophagus (Spechler & Goyal, 1986).

Extraesophageal manifestations of GERD include some relating to uncommon symptoms mentioned previously. Among these are asthma, posterior laryngitis, chronic cough, dental disease, and laryngeal cancer. It is usually hard to establish the association of any of these conditions with GERD in an individual patient. A discussion of the mechanisms by which GERD results in these problems is beyond the scope of this exercise.

4. The question refers to the nonpharmacological treatment of GERD, the components of which are well known to many clinicians. These relate to diet, personal habits, and positional changes (Rex, 1992). A mnemonic that participants may find useful when counseling a patient on the nonpharmacologic management of GERD is the nonsense phrase **F.M., S.W., T.A.B.L.E.** (FM and SW are, of course, the abbreviations for the radio modalities known as Frequency Modulation and Short Wave). The mnemonic is explained below:

FM/SW TABLE

F = Foods: Patients with GERD should be encouraged to decrease or eliminate their intake of fatty foods, alcohol, caffeine, chocolate, citrus juice, and peppermint, all of which are thought to promote reflux.

M = Meals: Patients should eat smaller meals, avoid meals close to bedtime, and remain upright for at least 2 hours after meals.

S = Smoking: Smoking, of course, is a health hazard for many reasons, and it is also thought to aggravate GERD.

W = Weight: Overweight patients should be encouraged to lose weight, as obesity commonly increases intra-abdominal pressure and, consequently, reflux.

T = Tight clothing: Tight clothing over the abdominal area should be avoided.

A = Aspirin: Aspirin and related medications should be avoided.

B = Bending: Bending or stooping over aggravates reflux symptoms in some patients and should be avoided.

L = Lozenges: Lozenges promote salivation and therefore make saliva available for neutralization of refluxed acid.

E = Elevate head of bed: This is a well-known simple intervention. The head of the bed is elevated on 15cm to 20cm blocks so that reflux is prevented by gravity.

Most of the nonpharmacological interventions mentioned above have not been carefully evaluated for effectiveness. There is objective evidence, however, for the effectiveness of elevation of the head of the bed. Harvey et al. (1987) studied the effects on reflux symptoms of *sleeping with the bed flat and taking placebo ranitidine pills, sleeping with the bed raised and taking placebo pills, taking ranitidine with the bed flat, and taking ranitidine with the bed raised.* Both ranitidine and raising the bed were found to be independently significantly effective in reducing symptoms and in reducing the extent of ulceration of the esophagus found on endoscopy. The combined effect of ranitidine and raising the bed was significantly greater than the sum of the individual effects. In the same study, both smoking and heavy alcohol consumption were found to **reduce** the effectiveness of ranitidine. The **relative** effectiveness of raising the bed, however, was far **greater** in smokers and in heavy alcohol consumers than in those who abstained from both. In summary, raising the head of the bed during sleep is a simple and very effective way of reducing both GERD symptoms and esophageal injury.

PART III

The Problem

You begin a discussion with Roger about what causes heartburn and what typically makes it worse. You discuss the nonpharmacological approach to GERD symptoms according to the FM/SW TABLE mnemonic. He appears very receptive to the specific suggestions. He says,

Well, I knew a lot of the things I do aren't good for you. I smoke like a chimney, drink like a fish, and eat like a lazy horse! I know I've really got to tackle all of that. That elevating the head of the bed stuff sounds pretty simple to do.

You tell Roger that although many of the lifestyle modifications you described are easier mentioned than implemented, the knowledge of what aggravates GERD may give him some control over his symptoms. "But what about pills, Doctor?" he says. "I have friends who buy pills for heartburn. They seem to work pretty well. Those antacids don't seem to solve the problem."

Questions

1. What are the main classes of pharmacological agents used to treat GERD?
2. Apart from pharmacotherapy and lifestyle modifications, are there any other treatments used for GERD?
3. What factor, especially in Roger's case, is important in determining the choice of pharmacotherapy?
4. What medication, if any, would you start at this point?
5. Are you concerned about Roger's hypertension and its present treatment?

Discussion

1. There are four main classes of medications used to treat GERD. The first category includes the **antacids** and **alginic acid.** Antacids increase the pH of gastric contents and are effective in providing symptomatic relief. Alginic acid is the active ingredient in Gaviscon™. It works by creating a barrier between refluxed gastric contents and the esophageal mucosa, and it is also effective in relieving symptoms (Rex, 1992).

The second category includes the **antisecretory agents.** The most commonly used of these are the **H2-receptor antagonists,** including cimetidine, ranitidine, famotidine, and nizatidine. They reduce the secretion of gastric acid and both provide symptomatic relief and promote esophageal healing. They are very widely used and are now available in nonprescription varieties in the United States.

The **proton pump inhibitors,** including **omeprazole** and **lanseprazole,** inhibit the hydrogen ion pump on the surface of parietal cells in the stomach. They are the most potent inhibitors of gastric acid secretion.

The third category of medications includes the **prokinetic agents,** such as *metaclopramide, bethanechol,* and the newer *cisapride.* These medications are able to improve esophageal clearance, increase LES pressure, and increase the rate of gastric emptying (Rex, 1992). Both *metaclopramide* and *bethanechol* are associated with serious side effects. Cisapride, on the other hand, is safe and effective.

The final category of pharmacologic GERD therapy includes **sucralfate,** which is presumably able to enhance the resistance of the esophageal mucosa to injury. Its effectiveness and safety are still being evaluated. With several other effective medications available, its role in the treatment of GERD is very limited at this time.

2. Surgical treatment of GERD, when performed by experienced surgeons, is effective in extremely refractory cases and often eliminates the need for long-term medical therapy (Marshall, 1995). Commonly employed operations include Nissen fundoplication and Belsey Mark IV repair. The details of these procedures are beyond the scope of this exercise. In a large randomized control trial in which surgical therapy was compared to various combinations of medical therapy, surgery was actually superior in improving symptoms and esophageal damage through up to 2 years of follow-up (Spechler & the Department of Veterans Affairs Gastroesophageal Reflux Disease Study Group, 1992). This study, however, was conducted prior to the widespread availability of the extremely effective proton pump inhibitors, making its results virtually obsolete.

3. In these days of rising health care expenses, cost is an extremely important factor in the choice of treatment of any kind. Roger has no health insurance and must pay all his own medical bills. The choice of antireflux therapy must certainly take this into consideration.

4. In a person first presenting with GERD symptoms, lifestyle modifications are universally recommended as part of the initial management plan (Beck & Pearson, 1993; DeVault & Castell, 1994; Pope, 1994; Rex, 1992). Symptoms can sometimes be managed with lifestyle modifications and antacids or over-the-counter H2-blocker medications alone. The decision to institute further pharmacotherapy is not always easy. Some discussion participants

may elect to educate Roger about lifestyle modifications and recommend the continued use of antacids. The patient's symptoms, however, are fairly severe and do have a significant impact on his life. For example, his sleep is disrupted. Further pharmacotherapy is likely to result in more rapid improvement, which the patient, who desires a "a quick fix," will definitely appreciate.

The choice of medication is another difficult decision. At the present time, for so-called uncomplicated reflux symptoms (i.e., reflux with no confirmed evidence of complications), a trial of an H2-blocker at conventional doses for 4 weeks is recommended by some as initial pharmacotherapy (Fennerty et al., 1996; Pope, 1994). Generic *cimetidine* is the least expensive of these agents. Split doses of H2-blockers provide greater relief of symptoms than a single daily dose (Marshall, 1995). This corresponds to cimetidine 400mg po bid.

5. Roger's blood pressure is elevated at this office visit. He is presently receiving treatment in the form of *diltiazem,* which may be inadequate. This is certainly a reason for concern. If Roger's blood pressure remains elevated on successive visits, a change in treatment may be needed.

The specific use of a calcium channel blocker raises another concern. Calcium channel blockers are known to reduce the *basal* or resting pressure of the LES. Indeed, for this reason calcium channel blockers are sometimes used to treat certain esophageal motility disorders. They are also commonly believed to aggravate reflux in patients with GERD (Beck & Pearson, 1993; Parkman & Cohen, 1995). As previously noted, most patients with GERD do not have a hypotensive LES. Furthermore, there are no actual studies to date that measure the impact of calcium channel blockers on reflux disease. Given this lack of evidence, there are only two clearly justifiable reasons to change Roger's antihypertensive medications. First, as noted above, the treatment effect may be inadequate. Second, calcium channel blockers are very expensive, with a cost to the pharmacist of $40 to $50 for 1 month's supply ("Drugs for Hypertension," 1995).

PART IV

The Problem

You tell Roger that "pills" may offer him substantial relief but certainly do not represent a "quick fix." You re-emphasize the importance of lifestyle modifications and prescribe cimetidine 400mg po bid. You ask Roger to return in 4 weeks to report on the status of his symptoms and his success in implementing lifestyle modifications.

Roger returns on schedule. He tells you,

I think I feel worse than before. I tried that elevating the head of the bed stuff and tried to eat smaller meals. I've tried cutting back on fat, but it isn't easy when you're a trucker. All they've got at those truck stops is grease. I cut back on drinking a lot. I still smoke a fair bit, but, Doc, I was hoping to get some relief by now. It doesn't seem like those pills are doing anything at all.

Roger's blood pressure is 130/80. The remainder of the physical examination is unchanged.

Questions

1. What special diagnostic procedures are sometimes employed in patients with GERD?
2. Describe how you would manage the case from this point.

Discussion

1. Several diagnostic tests are performed in select patients with GERD. The choice of test depends on the specific information desired (Fennerty et al., 1996). If the goal is to determine the presence of mucosal esophageal damage, **endoscopy** is appropriate. Endoscopy can also be used to determine the presence of esophageal strictures or hiatal hernia. In most patients presenting with dysphagia, however, a **barium swallow** is a simple and relatively inexpensive way to determine the presence of an esophageal stricture. If it is uncertain that GERD is the cause of a patient's symptoms, the appropriate test is **24-hour ambulatory pH monitoring.** This test measures the length of time the pH of the esophagus is low from refluxed acid. There are several other methods that are not commonly used to evaluate the integrity and function of the esophagus, but they seldom play a role in the assessment of GERD symptoms.

2. This is certainly not an easy question to answer. It is best to review the available options. The patient gives an initial classic history of heartburn, the primary symptom of GERD. He has not responded in any significant way to conventional doses of an H2-blocker or to lifestyle measures, which he appears to have implemented to some extent. One option is to continue the present treatment plan, meaning that the importance of lifestyle measures can be reviewed and the same dose of cimetidine

can be continued. Another alternative is to change the pharmacologic component of the treatment plan by either increasing the dose of cimetidine or switching to another class of medication. In patients with a suboptimal response to conventional empiric H2-blocker therapy, several authorities recommend further diagnostic testing to help confirm the diagnosis of GERD or to determine the extent of esophageal damage to guide further therapy. Beck and Pearson (1993) recommend endoscopy after a 4- to 8-week trial of H2-blockers, followed by 24-hour esophageal pH monitoring (depending on the endoscopic findings). Others also recommend endoscopic evaluation as the initial step after a trial of conventional empiric therapy (Pope, 1994; Rex, 1992). Whether this approach is cost-effective is uncertain at the present time. DeVault and Castell (1994) believe that initial empiric therapy is cost-effective and safe but that continuing empiric therapy for a prolonged period in a patient who initially fails to respond and in whom the diagnosis of GERD has not been confirmed is not prudent from the standpoint of cost, safety, or patient comfort.

The cost-effectiveness of performing endoscopy at this point in the case is one issue. The fact that Roger has no health insurance is another. The lump-sum cost of endoscopy may represent a considerable financial hardship. Ultimately, the best approach is to explain the role of diagnostic testing to him and to gauge his interest in endoscopy before making any further arrangements. The Medicare reimbursement for a diagnostic esophagogastroduodenoscopy (EGD) in 1994 was approximately $250.00 in the state of Florida (Larimore & Zuber, 1994). The cost to the patient, however, varies widely, and this specific information may be of value in helping Roger make a decision. See "The Rest of the Story," which follows.

The Rest of the Story

You tell Roger that he should not be discouraged by the lack of improvement in symptoms and that several other levels of treatment do exist. You commend him for implementing several lifestyle modifications and review the importance of these.

You tell Roger that further diagnostic testing may help confirm the diagnosis or detect damage to his esophagus that would require specific treatment. You explain the procedure of endoscopy to the best of your ability. Roger asks you several questions about whether it is painful, whether he will receive sedation, and whether there are any risks involved. You do your best to answer these but tell Roger he will also have the opportunity to direct questions to the gastroenterologist performing the procedure.

You tell the patient that endoscopy is expensive and that you understand that as he lacks health insurance, such an expense may be difficult to bear. He says, "Well, what are we talking about, Doc? A couple of hundred dollars?"

You call Dr. T. J. Roy, a Medford gastroenterologist, to whom you have previously referred several patients. Dr. Roy is sympathetic to Roger's situation. He tells you that the total fee for consultation and endoscopy is $425.00 but that some special financial arrangement can be made should that constitute a major financial burden.

Roger tells you, "Well, Doc, does it have to be soon? I'm turning 65 in 10 months, and I'd be covered by Medicare."

You tell Roger that 10 months is an excessive time for such evaluation, especially as empiric therapy would be expensive, might be risky, and could be ineffective in the interim. Roger says, "Well, OK, Doc. I'll go for it. I can afford it. I just thought there might be a way of not forking out the money." You ask Roger to direct questions of special financial arrangements to Dr. Roy and his staff. Dr. Roy is able to see Roger within 3 days.

PART V

The Problem

An EGD is performed by Dr. Roy. Roger continues lifestyle and cimetidine therapy. Dr. Roy faxes you a quick handwritten report of endoscopic findings, which reads as follows:

> Grade III esophagitis. No significant bleeding at present. Stomach and duodenum normal. Patient tolerated procedure well.

There are no recommendations for further diagnostic testing or treatment on Dr. Roy's report.

Questions

1. How is esophagitis classified?
2. How would you treat this condition in Roger's case?

Discussion

1. Esophagitis, as noted, is one of the complications of GERD. Esophagitis associated with microscopic changes including basal cell hyperplasia and mucosal infiltration with granulocytes and eosinophils can be described as *mild*. *Erosive esophagitis* refers to more severe, endoscopically visible damage characterized by friability, bleeding, exudates, and ulcers (Goyal, 1991). The American Society for Gastrointestinal Endoscopy (Richter, 1994) has a more precise classification system for macrosopic esophageal damage. *Grade 1* esophagitis is characterized by friable areas associated with red streaks. Patients with *Grade II* esophagitis have erosions that appear as whitish exudates surrounded by erythematous areas. *Grade III* esophagitis refers to severe damage in which ulcers with considerable depth appear.

2. Unresponsive GERD symptoms or documented esophageal damage requires intensification of initial empiric therapy. As always, lifestyle modifications should be encouraged. The most effective pharmacologic treatments for severe esophagitis are the proton pump inhibitors, which have a greater antisecretory effect than the H2-blockers (Kahrilas, 1996). It has been demonstrated that more than 80% of patients who receive omeprazole at a dose of 40mg/day for severe esophagitis experience healing within 12 weeks (Sontag, 1993). The concern over the high cost of PPI has recently been disputed in several studies. A decision analysis by Hillman, Bloom, Fendrick, and Schwartz (1992) demonstrated that *omeprazole* is more cost-effective than ranitidine therapy in patients with persistent gastroesophageal reflux disease when variables such as the risk of complications in unresponsive patients and the duration of treatment needed are taken into consideration.

The Rest of the Story

You ask Roger to return to your office to discuss further management. He returns and tells you, "That endoscopy was no picnic, but I survived." He has been using cimetidine as originally prescribed. You ask him how he is feeling. He tells you, "No better, Doc. I mean, I still have trouble sleeping because of terrible heartburn. I tried a lot of those 'lifestyle' things you talked about. Can't seem to quit smoking, though."

You discuss the results of the endoscopy with Roger. He is a little worried about the damage to his esophagus. He asks you, "That won't be permanent damage, will it?" You tell Roger that with proper treatment, the esophagus heals in most cases, and, furthermore, such treatment will likely lead to better relief of symptoms.

You ask Roger to discontinue the cimetidine and start him on omeprazole, 40mg po qday. You advise him that this medication will be considerably more expensive, but that it is more effective and will lead to fewer dangerous and expensive complications. Roger responds,

"Well, that endoscopy test is going to set me back a fair bit anyways. I guess I'll just have to fork out some more money. I hope this works, Doc." You tell Roger that the success rate with omeprazole is very high. You review lifestyle modifications once again and ask Roger to return in 4 weeks for follow-up.

PART VI

The Problem

Roger returns as scheduled and tells you he feels "absolutely great." He has been taking the omeprazole as prescribed and noticed a significant improvement in symptoms within a few days. "It's been gradually getting better and better, Doc. I mean, I feel almost normal for the first time in quite a while." When asked about his continued efforts to implement lifestyle modifications, Roger tells you, "Well, it's going OK. I sleep with the bed elevated. I don't eat at night. I stay away from booze and caffeine. To be honest though, I have been eating like a pig! You can't be perfect, you know!"

A blood pressure recorded at this visit is 120/90mmHg.

Questions

1. Roger seems to be "cured" of his symptoms. For how much longer would you recommend therapy with omeprazole?

Discussion

1. GERD symptoms and esophagitis have a very high relapse rate. Maintenance therapy is therefore recommended. Substantially reducing the dose of medication used during treatment or switching to a less potent agent is not usually effective in preventing relapse (Kahrilas, 1996). If Roger were switched back to cimetidine, for example, or if his dose of omeprazole were greatly reduced, symptoms and complications would be likely to reappear.

Klinkenberg-Knoll et al. (1994) have evaluated the efficacy of maintenance omeprazole therapy for 91 patients who initially failed a trial of H2-blockers but responded to omeprazole at a dose of 40mg/day. This is, of course, precisely Roger's situation. Of the 91 patients, 86 received a maintenance dose of 20mg of omeprazole daily. Of these patients, 47% experienced a recurrence of esophagitis, but all rehealed once the dose was doubled to 40mg/day. While being maintained at this higher dose, 7 of 40 patients who had already had a relapse had a second relapse and were switched to 60mg of omeprazole. This study reveals that higher maintenance doses of omeprazole are more likely to prevent relapse. Starting omeprazole at a lower maintenance dose, however, and adjusting it depending on the reappearance of symptoms, is an alternative strategy.

Klinkenberg-Knoll et al. (1994) addressed another issue associated with long-term use of omeprazole. Gastrin is a gut hormone that stimulates gastric secretion of acid. Omeprazole has been linked to **hypergastrinemia** and **gastric carcinoid** tumors in rats (Kahrilas, 1996). In their study, Klinkenberg-Knoll et al. found that a subgroup of patients receiving prolonged omeprazole therapy developed high gastrin levels. The incidence of micronodular hyperplasia and gastritis increased significantly with long-term therapy and was more pronounced in patients with high gastrin levels. No neoplastic changes were found in biopsy specimens of any of the patients in this study. The present consensus is that any risk of cancer with long-term omeprazole therapy is extremely low and that such therapy is safe (Fennerty et al., 1996; Marshall, 1995). It has been suggested that patients on maintenance therapy have their serum gastrin measured after 6 to 12 months. Those with abnormally high levels could be followed periodically by endoscopy and biopsy (Freston, 1994).

Conclusion

You tell Roger that you are delighted that he feels so well. You discuss the drawbacks and benefits of maintenance therapy with omeprazole. Roger has a great deal of confidence in this medication, as it has provided him with such excellent relief. "I know these pills cost an arm and a leg, but they are definitely worth it! Anyway, not too long to go before I get health insurance." You decide to begin with a maintenance dose of omeprazole of 20mg po qday and ask Roger to monitor his symptoms carefully so that a higher dose can be started if necessary.

Roger thanks you for all your help. You ask him to return to your office shortly to monitor his progress and for a periodic health assessment, including a discussion of cardiovascular risks and other issues. He agrees to return in a couple of weeks.

References

Beck, I. T., & Pearson, G. (1993, February). Heartburn and beyond: What you should do. *Patient Care,* 26-48.

Croog, S. H., Levine, S., Testa, M. A., Brown, B., Bulpitt, C. J., Jenkins, C. D., Klerman, G. L., & Williams, G. H. (1986). The effects of antihypertensive therapy on the quality of life. *New England Journal of Medicine, 314,* 1657-1664.

DeVault, K. R., & Castell, D. O. (1994). Current diagnosis and treatment of gastroesophageal reflux disease. *Mayo Clinic Procedures, 69,* 867-876.

Dimenas, E. (1993). Methodological aspects of evaluation of quality of life in upper gastrointestinal diseases. *Scandinavian Journal of Gastroenterology, 28*(Suppl. 199), 18-21.

Drugs for hypertension. (1995). *Medical Letter, 37,* 45-50.

Fennerty, B., Castell, D., Fendrick, M., Halpern, M., Johnson, D., Kahrilas, P. J., Leiberman, D., Richter, J. E., & Sampliner, R. E. (1996). The diagnosis and treatment of gastroesophageal reflux disease in a managed care environment. *Archives of Internal Medicine, 156,* 477-484.

Freston, J. W. (1994). Omeprazole, hypergastrinemia, and gastric carcinoid tumors. *Annals of Internal Medicine, 121*(3), 232-233.

Goyal, R. K. (1991). Diseases of the esophagus. In J. D. Wilson, E. Braunwald, K. J. Isselbacher, R. G. Petersdorf, J. B. Martin, A. S. Fauci, & R. K. Root (Eds.), *Harrison's principles of internal medicine* (12th ed., pp. 1226-1227). New York: McGraw-Hill.

Harvey, R. F., Hadley, N., Gill, T. R., Beats, B. C., Gordon, P. C., Long, D. E., MacPherson, R. I., & Tottle, A. J. (1987). Effects of sleeping with the bed-head raised and of ranitidine in patients with severe peptic oesophagitis. *Lancet, 2,* 1200-1203.

Hillman, A. L., Bloom, B. S., Fendrick, A. M., & Schwartz, J. S. (1992). Cost and quality effects of alternative treatments for persistent gastroesophageal reflux disease. *Archives of Internal Medicine, 152,* 1467-1472.

Kahrilas, P. J. (1996). Gastroesophageal reflux disease. *Journal of the American Medical Association, 276*(12), 983-988.

Klinkenberg-Knoll, E. C., Festen, H.P.M., Jansen, J.P.M.J., Lamers, C.B.H.W., Nelis, F., & Snel, P. (1994). Long-term treatment with omeprazole for refractory reflux esophagitis: Efficacy and safety. *Annals of Internal Medicine, 121*, 161-167.

Larimore, W. L., & Zuber, T. J. (1994). Coding and reimbursement for gastrointestinal endoscopic procedures in primary care. *Journal of Family Practice, 39*(2), 153-159.

Marshall, J. B. (1995). Severe gastroesophageal reflux disease. *Postgraduate Medicine, 97*(5), 98-106.

Parkman, H. P., & Cohen, S. (1995). Heartburn, regurgitation, odynophagia, chest pain and dysphagia. In W. S. Haubrich, F. Schaffner, & J. E. Berk (Eds.), *Bockus gastroenterology* (pp. 30-40). Philadelphia, PA: W. B. Saunders.

Pope, C. E. (1994). Acid-reflux disorders. *New England Journal of Medicine, 331*(10), 656-660.

Rex, D. K. (1992). Gastroesophageal reflux disease in adults: Pathophysiology, diagnosis and management. *Journal of Family Practice, 35*(6), 673-681.

Richter, J. E. (1994). Gastroesophageal reflux disease. *ASGE Clinical Update, 1*(4), 1-5.

Sontag, S. J. (1993). Gastroesophageal reflux disease. *Alimentary Pharmacological Therapy, 7*, 293-312.

Spechler, S. J., & the Department of Veterans Affairs Gastroesophageal Reflux Disease Study Group. (1992). Comparison of medical and surgical therapy for complicated gastroesophageal disease in veterans. *New England Journal of Medicine, 326*, 786-792.

Spechler, S. J., & Goyal, R. K. (1986). Barrett's esophagus. *New England Journal of Medicine, 315*, 362-371.

Velanovich, V., Vallance, S. R., Gusz, J. R., Tapia F. V., & Harkabus, M. A. (1996). Quality of life scale for gastroesophageal reflux disease. *Journal of the American College of Surgeons, 183*, 217-224.

Weinberg, D. S., & Kadish, S. L. (1996). The diagnosis and management of gastroesophageal reflux disease. *Medical Clinics of North America, 80*(2), 411-428.

Appendix: Gastroesophageal Reflux Data Sheet

Questions about symptoms (circle one for each question)	Scale					
1. How bad is the heartburn?	0	1	2	3	4	5
2. Heartburn when lying down?	0	1	2	3	4	5
3. Heartburn when standing up?	0	1	2	3	4	5
4. Heartburn after meals?	0	1	2	3	4	5
5. Does heartburn change your diet?	0	1	2	3	4	5
6. Does heartburn wake you from sleep?	0	1	2	3	4	5
7. Do you have difficulty swallowing?	0	1	2	3	4	5
8. Do you have pain with swallowing?	0	1	2	3	4	5
9. If you take medication, does this affect your daily life?	0	1	2	3	4	5
10. How satisfied are you with your present condition?	Very satisfied	Satisfied	Neutral	Dissatisfied	Very dissatisfied	Incapacitated

SOURCE: Velanovich et al. (1996, p. 218). Used by permission.
NOTE: 0, no symptoms; 1, symptoms noticeable but not bothersome; 2, symptoms noticeable and bothersome but not every day; 3, symptoms bothersome every day; 4, symptoms affect daily activities; 5, symptoms are incapacitating—unable to do daily activities.

9. INFANTILE DIARRHEA

Francine St. George

Goal: The goal of this exercise is to assess and develop
the participants' understanding of the management
of acute diarrhea in a young child.

Specific Objectives: Upon completion of this exercise, each participant should be able to accomplish the following:

1. Obtain a thorough, pertinent history from a parent with a child with acute diarrhea.
2. Assess a young child with diarrhea for dehydration.
3. Explain the indications for oral rehydration therapy (ORT) and how this therapy works.
4. List at least five common causes of acute infectious pediatric diarrhea.
5. Explain how the parasite *Giardia lamblia* is spread, treated, and controlled.

PART I

The Patient

Social History

The St. Georges of Kapuskasing have always been a deeply troubled and tragic family. Bonnie is the oldest of three children born to Elmer and Faith St. George. Elmer was a violent man who physically abused both his wife and children and sexually abused Bonnie's younger sister Doris. He spent much of his life in and out of prisons throughout northern Ontario, incarcerated for such varied offences as rape, brawling, and driving while under the influence of alcohol. Elmer was a man with no friends and many enemies. In the end, it was his alcoholism that finished him off. Shunned by his family, Elmer died alone in a hospital in Kapuskasing of liver failure, at the age of 47.

Bonnie's mother Faith is a subdued, 50-year-old woman who lives with her two younger children, Doris, 18 years old, and Mack, 14, in a small cottage outside Kapuskasing. Though never the criminal her husband was, Faith has never been a responsible parent. When the children were little, she would leave them unattended at home while she left to play cards or bingo with her friends. Worse still, she would often leave them in the care of Elmer. A year after Elmer's death, a concerned social worker paid a visit to the St. George household in the dead of the northern Ontario winter to find no one home except Mack, then just 9 years old, shivering uncontrollably and hugging a radiator that emanated no heat, as Faith had carelessly turned it off prior to one of her usual outings. The shocked social worker immediately took young Mack into the care of the local children's aid agency, and Faith was charged with child abuse in the form of neglect. Several months later, Mack was reunited with his family after Faith was forced to attend a special parenting program.

As the St. George children grew older, they became better able to look after their own needs and relied less on their incompetent parents. They also received help from their neighbors, other relatives, and the community as a whole. As a teenager, Bonnie took on the role of parent to Doris and especially Mack while her mother often left the home for several days at a stretch. Bonnie's "Uncle" Edison, a kind and gentle man who was only a distant relative of the St. Georges, often provided the support the children needed. He drove them to school and bought them groceries. In a community that enthusiastically celebrates Christmas, Faith usually neglected to buy her children any gifts, preferring to spend the money she received through government social assistance on beer and cigarettes. Uncle Edison would invite the children to spend Christmas with his family. His generosity won the hearts of the St. George children; Bonnie and her siblings love Edison very much.

Bonnie became involved with Rick Abson, 25, 2 years ago. Rick has also had a difficult family life. The couple decided to leave their troubles in Kapuskasing behind and start a new life in the south. The Akwesasne Mohawk Reserve, straddling the U.S.-Canadian border near Cornwall, Ontario, became their home. Soon after the birth of their daughter, Francine, Rick left Akwesasne for a high-paying job in Syracuse, New York. Bonnie has not seen or heard from him in nearly 8 months and does not expect him to return to carry on his duties as a parent or to contribute financially to her or Francine's well-being.

Bonnie and Francine live in a trailer on the Akwesasne Reserve, which they rent with money received from the government. Bonnie completed ninth grade prior to leaving Kaspuskasing. Aside from working as a baby-sitter on the reserve from time to time, she has never been employed. Despite a tragic family life, poverty, and abandonment, she is a resilient young woman and a very conscientious mother. You have been her primary care physician since she arrived in Akwesasne. She has never missed an appointment, either for herself or for Francine.

Elmer St. George was part Cree Indian and part Irish-Canadian. Both Faith's and Rick Abson's families are of Mohawk descent, originally from southern Quebec.

Past Personal and Family Medical History

Bonnie has been your patient for nearly 2 years. You provided her with prenatal care and were involved in the uncomplicated spontaneous vaginal term delivery of Francine, her first and only child.

You have been seeing Francine on a regular basis since birth, almost always for routine pediatric care. You encouraged Bonnie to breast-feed Francine, but she found it difficult and inconvenient and provided her daughter with iron-fortified formula instead. Francine was brought in by her mother on two occasions with upper respiratory symptoms that resolved quickly. She is a healthy child who is growing normally and reaching all developmental milestones. Her immunizations are up to date.

Bonnie has never smoked. She used to drink heavily on weekends but discontinued this practice during her pregnancy and has not resumed. She is a healthy but obese young woman.

Rick Abson suffers from mild asthma. To the best of Bonnie's knowledge, he is otherwise healthy.

The Problem

You are a family physician in a solo practice in the small city of Cornwall, Ontario. Francine St. George, an 18-month-old girl, is brought to your office on a warm September day by her mother, Bonnie. Bonnie tells you that Francine has had roughly 10 episodes of watery diarrhea over the past 24 hr. She has had no vomiting or fever.

Questions

1. The chief complaint is diarrhea of 1 day's duration. What additional components of the history would you like to obtain?
2. How would you perform a focused physical examination of Francine?
3. Would you like to obtain any laboratory investigations at this time?

Discussion

1. Diarrhea is an extremely common problem that can often have serious consequences, especially in developing countries. The World Health Organization (WHO), which is a leader in the international effort to treat and prevent the complications of diarrhea in children, has prepared an extensive practice guideline for health care providers upon which much of these suggested responses are based (WHO, 1993). Included in this guideline are the important facts to obtain from the history. Obvious questions include the **duration of diarrhea** and the **presence of other symptoms or signs** such as **fever, vomiting, cough, rashes,** and so on. The **pre-illness feeding pattern** should be ascertained, as well as **foods and liquids taken during the illness.** The **immunization and medication history** should be obtained. It is important to ask about **blood in the stool,** a sign of shigellosis, which

can be treated with antibiotics (WHO, 1993). A **travel history** and **family history of chronic diarrhea** is also recommended (Havener, Meis, & Graber, 1990; Meyers, 1995). Some of these points have already been addressed. The presence of decreased or absent voiding or voiding of very dark urine is a sign of significant dehydration and should be ascertained (Meyers, 1995).

2. The focus of the physical examination is the assessment of the child for signs of dehydration—the most common and serious consequence of diarrhea. These signs are likely to be very familiar to most discussion participants. The child's general condition; eyes, mouth, and tongue; and skin should be examined. The child's thirst should be gauged by his or her eagerness to take in fluids (WHO, 1993). The physical signs and corresponding degree of dehydration are summarized in Figure 9.1.

Dehydration	LOC	Eyes	Tears	Mouth/Tongue	Thirst	Skin	Percentage of Body Weight Loss	Fluid Deficit (mL/kg)
None	Alert	Normal	Present	Moist	Normal	Pinch retracts immediately	< 5	< 50
Some	Irritable	Sunken	Absent	Dry	Thirsty	Pinch retracts slowly	5-10	50-100
Severe	Lethargic or unconscious	Very sunken	Absent	Very dry	Drinks poorly	Pinch retracts very slowly	> 10	> 100

SOURCE: Adapted from WHO (1993).

Figure 9.1 Physical Signs and Corresponding Degree of Dehydration

Missing from the signs above is *capillary refill time*, which has been studied by Saavedra, Harris, Song, and Finberg (1991). In their study, the mean capillary refill time in 30 normal infants 2 to 24 months old was determined after enough pressure was applied to the tip of a finger of each patient to blanch the nailbed. Infants with varying degrees of dehydration were then evaluated in the same manner. From this, it was determined that a capillary refill time of less than 1.5 s strongly indicates a fluid deficit of 50mL/kg or less, 1.5 s to 3.0 s corresponds to 50 and 100mL/kg, and more than 3.0 s corresponds to greater than 100mL/kg. Although the capillary refill time may be a reliable sign of the degree of dehydration, it is hard to imagine that standardization of the technique is not a problem. There is, of course, no danger to adding this sign to those in Figure 9.1 to help support the diagnosis of a particular degree of dehydration.

Beyond the examination for dehydration, the physical examination should include the patient's vital signs and weight. Any available stool should be examined for the presence of blood (WHO, 1993).

3. Extensive laboratory evaluation is not needed in the outpatient management of infantile diarrhea. Leung and Robson (1989) point out, however, that monitoring of stool, urine, and serum electrolytes plays a role in the *inpatient* management of children with diarrhea and severe dehydration. Adelman and Solhung (1996) point out that laboratory tests can be useful in pinpointing the type and severity of dehydration but that the clinical evaluation of the patient is of extreme importance, and management should not be delayed pending the results of lab tests. The WHO (1993) does not encourage measurement of serum electrolytes, as such results rarely provide helpful information and, furthermore, may be misinterpreted, leading to mismanagement.

If a urine sample is available, the urine specific gravity can be easily measured (Adelman & Solhung, 1996; Leung & Robson, 1989). In previously healthy children, a specific gravity of >1.020 suggests some degree of dehydration. You may elect to perform this simple, inexpensive test.

PART II

The Problem

Bonnie tells you that apart from diarrhea, Francine has had no cough, rashes, rhinorrhea, tugging of ears, or other symptoms. She has been irritable and inconsolable for the past day. Prior to her illness, Francine was fed a good mix of vegetables, cereals, milk, and meats. Since the diarrhea began, Bonnie, based on the advice of a friend who lives on the reserve, has been giving Francine only apple juice in the form of several small cups a day. Francine has been drinking this eagerly.

Bonnie has noticed no blood in her daughter's watery stools. She tells you that she is not sure of Francine's voiding pattern nor the appearance of her urine, as her diapers are frequently soaked with diarrhea.

Bonnie is unaware of any family history of chronic diarrhea in either her or Rick Abson's families. Neither she nor Francine have been outside the reserve for several weeks.

Your physical examination is summarized below:

Gen: Somewhat irritable, alert child
    Temp = 37.3°C aural; RR = 30/min; P = 100/min; Wt. = 10.5kg
HEENT: eyes—somewhat sunken; Child cries throughout examination with no tears evident
    mouth and tongue—dry
Resp: Chest clear/normal breath sounds
Skin: Pinch retracts normally
    Capillary refill time = 2.0 s
Abdomen: no distension/no masses/slightly hyperactive bowel sounds

Bonnie offers Francine her bottle of apple juice during the examination, which Francine takes enthusiastically.

Questions

1. Why is Bonnie's choice of apple juice for Francine inappropriate?
2. What is oral rehydration therapy?
3. What are the most common causes of acute infantile diarrhea?
4. Are antidiarrheal or antimicrobial medications routinely used to treat diarrhea?
5. Describe your management of the case from this point.

Discussion

1. Fluid should be consumed during episodes of acute diarrhea to provide rehydration and to replace ongoing fluid loss through the impaired gut. During episodes of diarrhea, the coupled transport of sodium and glucose across the gut wall is a mechanism that normally remains intact. Movement of glucose across the brush border cells that line the intestine is driven by the sodium gradient across the cells

(Ghishan, 1988). Water follows this coupled transport of electrolytes through osmosis. The ideal solution for children with diarrhea in whom the aim is rehydration would contain both sodium and glucose (or other carbohydrate) in proportions that maximally take advantage of this coupled transport mechanism. Apple juice is rich in sugar and low in sodium. The excess carbohydrate leads to the osmotic retention of water in the gut and consequent loss of fluids and electrolytes (Goepp & Katz, 1993). It is therefore not an appropriate choice for fluid therapy during episodes of acute diarrhea.

2. *Oral rehydration therapy* (ORT) is the fluid and electrolyte component of treatment for diarrhea. It is designed to provide rehydration and replace ongoing fluid losses. It has been available for many years and has been used throughout the world. Its enormous impact on global health is well known. ORT is essentially the provision of a special fluid solution that takes advantage of the previously described coupled transport mechanism. A number of ORT solutions are available. The most widely used is that from the World Health Organization, which is provided in the form of packets; the contents are to be mixed in a liter of water. Each liter contains 20gms of glucose, 3.5gms of sodium chloride, 1.5gms of potassium chloride, and either 2.9gms of the salt trisodium citrate or 2.5gms of sodium bicarbonate. Commercially available rehydration solutions include the popular *Rehydralyte*™. The American Academy of Pediatrics (AAP) recommends that all solutions used for oral rehydration have a final carbohydrate-to-sodium ratio of less than 2 to 1 (Mauer et al., 1985). The WHO (1993) recommends a lower ratio of 1.4 to 1.

Despite the enormous body of evidence supporting the use of appropriate oral rehydration solutions in the therapy of acute diarrhea, it is interesting to note that its use is widespread in many developing countries but still has not been wholeheartedly embraced in North America. A survey of 230 community-based American pediatricians, 112 chairpersons of pediatric departments, 89 pediatricians attending a postgraduate course, and 38 pediatric residents revealed that the usage rate of ORT solutions conforming to the AAP recommendations was less than 30% (Snyder, 1991). The reasons for this have been explored by Reis, Goepp, Katz, and Santosham (1994), who surveyed 104 American community pediatricians through a knowledge-attitudes-practice (KAP) questionnaire. It was revealed that most physicians do have a good knowledge of ORT but often do not prescribe it because it is inconvenient to administer compared to IV fluid therapy. Poor remuneration for ORT therapy with accompanying teaching (compared to IV therapy) was also seen as a barrier. Moreover, the cost of oral rehydration solutions in the United States and Canada, unlike that in developing countries, is relatively high. Of the pediatricians surveyed, 15% felt that ORT was too expensive for their patients.

3. The prevalence of various causes of acute diarrhea in infants obviously varies with location, living conditions, and season. Most acute diarrhea is caused by infectious agents. Among these, viruses are most common. In the United States, **rotavirus** is the most common viral cause, followed by **Enteric adenovirus** and **Norwalk agent** (Mehta & Lebenthal, 1994). Common bacterial causes of infantile diarrhea include **salmonella** and **Campylobacter jejuni.** The most common parasitic

cause in the United States is **Giardia lamblia** (Seidel, 1993). The most common infectious agents in developing countries differ somewhat from those in North America.

It is important to note that Bonnie and Francine belong to the Canadian native population, among which infantile diarrhea is an important cause of morbidity and mortality (Nutrition Committee, 1994). Diarrheal disease is also an enormous problem among Native American children in the southwestern United States. Santosham et al. (1995) have studied the prevalence of various causes of diarrhea among the White Mountain Apaches of Arizona. The most common diarrheal pathogens were *rotavirus, enterotoxigenic E. coli, shigella,* and *campylobacter.*

4. Most cases of acute infantile diarrhea are self-limited. Antimicrobial medications are not indicated unless a specific microbial cause is identified. Antidiarrheal medications are often used, but the WHO (1993) states clearly that there is no evidence of their practical benefit in the treatment of children with acute diarrhea. Indeed, some of them can be dangerous. Despite this, pharmaceutical companies continue to market medications such as *Kaopectate*™ (recommended for children with acute diarrhea over the age of 3 years). Lexchin (1994) has recommended that all companies making antidiarrheal medications cease to list them as indicated for acute diarrhea in children and be required to state that ORT is the best treatment. It should be noted, however, that there is evidence for the benefit of *bismuth subsalicylate* in the treatment of acute pediatric diarrhea. Soriano-Brucher et al. (1991) assessed the impact of bismuth sub-

salicylate in treating infants of 4 to 28 months with acute diarrhea in a randomized, double-blind, placebo-controlled trial. Bismuth salicylate solution was associated with decreased stool frequency and stool weight, improved stool consistency, shortened duration of illness, and improvement in clinical well-being. Use of bismuth salicylate, unfortunately, is complicated by the inconvenience of its administration. Soriano-Brucher et al. administered bismuth salicylate solution at a dose of 1.14mL/kg five times daily.

5. A review of what is known thus far about Francine and her illness is warranted. She was previously a healthy 18-month-old girl with a 1-day history of bloodless diarrhea unaccompanied by other symptoms. She is fully immunized and is taking no medications. She normally consumes a healthy, varied diet but has been taking only apple juice, a high sugar/low sodium drink, since the diarrhea began. The child has not traveled outside her immediate environment. Francine's frequency and quantity of voiding are uncertain. The physical examination is consistent with *some* dehydration—corresponding to a fluid deficit of 50-100mL/kg. Under such circumstances, the WHO (1993) recommends initial administration of ORT within the supervised environment of a health care facility. This corresponds to *WHO Treatment Plan B.*

There are a number of equations used for calculating the amount of oral rehydration fluid needed. For children of 12 to 23 months weighing 8 to 10.9kg and with 5% to 1% dehydration, 600 to 800 mL of solution is recommended by the WHO over the first 4 hr of therapy. The Canadian Pediatric Society (Nutrition Committee, 1994) recommends 20mL/kg over the 1st hr followed by 15 to 20 mL/kg/hr for the next 6 to 8 hr. A child should be assessed frequently during this period for his or her ability to take in rehydration solution. A complete re-assessment for hydration status is recommended after 4 hr.

PART III

The Problem

You explain to Bonnie that Francine is suffering from some dehydration and that correction of this problem is the immediate priority. You provide 700mL of WHO rehydration solution, which you instruct Bonnie to give her daughter by cup, slowly over 4 hr, in a separate room in your office. Bonnie has no objection to staying in the immediate vicinity of the clinic. You tell her that you will check in on her and Francine from time to time.

Your periodic assessments during this rehydration period reveal that Francine takes the oral rehydration solution (ORS) readily. After 4 hr you return for a complete re-assessment. Francine has taken the entire amount of ORS. She is alert but still somewhat irritable. Her eyes are only slightly sunken. Her mucous membranes appear moist. She continues to take ORS when offered. The child's skin turgor remains normal, and her capillary refill time is now 1.5 s.

Examination of Francine's diaper reveals that she continues to have diarrhea. It does appear that she has passed a small amount of clear, dark urine.

Questions

1. How would you continue to manage this case?

Discussion

1. Francine's hydration status has improved dramatically—an expected result, given the proven efficacy of ORT. In these circumstances, the child can be sent home with her mother, where home therapy with ORT can be continued.

It has been advocated that the solution used to replace ongoing losses, or *maintenance* solution, be lower in sodium than that used in the rehydration phase (40 to 60 mEq of Na in maintenance solution vs. 90 mEq sodium in WHO-ORS) (Havener et al., 1990; Meyers, 1995). It should be noted that most commercially available rehydration solutions in the United States and Canada are lower in sodium than the WHO solution. *Rehydralyte,* for example, contains only 75 mEq of sodium. Cohen et al. (1995) have successfully used two low-sodium solutions, containing 45 and 50 mEq of sodium, for both rehydration and maintenance, respectively, in 60 infant boys with mild or moderate dehydration. An alternative to using a low-sodium maintenance preparation is simply to alternate administration of high-sodium solutions with water or other low-salt fluids (Nutrition Committee, 1994). Indeed, ORT need not even be administered in the form of ORS at home (WHO, 1993). In addition to ORS, acceptable fluids include salted drinks, such as salted rice water and vegetable or chicken soup with salt. Fluids that do not contain salt, such as plain water, can also be given. Soft drinks, sweet juices, and so on should be avoided for reasons discussed earlier. As a general rule, the child should be given as much fluid as he or she wants (WHO, 1993), but roughly 50 to 100 mL of fluid is needed to replace losses after each diarrheal stool in children under 2 years.

It is a common practice in many societies, and even in various health care environments, to withhold regular feeds from patients with diarrhea. Fasting has been shown to have a negative impact on the child's overall nutritional status and actually prolong the course of diarrhea (Havener et al., 1990). Early refeeding upon correction of dehydration (Subcommittee on Nutrition and Diarrheal Diseases Control, National Research Council, 1985;

WHO, 1993) is the recommended practice. The child's usual diet is acceptable for this purpose (Richards, Claeson, & Pierce, 1993). There is no evidence that withholding of milk, diluting feeds, or prescribing a traditional BRAT diet (bananas, rice, applesauce, tea/toast) is beneficial during refeeding (Meyers, 1995; Richards et al., 1993).

Bonnie should be sent home with clear instructions on how to care for Francine. She should be made aware of the signs and symptoms of dehydration and should be asked to contact her physician should these develop. Passage of many watery stools, repeated vomiting, fever, blood in the stool, or no improvement in diarrhea after 3 days are all reasons to seek the help of a physician (WHO, 1993). Bonnie needs to understand that the recommended dietary and fluid therapy is not a cure for diarrhea but rather a way to prevent its complications. Informative patient education materials can be provided (Goepp & Katz, 1993).

PART IV

The Problem

You instruct Bonnie to begin refeeding her daughter with the same good variety of foods she was taking prior to her illness. You have several sample bottles of *Pedialyte,*™ a popular maintenance solution, in your office, which you provide to Bonnie at no cost. You tell her to give Francine as much Pedialyte as she wants. You give Bonnie some patient information sheets on diarrhea in children (Goepp & Katz, 1993), which you review carefully with her, making special note of the signs of dehydration. You ask her to call you should Francine develop very large, watery stools, repeated vomiting, fever, or blood in her stool.

You ask Bonnie to call you should the diarrhea persist after 3 days. You also tell her that you are available any time to address any concerns or answer any questions she may have.

Bonnie calls and asks to see you 3 days later. She tells you that Francine is no longer irritable and has been drinking Pedialyte, eating, and voiding normally. Unfortunately, though her diarrhea has improved, she still has had small amounts of bloodless watery diarrhea five or six times daily for the past 2 days. She has manifested no fever, vomiting, or other symptoms.

Interestingly, two other children Bonnie has been caring for in her home have also developed diarrhea over the past 3 days.

On physical examination, Francine is playful and alert. She shows no signs of dehydration. Her weight is 11.0kg.

Questions

1. Francine's diarrhea has now persisted for 4 days. Would you now like to obtain any laboratory investigations?
2. Describe your further management from this point.

Discussion

1. The answer to this question is complicated by the fact that two other children cared for in the same home have developed diarrhea. There is no need to obtain serum electrolytes or urine specific gravity, as, clinically, Francine's hydration status is normal. The question is whether investigations are warranted to identify the cause or causes of Francine's diarrhea. The presence of a bacterial or parasitic pathogen as a cause of diarrhea may change management from simple maintenance of fluid balance until symptoms disappear to active antimicrobial therapy.

Leung and Robson (1989) recommend that stool be examined in all children in whom diarrhea persists "for more than a few days or when a parasitic cause is suspected." "More than a few days" is clearly ambiguous. The WHO (1993), for example, defines "persistent diarrhea" as diarrhea that lasts at least 14 days, which is often associated with malnutrition and serious intestinal or nonintestinal infections.

Stool cultures, used to identify pathogenic stool bacteria, can be obtained from children with diarrhea. They are not routinely recommended, as most cases of infantile diarrhea are self-limited and viral in origin (Meyers, 1995; WHO, 1993). Stool cultures and examination for ova and parasites are expensive and are frequently inappropriately ordered in some settings (Siegel, Edelstein, & Nachamkin, 1990). Dewitt, Humphrey, and McCarthy (1985), in a prospective study of children under the age of 4 years with diarrhea, determined which historical variables, physical examination findings, and simple laboratory tests are predictive of a bacterial cause of diarrhea. It was found that **abrupt onset of diarrhea, no vomiting prior to onset of diarrhea, and more than four stools per day** was the best combination of any historical variables or physical examination findings in predicting which patients had diarrhea caused by pathogenic bacteria. This three-item "decision rule" was found to have a sensitivity of 96%, specificity of 40%, positive predictive value of 28%, and negative predictive value of 85%.

The presence of stool polymorphonuclear cells has long been used as a *screening* test, or factor predictive of bacterial diarrhea. The study by Dewitt et al. (1985) confirms the utility of this test. It was found to be 85% sensitive, 88% specific, with a positive predictive value of 59%, and a negative predictive value of 97%. This screening test, therefore, was a better predictor of bacterial diarrhea than any combination of historical or physical examination variables. Dewitt et al. point out that a useful stepwise strategy is first to apply the three-item decision rule and then to examine the stool for polymorphonuclear cells only in patients in whom the decision rule predicts a bacterial cause of diarrhea.

Francine's diarrhea did begin abruptly, was not associated with preceding vomiting, and does consist of more than four stools daily. On this basis, there is an elevated probability of bacterial diarrhea. Examination of the stool for polymorphonuclear cells is certainly justifiable on these grounds. A positive result can be followed by stool cultures.

Stool is easily examined for polymorphonuclear leukocytes by placing a very small amount on a slide and adding a drop of saline or methylene blue (Meyers, 1995).

The possibility of a parasitic cause of Francine's diarrhea cannot be dismissed.

Diarrheal disease of parasitic origin, particularly *Giardia lamblia,* is common in day care facilities. Bonnie does not run a formal day care center, but the factors that predispose children to various causes of diarrhea in day care centers, such as easy person-to-person transmission of infectious agents and fecal contamination of chairs, tables, and so on, likely exist in her home. On these grounds, sending a couple of fresh stool samples for ova and parasites is reasonable.

2. Francine's hydration status is adequate. Dehydration is still a concern, and the same fluid and nutritional management should continue. Bonnie should be informed once again about the signs and symptoms of dehydration. She should be advised to contact her physician should she have any questions or concerns. Stool samples can be provided when convenient but preferably as soon as possible. Close follow-up should be arranged.

PART V

The Problem

You inform Bonnie that her daughter shows no signs of dehydration and that she should continue with regular feeds and maintenance solution. You tell her that it would be valuable to obtain a stool sample because Francine's diarrhea has persisted for some time and her clinical history is consistent with a possible bacterial cause of diarrhea. Furthermore, the fact that two other children in the same environment have developed diarrhea makes you suspicious of an outbreak of potentially treatable infectious diarrhea in the day care setting. You review the signs and symptoms of dehydration and ask Bonnie to contact you should she have any questions or concerns.

Francine has a small, watery bowel movement just as she and Bonnie are about to leave. You obtain a stool sample. Examination under a microscope does not reveal a significant number of polymorphonuclear leukocytes. Realizing that the negative predictive value of this test is extremely high (97%), you decide not to send samples for culture. You are still concerned about a parasitic cause of diarrhea, and you send this and another stool sample provided the next day to a local laboratory for ova and parasites examination (O+P). You call Bonnie that day to inquire about Francine's condition. Bonnie tells you that Francine continues to have a small watery bowel movement every 4 to 6 hr but has been eating, drinking, and voiding normally. She remains playful and alert. Bonnie also tells you that she spoke to the mother of one of the other children with diarrhea, a 4-year-old boy, who has precisely the same clinical picture—frequent watery stools without preceding vomiting and unaccompanied by fever or other symptoms.

The next day, the result of the O+P examination is faxed to your office. It reads,

Numerous Giardial cysts in both stool samples. No trophozoites seen. No other parasites identified.

Questions

1. What is *Giardia lamblia,* and how is it generally spread?
2. How would you treat Francine's Giardiasis?
3. How would you manage the presumed outbreak of this disease in Bonnie's home?

Discussion

1. *Giardia lamblia* is a pathogenic intestinal protozoan parasite that inhabits the proximal small intestine. It exists in two forms: trophozoites and cysts. Trophozoites are found in the duodenal fluid of infected individuals and in loose stools, but not usually in formed stools. They are relatively delicate and do not survive long in the external environment. Cysts are much tougher and can survive in water for several months. Ingestion of cysts is the primary mode of transmission of *Giardia.* Diarrhea, abdominal cramping, and, occasionally, fever follow after an incubation period of 1 to 3 weeks. As many as two thirds of infected individuals have no symptoms whatsoever (Weller, 1996).

In addition to diagnosis by microscopic examination, there are now several enzyme-linked immunosorbent assay tests (ELISA) for *Giardia* that are highly sensitive and specific (Seidel, 1993).

As previously noted, Giardiasis is extremely common in day care facilities, where it is spread by the fecal-oral route (Pickering, Woodward, DuPont, & Sullivan, 1984). Fecal contamination is common in the day care environment (Laborde, Weigle, Weber, Sobsey, & Kotch, 1994). *Giardia lamblia* is also spread by consumption of contaminated water and food, male homosexual contact, and swimming in contaminated pool water (Gray, Gunnell, & Peters, 1994).

2. Quinacrine HCL, metronidazole, and furazolidone are commonly used to treat Giardiasis. Quinacrine and metronidazole are equally effective in eradicating the organism and are slightly more effective than furazolidone (Seidel, 1993). It should be noted, however, that metronidazole is not approved for the treatment of Giardiasis in the United States. Quinacrine is extremely bitter tasting and should be combined with another more palatable substance. It is also associated with vomiting and abdominal upset. It is usually given at a dose of 7mg/kg per day in three divided doses for 1 week.

Furazolidone is generally better tolerated by children, although it is also associated with vomiting, abdominal upset, and, occasionally, skin rashes. It is available in a suspension, making it convenient to administer. It is given in doses of 6mg/kg/day divided qid for 10 days (Sanford, Gilbert, & Sande, 1996).

3. An effort must be made to prevent the spread of *Giardia lamblia* from Bonnie's home to the surrounding community. In many jurisdictions, including the province of Ontario, cases of Giardiasis must be reported to public health authorities. There is no question, of course, that the two other children who developed diarrhea need to be evaluated for Giardiasis. Either Bonnie or her physician need to contact their respective parents for this purpose. Furthermore, many infected individuals are asymptomatic and develop no sequelae from such asymptomatic infections. Other children recently cared for in Bonnie's home should be tested, depending on the selected treatment strategy, as discussed later. Bonnie herself can also be tested, as well as any other adults who have spent an extended period in her home.

Bartlett et al. (1991) have studied the effectiveness of three different strategies to control the prevalence of *Giardia lamblia* in the day care setting. The first strategy involved the exclusion and treatment of symptomatic and asymptomatic infected children; the second, exclusion and treatment of symptomatic children only; and the third, exclusion and treatment of symptomatic infected children and treatment without exclusion of asymptomatic infected children. At the end of a 6-month follow-up, no strategy was associated with a significantly lower prevalence of *Giardia*, although each strategy reduced the prevalence to a level lower than at the outset of the trial. Given that nontreatment and no exclusion of asymptomatic individuals is as effective a strategy as the others, the decision not even to test asymptomatic individuals is justifiable. Strict exclusion of children from day care is not only of questionable value but is expensive, as parents often lose time from work and other activities. Cody, Sottnek, and O'Leary (1994) recommend thorough cleansing of potentially contaminated surfaces in day care (e.g., chairs, tables, etc.) with soap or detergent as a relatively inexpensive and effective strategy to control transmission of *Giardia*. A reasonable starting point for Bonnie's physician is to recommend to her that she thoroughly cleanse any areas potentially contaminated with feces prior to resuming the care of children in her home.

Conclusion

You tell Bonnie that her daughter has been infected by *Giardia lamblia* and briefly review the nature of this infection and how it is spread. You tell her that this is an extremely common infection in many day care centers and that it is important for her thoroughly to wash all surfaces potentially contaminated with stool on a regular basis to control its spread.

Bonnie provides the names of the other two children who have developed diarrhea. You call their parents and explain that they may have been infected by *Giardia*. You advise them to seek the help of their physicians with this information if they have not already done so.

You prescribe an appropriate dose of furazalidone for Francine.

Francine's diarrhea gradually stops over the next 2 days. She and Bonnie return to your office for follow-up 3 days after beginning treatment. Francine shows no signs of dehydration. Her diarrhea has stopped. You advise Bonnie to continue the full course of treatment. You remind her of your continued availability should she have any questions or concerns or should Francine become ill once again.

References

Adelman, R. D., & Solhung, M. J. (1996). Pathophysiology of body fluids and fluid therapy. In R. E. Behrman, R. M. Kliegman, A. M. Arvin, & W. E. Nelson (Eds.), *Nelson textbook of pediatrics* (15th ed., pp. 206-210). Philadelphia, PA: W. B. Saunders.

Bartlett, A. V., Englender, S. J., Jarvis, B. A., Ludwig, L., Carlson, J. F., & Topping, J. P. (1991). Controlled trial of Giardia lamblia: Control strategies in day care centers. *American Journal of Public Health, 81*, 1001-1006.

Cody, M. M., Sottnek, H. M., & O'Leary, V. S. (1994). Recovery of Giardia lamblia cysts from chairs and tables in child day-care centers. *Pediatrics, 94*(6, Part 2), 1006-1008.

Cohen, M. B., Mezoff, A. G., Laney, D. W., Bezerra, J. A., Beane, B. M., Drazner, D., Baker, R., & Moran, J. R. (1995). Use of a single solution for oral rehydration and maintenance therapy of infants with diarrhea and mild to moderate dehydration. *Pediatrics, 95*(5), 639-645.

DeWitt, T. G., Humphrey, K. F., & McCarthy, P. (1985). Clinical predictors of acute bacterial diarrhea in young children. *Pediatrics, 76*, 551-556.

Ghishan, F. K. (1988). The transport of electrolytes in the gut and the use of oral rehydration solutions. *Pediatric Gastroenterology, 35*(1), 35-50.

Goepp, J. G., & Katz, S. A. (1993). Oral rehydration therapy. *American Family Physician, 47*(4), 843-848.

Gray, S. F., Gunnell, D. J., & Peters, T. J. (1994). Risk factors for giardiasis: A case-control study in Avon and Somerset. *Epidemiology and Infection, 113*, 95-102.

Havener, S., Meis, S., & Graber, M. A. (1990). Vomiting/diarrhea/dehydration. In M. A. Graber, R. J. Allen, & B. T. Levy (Eds.), *University of Iowa family practice handbook. Chapter 10: Pediatrics* (Section 2). Iowa City: University of Iowa. (http://indy.radiology.uiowa.edu/Providers/Clin Ref/FPHandbook/03.html; accessed December 7, 1996)

Laborde, D. J., Weigle, K. A., Weber, D. J., Sobsey, M. D., & Kotch, J. B. (1994). The frequency, level, and distribution of fecal contamination in day-care center classrooms. *Pediatrics, 94*(6, Part 2), 1008-1011.

Leung, A. K., & Robson, W.L.M. (1989). Acute diarrhea in children: What to do and what not to do. *Postgraduate Medicine, 86*(8), 168-174.

Lexchin, J. (1994). Agents against pediatric diarrhea. Assessing the information companies supply to Canadian physicians. *Canadian Family Physician, 40*, 2082-2087.

Mauer, A. M., Dweck, H. S., Finberg, L., Holmes, F., Reynolds, J. W., Suskind, R. M., Woodruff, C. W., & Hellerstein, S. (1985). American Academy of Pediatrics Committee on Nutrition: Use of oral fluid therapy and posttreatment feeding following enteritis in children in a developed country. *Pediatrics, 75*, 358-361.

Mehta, D. I., & Lebenthal, E. (1994, March). New developments in acute diarrhea. *Current Problems in Pediatrics, 23*(3), 95-107.

Meyers, A. (1995). Modern management of acute diarrhea and dehydration in children. *American Family Physician, 51*(5), 1103-1117.

Nutrition Committee, Canadian Paediatric Society. (1994). Oral rehydration therapy and early refeeding in the management of childhood gastroenteritis. *Canadian Journal of Paediatrics, 1*(5), 160-164.

Pickering, L. K., Woodward, W. E., DuPont, H. L., & Sullivan, P. (1984). Occurrence of Giardia lamblia in children in day care centers. *Journal of Pediatrics, 104*, 522-526.

Reis, E. C., Goepp, J. G., Katz, S., & Santosham, M. (1994). Barriers to use of oral rehydration therapy. *Pediatrics, 93*(5), 708-711.

Richards, L., Claeson, M., & Pierce, N. F. (1993). Management of acute diarrhea in children: Lessons learned. *Pediatric Infections and Disease Journal, 12*, 5-9.

Saavedra, J. M., Harris, G. D., Song, L., & Finberg, L. (1991). Capillary refilling (skin turgor) in the assessment of dehydration. *American Journal of Diseases of Children, 145*, 296-298.

Sanford, J. P., Gilbert, D. N., & Sande, M. A. (1996). *The Sanford guide to antimicrobial therapy.* Dallas, TX: Antimicrobial Therapy Inc.

Santosham, M., Sack, R. B., Reid, R., Black, R., Croll, J., Yolken, R., Aurelian, L., Wolff, M., Chan, E., Garrett, S., & Froehlich, J. (1995). Diarrheal diseases in the White Mountain Apaches: Epidemiologic studies. *Journal of Diarrhoeal Disease Research, 13*(1), 18-28.

Seidel, J. (1993). Giardiasis. *Pediatrics in Review, 14*(7), 284-285.

Siegel, D. L., Edelstein, P. H., & Nachamkin, I. (1990). Inappropriate testing for diarrheal diseases in the hospital. *Journal of the American Medical Association, 263*(7), 979-982.

Snyder, J. D. (1991). Use and misuse of oral therapy for diarrhea: Comparison of US practices with American Academy of Pediatrics recommendations. *Pediatrics, 87*(1), 28-33.

Soriano-Brucher, H., Avendano, P., O'Ryan, M., Braun, S. D., Manhart, M. D., Balm, T. K., & Soriano, H. A. (1991). Bismuth subsalicylate in the treatment of acute diarrhea in children: A clinical study. *Pediatrics, 87*(1), 18-27.

Subcommittee on Nutrition and Diarrheal Diseases Control, National Research Council. (1985). *Nutritional management of acute diarrhea in infants and children.* Washington, DC: National Academy Press.

Weller, P. F. (1996, June). Protozoan infections. In D. C. Dale & D. D. Federman (Eds.), *Infectious diseases* (chap. 34). New York: Scientific American, Inc. (Retrieved from SAM-CD April 9, 1997)

World Health Organization. (1993). *The treatment of diarrhea: A manual for physicians and other senior health workers* (WHO/CDD/SER/80.2, Rev. 3). Geneva: Author. (http://www.who.ch/ programmes/cdr/pub/cdd/textrev4.htm; accessed April 24, 1997)

10. FAILURE TO THRIVE,

OR GROWTH DEFICIENCY

Lindsay Clarke

Goal: The goal of this group discussion exercise
is to familiarize participants with the evaluation of the
problem of growth deficiency in an infant.

Specific Objectives: Upon completion of this exercise, each participant should be able to accomplish the following:

1. Use a standardized growth chart to determine whether a child has "failure to thrive" and to determine the pattern and degree of malnutrition.
2. Describe a framework for evaluation of failure to thrive that accounts for nutritional, medical, psychosocial, and developmental factors.
3. Describe a systematic approach to the evaluation of "chronic cough" in a young child.
4. Describe three frequent presenting features of cystic fibrosis, as well as the way in which this disease is diagnosed.

PART I

The Patient

Social History

Lindsay Clarke is a 7-month-old baby girl who lives with her mother, Tina, 19 years old, and her mother's boyfriend, Russell, 26, in a mobile home in northwestern Arizona. Lindsay was born in Odessa, Texas, where Tina grew up. A high school dropout, Tina was living with her parents, Jan and Brendan Clarke, and dating Ryan Voeller, 19, when she became pregnant with Lindsay. When Ryan learned of Tina's pregnancy, he immediately absolved himself of all responsibility and broke off their relationship. He has since acknowledged that he is Lindsay's father, but he plays no role in either Tina's or his daughter's life. Tina has had a strained relationship with her parents for several years. A deeply religious couple, Jan and Brendan found coping with Tina's out-of-wedlock pregnancy extremely difficult. Frequent disputes eventually led Tina to leave her family's home 3 months before Lindsay was born. She moved in with her friend, Gertrude.

Tina describes Gertrude as a "party animal." Jan and Brendan were less kind and described their daughter's roommate as "reckless, insane, and promiscuous." It was at a raucous party at Gertrude's apartment that Tina first met Russell, a somewhat withdrawn, rugged-looking young man, who worked in an auto parts store and referred to himself as a "combat enthusiast." According to Tina, "Russ had this aura about him. I was crazy about him from the start." On the other hand, Russell at first had no interest in Tina, who at the time was 8 months pregnant.

Lindsay was born during this chaotic time in Tina's life. Her arrival, however, brought a newfound tranquility to the Clarke household. Gertrude had no tolerance for a baby in her apartment and told Tina to leave. By contrast, no longer troubled by their daughter's "untraditional" passage to motherhood, Jan and Brendan quickly became doting grandparents. Tina and Lindsay moved back home. The Clarkes provided mother and daughter with a newly furnished bedroom, complete with crib. On the few occasions that Lindsay left Tina's arms, Lindsay found herself in the gentle embrace of one of her grandparents. Brendan describes his granddaughter as "absolutely precious and irresistible."

Tina met Russell on a few other occasions, and before long the two engaged in an intimate relationship. Russell, who always referred to Lindsay as "the baby," was not too interested in fatherhood and valued his independence. Two months after Lindsay was born, he quit his job at the auto parts store and left abruptly for Arizona to pursue a career as a "bounty hunter." Tina was despondent, and the Clarke household was once again thrown into turmoil as she insisted repeatedly on leaving with Lindsay, against her parents' wishes, to start a new life with Russell in Arizona. One evening, a fierce argument with Brendan led Tina to pick up her baby and storm out of her parents' home. She boarded a bus that night and spent the early morning hours shivering in a bus station in El Paso. Eventually Tina made her way to Arizona with her daughter, where she found Russell living alone in a small rented trailer.

Russell was at first troubled by Tina and Lindsay's unannounced arrival. He had had a difficult couple of months. His attempt to become a bounty hunter had not worked out. He had applied successfully for welfare but spent much of his money on combat magazines and army surplus supplies. He ate poorly and irregularly, often relying on the hospitality of others in the trailer park for meals. All in all, he was ill prepared to host his "girlfriend" and her daughter. Nevertheless, it would have taken an exceptionally cruel individual to turn Tina and Lindsay away when they looked so cold, tired, and desperate. Tina and Lindsay moved in, and Russell soon forgot his difficulties as he and Tina rekindled their relationship. The couple, now with a need to provide diapers, baby food, and other items, was desperately short of money. Tina reluctantly called her parents and asked them for a "loan" of $1,000. At first they refused and insisted that she return home at once. Tina made it clear that that would not happen. Worried about their daughter and granddaughter's well-being, after a couple of days of contemplation, the Clarkes wired their daughter the money. A few days later Tina applied for welfare and enrolled in a WIC (Women, Infants, Children) program.

It became obvious that the tiny trailer originally intended for one could not accommodate a small family. Tina, Lindsay, and Russell moved into a much larger, comfortable, well-furnished mobile home soon after Tina's welfare application was approved.

Tina and her parents are Southern Baptists. Russell belongs to no organized religion. Brendan Clarke traces his family's roots to England and Norway. His great-great-great-grandfather came to Texas from Ohio just before the Civil War. Jan's family came to Texas from Ireland in the 1840s. Tina believes Ryan Voeller's family to be primarily of German origin.

Past Personal and Family Medical History

Lindsay is Tina's first child. She was born at 39 weeks' gestation by spontaneous vaginal delivery at a birth weight of 3,250g. Tina describes no medical problems during her pregnancy nor during labor, delivery, or the postnatal period. She gained approximately 13kg during her pregnancy. She has never drunk alcohol, smoked, or used any illicit drugs. Tina took multivitamin tablets while pregnant but then, as now, used no other medications. Russell neither smokes nor drinks.

Lindsay was seen on a regular basis by her pediatrician, Dr. Thurman Wood of Odessa, Texas, until she was 6 months old. Dr. Wood administered her regular 2-, 4-, and 6-month vaccinations. At 4 months, Lindsay was admitted to the hospital for 3 days with a diagnosis of pneumonia. According to Tina, Dr. Wood was concerned about her growth at her 6-month checkup. In Tina's words,

> Lindsay seems so skinny to me. Dr. Wood told me she wasn't gaining weight that well. He told me we would watch things for a while and to return for a 7-month checkup. Well, then my life turned upside down. I missed that appointment.

Lindsay has been breast-fed since birth. Tina attended a breast-feeding clinic in Odessa for young mothers, at which she was told that her technique was "excellent" and that Lindsay was feeding well. Tina has been introducing bottled baby foods at a rate of roughly one new variety per week, which Lindsay seems to enjoy very much.

Tina tells you that her parents, Brendan, 50, and Jan, 46, are in perfect health. She has a younger brother, Robert, 16, who has no significant health problems.

Tina is not too familiar with Ryan Voeller's health. She believes that he is "perfectly healthy" even though he smokes cigarettes heavily. Tina does know that Ryan had an older brother who died 3 years ago at the age of 18 with "some sort of lung problem."

The Problem

You are the only physician in the remote northwestern Arizona community of Hackberry. Your practice has a large catchment area, including a nearby Native American reservation.

Age	Weight (kg)	Recumbent Length (cm)	Head Circumference (cm)
Birth	3.25	48.0	33.5
2 Weeks	3.30	50.2	34.0
1 Month	3.80	53.0	37.0
2 Months	4.82	55.4	38.2
3 Months	5.20	59.5	39.5
4 Months	5.35	61.0	41.2
6 Months	5.50	62.0	42.3

Figure 10.1.   Growth Chart for Lindsay Clarke

There is a community hospital approximately 40 km away that has a fairly complete array of diagnostic facilities and specialist services. Tina Clarke brings her 7-month-old daughter to your office and tells you, "I was supposed to have a growth check on Lindsay. She's kind of small for her age. My doctor in Texas told me I should have her checked out."

You begin your assessment with some measurements to confirm Tina's concerns. Lindsay weighs 5.65kg. Her recumbent length is 62.5cm. Her head circumference is 43.2cm. You decide that more data are required to get a complete picture of Lindsay's growth. With Tina's permission, you call Dr. Wood in Texas. He tells you that he was concerned about Lindsay's missed appointment. His secretary faxes you a copy of records of Lindsay's clinic visits up until Lindsay was 6 months old (see Figure 10.1).

Questions

1. Using the charts in Figures 10.2 and 10.3, plot Lindsay's weight, length, head circumference, and weight per length using the data previously given.
2. Define "failure to thrive." Does Lindsay have this condition?

Discussion

1. See "The Rest of the Story," which follows this section, for Lindsay's completed growth chart.

2. The term "failure to thrive," first used at the turn of this century (Schwartz & Abegglen, 1996), is somewhat ambiguous. It refers to children who are underweight, stunted, and often undernourished. Some advocate "growth deficiency" as a more precise and meaningful term

(Bithoney, Dubowitz, & Egan, 1992). Universal criteria for failure to thrive are not available. There is agreement, however, that this diagnosis should be made on the basis of anthropometric measurements only (Drotar, Malone, & Devost, 1985) rather than a combination of measures of growth and assessment of development and behavior. There is no consensus as to which anthropometric measures should be

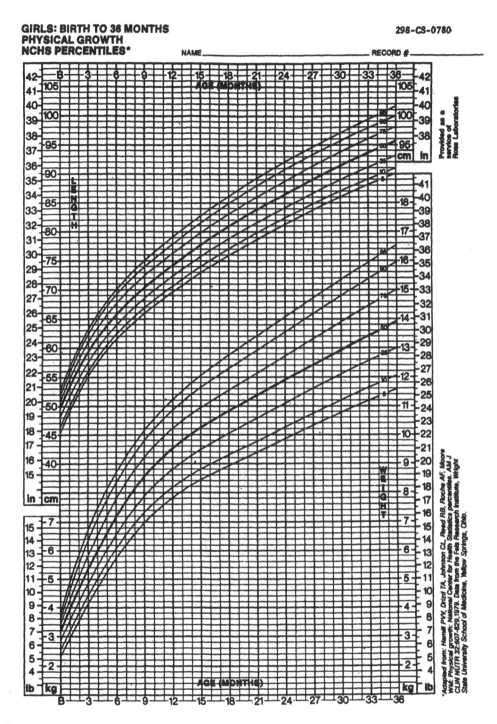

Figure 10.2   National Center for Health Statistics Pediatric Growth Chart: Expected Weight and Length Percentiles for Girls

SOURCE: Department of Health, Education and Welfare, Public Health Service Health Resources Administration, National Center for Health Statistics, and the Centers for Disease Control. Used with permission of Ross Products Division, Abbott Laboratories, Columbus, OH 43216, from National Center for Health Statistics Growth Charts. © 1982 Ross Products Division, Abbott Laboratories.

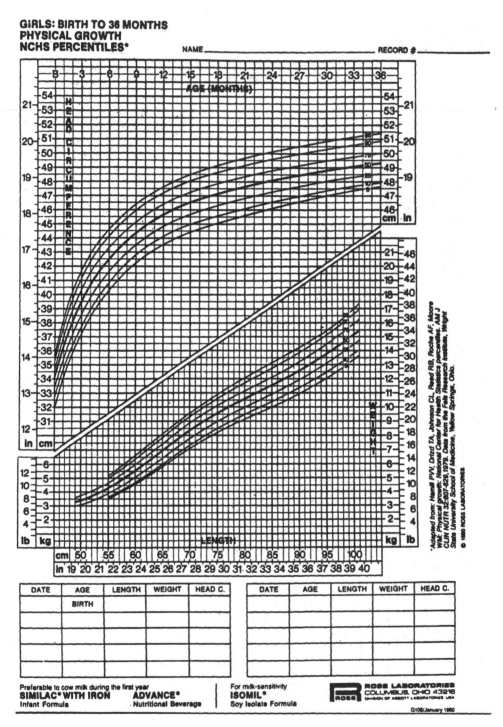

Figure 10.3   National Center for Health Statistics Pediatric Growth Chart: Expected Head
Circumference and Weight for Length Percentiles for Girls

SOURCE: Department of Health, Education and Welfare, Public Health Service Health Resources Administration, National Center for
Health Statistics, and the Centers for Disease Control. Used with permission of Ross Products Division, Abbott Laboratories, Columbus,
OH 43216, from National Center for Health Statistics Growth Charts. © 1982 Ross Products Division, Abbott Laboratories.

used to define failure to thrive. Anthropometric criteria can be divided into those that measure **growth velocity** and those that measure **attained growth.** A child under 5 months of age who fails to gain weight for 10 or more days, for example, can be said to have an abnormal growth velocity and therefore failure to thrive (Viteri, 1981). The crossing of two major percentile lines on a standardized growth chart is another way by which failure to thrive can be diagnosed by velocity criteria (Leung, Robson, & Fagan, 1993).

Attained growth is usually plotted in terms of **weight, recumbent length, and head circumference** on the widely available growth charts developed by the National Center for Health Statistics (NCHS), which allow for comparison with other children of the same age in the American population. Weight is the first parameter that deviates from normal in a child with failure to thrive. Length or height fails to increase only if malnutrition persists for an extended period. With these facts in mind, the following conclusions can be made: Depressed **weight for age** can be due to both acute or chronic insults. Depressed **weight for length** alone usually suggests acute malnutrition. Depressed **length for age** represents a more chronic problem. Depressed **weight for length** accompanied by depressed **length for age** suggests acute malnutrition superimposed on chronic malnutrition. Head circumference is affected only in very severe cases of malnutrition (Leung et al., 1993). For practical purposes, failure to thrive is often defined as a growth pattern in which *weight* is persistently below the 5th percentile for age (Bithoney et al., 1992).

Analysis of Lindsay's growth chart reveals that her rate of weight gain began to decrease at approximately 3 months of age. Her present weight for her age is well below the 5th percentile. Her gain in length began to drop off around 4 months of age. Her present length is around the 5th percentile for age. According to the definition described above, Lindsay certainly has failure to thrive. Both Lindsay's height and weight have crossed two major percentile lines on the growth chart. She can therefore be diagnosed with failure to thrive on the basis of velocity criteria as well.

The Rest of the Story

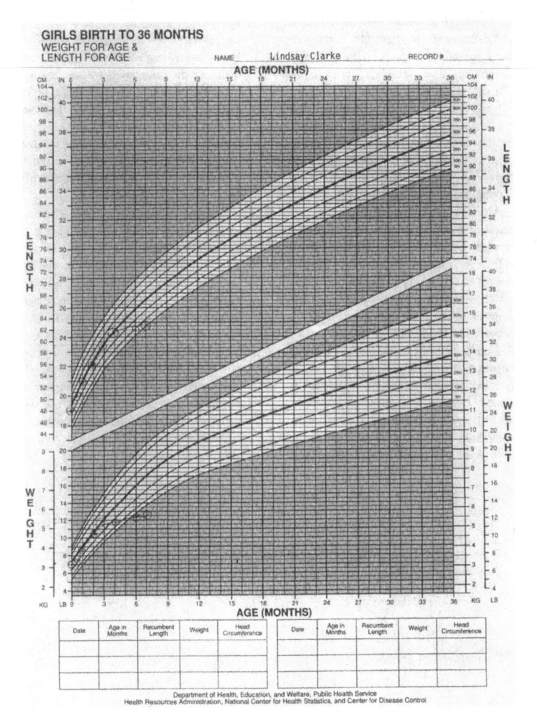

Figure 10.4   Lindsay Clarke's Weight and Length Chart

SOURCE: Used with permission of Ross Products Division, Abbott Laboratories, Columbus, OH 43216, from National Center for Health Statistics Growth Charts. © 1982 Ross Products Division, Abbott Laboratories.

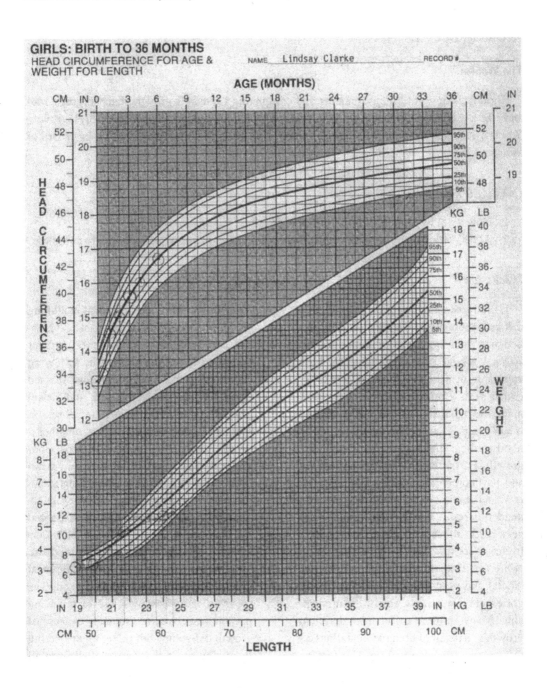

Figure 10.5 Lindsay Clarke's Head Circumference and Weight for Length Chart

SOURCE: Used with permission of Ross Products Division, Abbott Laboratories, Columbus, OH 43216, from National Center for Health Statistics Growth Charts. © 1982 Ross Products Division, Abbott Laboratories.

PART II

The Problem

Upon finishing your measurements and completing Lindsay's growth chart (Figures 10.4 and 10.5), you inform Tina that Dr. Wood was right in being concerned about the baby's growth. You tell Tina that Lindsay will require further evaluation to determine the cause or causes of her small size.

Questions

1. How would you approach the problem of failure to thrive in general?
2. At this office visit, what elements of an overall assessment would you like to complete?

Discussion

1. Failure to thrive is often an extremely difficult problem to evaluate. It is a particularly daunting task for a single physician working in a small town. A team approach, in which a physician works together with a nutritionist, social worker, medical specialist, and others, is preferred if it is possible. Virtually any serious childhood medical illness can lead to deficient growth. Furthermore, a number of social and psychological variables such as poverty and mother-child bonding can independently result in failure to thrive and are very hard to assess. The causes of failure to thrive are traditionally divided into *organic* (medical illnesses) and *nonorganic* (social and psychological). The two categories are not always easily distinguishable. Many children suffer from deficient growth as a result of both medical illnesses and psychosocial deprivation. This fact led to the creation of a third category: *mixed* failure to thrive (Casey, 1983).

There is an immense number of descriptions in the medical literature of how to approach the child with failure to thrive. Most use the traditional categorization described above as a starting point in making an assessment. This categorization, however, has recently fallen into disfavor among many pediatricians. The following discussion is based on the elegant revised approach described by Frank and Zeisel (1988). Malnutrition is the ultimate reason that most children fail to thrive, whether it be the result of inadequate intake, poor absorption of nutrients, or increased metabolic needs. Rather than attempting to determine whether growth deficiency is organic or nonorganic, the approach favored by Frank and Zeisel involves consideration of all (a) **nutritional,** (b) **medical,** (c) **psychosocial,** and (d) **developmental** factors that have led to malnutrition. The focus of the workup is not so much on pinpointing one or several causes of growth deficiency but rather on correcting the malnutrition that has resulted from all the factors above. There is a separate approach to each of the four areas of concern.

Nutritional Factors. Evaluation of nutritional factors involves three principal tasks. First, *anthropometric measures need to be interpreted.* This has already been done to some extent. Next, a *dietary assessment* should be made. Finally, *changes in the diet* need to be made to promote "catch-up growth."

It has been determined that Lindsay definitely has failure to thrive. The type of growth deficiency, which may help identify the pattern of malnutrition, is very important to discover. Lindsay has depressed *weight per age.* Her *length per age* is presently at the 5th percentile and has recently crossed two major percentile lines. Her *weight per length* has similarly crossed two percentile lines. This pattern suggests acute, superimposed on chronic, malnutrition. Beyond the actual pattern of insult, it is also important to determine the severity of malnutrition. This is usually done using the **Gomez Criteria** (Gomez et al., 1956), whereby a child's **weight per age** is divided by the **median (50th percentile)** weight of children at that age. A weight of 90% to 100% of the median indicates no malnutrition; 75% to 85%, Grade I or mild malnutrition; 60% to 74%, Grade II or moderate malnutrition; and < 60%, Grade III or severe malnutrition, necessitating immediate hospitalization. Lindsay's present weight is 5.65kg. The median weight for a 7-month-old girl is 7.73kg. Lindsay's weight is 73% of the median. She therefore has borderline mild-moderate malnutrition.

A dietary assessment, either in the form of a 24-hour dietary recall or a 7-day food frequency inventory, should be made by a nutritionist or other qualified professional. As much of Lindsay's nutrition comes in the form of breast milk, another assessment of Tina's breast-feeding technique may be a good idea. In many parts of North America, resources are available for this purpose. It may be hard to get a nutritional and/or breast-feeding assessment in a remote rural community.

Making dietary adjustments to promote catch-up growth in a young child is usually beyond the scope of a busy family physician and is best accomplished by an experienced nutritionist. You should, however, understand the essential principles of nutritional rehabilitation. The number of calories required daily to promote catch-up growth can be estimated through the following formula (MacLean, de Romana, Masse, et al., 1980):

$$\frac{kcal}{kg} = \frac{\frac{120 kcal}{kg} \times median\ weight\ for\ current\ height}{Current\ weight\ (kg)}.$$

The resulting daily caloric intake provides 1.5 to 2 times the amount normally required in a healthy, growing child of the same age. The high intake should be continued until previous growth percentiles are attained.

Medical Factors. There are four main priorities in assessing the impact of medical illness on growth: (a) assessing the impact of perinatal risks, (b) identifying and treating the cycle of infection and malnutrition, (c) determining the impact of any chronic illness on growth, and (d) obtaining laboratory tests in an appropriate fashion.

Lindsay's perinatal history has already been provided. She was born at term to a healthy young mother who used no drugs, alcohol, or significant medications during pregnancy. There is no indication of a problem in the intrapartum period. Lindsay was normal in size and, indeed, appeared to grow at a normal rate until approximately 3 months of age.

The **Infection-Malnutrition cycle** refers to a process in which a young child suffers frequent episodes of otitis media, gastroenteritis, respiratory illness, or other infectious diseases. Such infections decrease appetite but increase metabolic demands, often leading to growth deficiency. This in turn impairs immune function, making the child more susceptible to further infections and thus completing the cycle. This process can be interrupted by promptly treating infections and prescribing a diet that meets the child's metabolic needs at all times.

A vast number of different childhood chronic illnesses can lead to failure to thrive. Identifying a chronic illness responsible for growth deficiency is often an enormous challenge. A thorough review of systems should be performed, followed by a focused physical examination.

The use of diagnostic laboratory tests is very controversial. In a review of hospital records of 122 infants admitted for workup of failure to thrive, Berwick, Levy, and Kleinerman (1982) found that an average of 40 laboratory tests were ordered per infant. Surprisingly, only 0.8% of all tests showed an abnormality that contributed *diagnostically*. A negative laboratory test can of course often be helpful in ruling out a particular condition. Furthermore, some tests can be used to determine the severity of the possible effects of malnutrition (e.g., a CBC to determine the severity of anemia). These considerations aside, there are no uniform recommendations on which screening laboratory tests to perform in all children with failure to thrive. It is reasonable to use the laboratory as a resource to confirm a suspicion raised during the review of systems and physical examination rather than as a screening tool (Bithoney et al., 1992).

Psychosocial Factors. In most cases of failure to thrive, no medical or "organic" cause can be identified, and growth deficiency is attributed to so-called psychosocial factors (Sills, 1978). Although Frank and Zeisel (1988) do not favor this dichotomy as a way of understanding failure to thrive, they nevertheless emphasize the consideration of psychosocial factors in all such cases. In a case such as Lindsay's, in which her young mother has recently been through quite turbulent changes and has left behind a relatively stable support system for uncertain, relatively isolated social circumstances, most clinicians would implicate psychosocial factors as at least partly causative in failure to thrive. Frank and Zeisel divide the **psychosocial** management of failure to thrive into (a) assessing the role of poverty, (b) identifying family dysfunction, (c) identifying feeding disorders, (d) identifying child abuse, and (e) providing interventions that target any of the previous problems. These are not simple tasks and are best accomplished through a multidisciplinary approach. A social worker, for example, is likely to be much better equipped to determine if Tina is having difficulty providing enough nutritional support for her daughter due to poverty. A breast-feeding assessment as indicated previously, completed by an individual with experience in the field, may identify a feeding problem. The vast majority of children with failure to thrive do *not* experience abuse at the hands of their caretakers. If abuse is suspected, however, it is imperative that the physician alert the proper authorities to ensure safety, as well as address the medical and psychological impact of abuse.

Family dysfunction can be identified and qualified through a number of formal mechanisms. The Home Observation for Measurement of the Environment (HOME), for example, is an inventory of information that provides a picture of the interaction between mother and child (Casey, Bradley, & Wortham, 1984). It is routinely divided into six subscales: *(a) emotional and verbal responsivity of mother, (b) acceptance of child, (c) organization of the physical and temporal environment, (d) provision of appropriate play materials, (e) maternal involvement with child, and (f) opportunities and variety in daily stimulation.* Each category includes a number of scored items such as "mother caresses or kisses child at least once during visit" under *emotional and verbal responsivity of mother.* This complex tool is supposedly a reliable measure of maternal-child dysfunction (Bradley & Caldwell, 1981), although it is hard to imagine that it is not prone to the subjective biases of the administering party. In any case, such measures of family dysfunction are generally used by highly qualified and experienced individuals whose help would probably be unavailable in the remote community in which Tina and Lindsay live. A simple home visit in which the general living conditions are observed, together with the way in which the members of the household interact with one another, may provide a great deal of understanding about the impact of psychosocial factors on Lindsay's growth deficiency.

Developmental Factors. **Developmental** problems are normally not included in the definition of failure to thrive. Never-

theless, disordered development can be the cause or consequence of growth deficiency, and a formal developmental assessment is recommended for all children with failure to thrive (Frank & Zeisel, 1988). The commonly employed Denver Developmental Screening Test is not a sufficiently sensitive measure of development in children with growth deficiency (Bithoney et al., 1992). More accurate tests, such as the Bayley Scales of Infant Development (Snow, 1989), are usually employed. A discussion of these is beyond the scope of this exercise. Special interventions beyond correcting malnutrition, such as family therapy, are available to help restore normal development.

2. The preceding discussion provides a framework for an overall approach to failure to thrive. Many of the components of this approach cannot be effectively completed by a family physician. Furthermore, in Tina and Lindsay's present location, ancillary health services are undoubtedly limited. Consequently, this imposes a limit on professionals who can form a multidisciplinary team. What is needed is an agenda for this office visit that will at least partly fulfill the requirements of a complete evaluation. It may be wise to find out what other services are available within a reasonable distance, such as social work, breast-feeding assessment, pediatric specialists, and so on. A thorough medical evaluation can be completed in the office. Part of the nutritional assessment, namely determination of the degree of malnutrition based on anthropometric measurements as described above, can also be done. As mentioned, a simple home visit made by the physician provides a great deal of understanding of the role of psychosocial factors in failure to thrive and can be arranged at this time.

PART III

The Problem

You tell Tina that, based on your measurements, Lindsay is suffering from borderline moderate malnutrition. From what you know about Lindsay's perinatal history, you decide that there was no problem that could have contributed to her present failure to thrive. Apart from her one admission for pneumonia, Tina tells you that, to the best of her knowledge, Lindsay has had no ear or eye infections or any episodes of gastroenteritis. Indeed, a review of systems reveals no reflux, vomiting, or diarrhea. Lindsay has been having thin, yellow stools roughly three times daily since birth. She has been voiding normally. There is no history of rashes or skin infections. During the day, according to Tina, Lindsay is a "playful" baby who has a voracious appetite. She is breast-fed roughly every 4 hours. In addition, Lindsay receives baby food by cup during regular meals with Tina and Russell.

Tina tells you that Lindsay appears to "cough all the time." The cough is particularly bad at night. In Tina's words,

> Lindsay has been coughing more or less since she was born. I took her to the doctor lots of times. He said she would be OK and that she didn't have a fever and not to be worried. Of course, one time, she wound up in the hospital with pneumonia. I got worried after that—she just kept coughing, but Dr. Wood told me she was just prone to colds.

To the best of her mother's knowledge, Lindsay's cough is not accompanied by fever, rhinorrhea, irritability, or feeding problems. "It's a really wet-sounding cough, but she seems to be OK besides that."

Your physical examination reveals the following:

Gen: Playful, smiling baby, very thin looking; afebrile

Skin: No rashes, jaundice, bruising, or other lesions

HEENT: Normal fontanelles; normal ears, nose, throat, and palates

   Follows object with eyes through 180 degrees; turns head to localized sounds

Resp: No chest deformities; normal respiratory rate; normal breath sounds; no adventitious sounds; no cyanosis or clubbing; patient coughs occasionally during examination

CVS: Pulse = 100/min; normal heart sounds; no murmurs; normal femoral pulses

Abdomen: Normal bowel sounds; no masses

GU: Normal genitalia

MSK: normal hips

Neuro: Gen: playful, alert baby

   good body tone

   sits unassisted

   grasps object without difficulty

Questions

1. The review of systems reveals chronic cough. Are you concerned about this?
2. What are the most common causes of chronic cough in infants?
3. How would you further evaluate Lindsay's cough?

Discussion

1. Chronic cough can represent a number of conditions, some of them quite serious. It definitely deserves further evaluation.

2. Like failure to thrive, chronic cough is a problem with an enormous number of potential causes. The most common causes, however, are recurrent viral infections and reactive airway disease initiated by viral infections (Kamei, 1991). Other common causes include allergies, irritation from environmental stimuli such as smoke, and infections such as chlamydial pneumonitis and tuberculosis. Less common but more serious causes include foreign body aspiration, interstitial pneumonia, conditions of inadequate mechanical clearance such as cystic fibrosis and the immotile cilia syndrome, and congenital anomalies such as tracheoesophageal fistula.

3. Kamei (1991) describes a clear approach to discussing chronic cough that participants may find useful. The history includes questions about overall well-being, growth, medications, immunizations, fever, and maternal health. This has already been provided. The quality of the cough sometimes helps with the diagnosis. A dry, croupy cough is usually associated with upper airways disease. The chronology of the cough is also useful. Cough that occurs after feedings may be due to reflux disease or to a tracheoesophageal fistula. Cough that is due to foreign body aspiration sometimes first manifests itself as a choking episode. The family history sometimes provides useful information. A family history of asthma or atopy, for example, makes the diagnosis of reactive airways disease in the infant more likely.

The physical examination should focus on the general health of the child through measurements of weight and so on, which has been done in this case. The pulmonary exam should include identification of chest deformities (e.g., barrel-shaped chest), tachypnea, clubbing, and cyanosis, in addition to auscultatory findings. The child should be examined as well for signs of atopy, such as eczema. Much of this physical examination has been performed.

Beyond the history and physical examination, further evaluation is needed in children who have chronic cough **accompanied by signs of serious disease,** such as **failure to thrive, history of pneumonia, or hemoptysis.** Lindsay, therefore, qualifies for further evaluation. This is an uncommon situation. Most cases of chronic cough can be observed or treated empirically with bronchodilators if reactive airways disease is a possibility. Kamei (1991) suggests a TB test and CXR to further evaluate chronic cough, as well as a CBC, which may provide several useful clues. A lymphocytosis may suggest pertussis; a lymphopenia, an immune disorder or viral infection. Eosinophilia accompanies many allergic disorders and chlamydia pneumonia. Anemia is consistent with serious chronic diseases such as cystic fibrosis or pulmonary hemosiderosis. Anemia, however, is a relatively nonspecific finding, as it may also be the result of failure to thrive and malnutrition in general.

See "The Rest of the Story," which follows.

The Rest of the Story

You come to learn that the services of a social worker, Joanna Fernandez, are available at the closest community hospital, in Kingman, Arizona. You call Joanna, who tells you she would be happy to see Tina and Lindsay within the next couple of days and to determine whether they are in need of help in purchasing food and other supplies. A nurse at the hospital has several years of experience in making breast-feeding assessments and would be happy to join the multidisplinary team involved in this case. There is a nutritionist available at the community hospital, but she has little experience with children and tells you she would be uncomfortable making a nutritional assessment in this case. Dr. Paul Lowry, a pediatrician, also works at the community hospital, and he tells you he would be happy to provide whatever help he can, including help with nutritional rehabilitation. He is also able to provide a formal developmental assessment sometime in the near future. There are, unfortunately, no pediatric subspecialists in the vicinity. You ask Tina and Lindsay to drive to Kingman to have some lab tests done that will help assess Lindsay's cough. A CXR and TB test (PPD) are obtained. The CXR is read as normal by a radiologist. The CBC reveals a hemoglobin of 5.5mM (8.9g/dL), with hypochromic, microcytic indices and no other abnormalities.

With Tina and Russell's permission, you make a home visit to assess the social and psychological function of the household in a general manner. Your account of that visit reads as follows:

I drove to the trailer park in the morning. The streets had no names, and all in all it was somewhat of a disorganized place, with all sorts of trailers dispersed among larger mobile homes. However, I found the mobile home in which I was interested without much difficulty. I recognized the old Chevy Malibu in which Tina and Lindsay came to my office. I knocked on the screen door, and a tall, thin young man in a baseball cap, T-shirt, and jeans emerged. "You must be Russell!" I said. He nodded his head in agreement. "I'm the doctor looking after Tina and Lindsay." Russell stepped aside, letting me enter his home.

The mobile home, which looked quite dusty and weathered on the outside, actually had a freshly renovated interior. The place was spotlessly clean and appeared to be well furnished. Tina was sitting in a recliner watching television. "Hi, Doctor. Thanks for stopping by. Lindsay's in her crib. I'll go get her." I asked Tina if Lindsay had a nice crib. She offered to show it to me and led me into the main bedroom in which all three members of the household sleep. Lindsay was lying on her back, looking quite content and cheerful, attempting to grasp the rotating toy that circled above. The bedroom was, like the living room, clean and well furnished. In the closet was a supply of diapers and baby powder. Tina picked Lindsay up and we walked out of the bedroom together.

"I wanted to see if everything was all right in your home," I told Tina. Russell remained aloof.

"Well, Doctor, things are pretty good," Tina said. "We're doing OK for money. Things are a bit more stable now. I can't complain. How were those test results?"

"Well, the CXR looks fine. The blood test shows that Lindsay has a mild anemia; in other words, her blood count is a little low. That really isn't surprising in children who are undernourished."

"Well, is that serious?"

"Well, anemia is often just a sign of some other disease going on. That's what we have to investigate further. I have to take a look at Lindsay to read her TB test." I read Lindsay's skin test as negative. I tried to engage Russell in conversation. "Russell, how are you doing? How are you adjusting to the changes?"

"I'm OK, Doctor. Takes a bit of getting used to." Russell spoke in an almost imperceptible soft voice and with a near-blank expression on his face. Tina told me that she had spoken to her parents recently and that they were very concerned about her and Lindsay. She told them she was doing quite well but did miss home terribly. At that point, the telephone rang.

"Russ, can you take Lindsay? It's probably for me." Tina handed the baby to her boyfriend. He held her snugly in his arms, and for the first time I saw a smile on his face as he teased the playful child. "Russ is great with the baby," Tina said, as she walked to answer the phone. "At first he was uncomfortable around her—now he loves her." As Tina answered her call, I asked Russ if it was OK if I took a look around. He had no objection. I went to the kitchen. The refrigerator was well stocked with an enormous number of frozen dinners, hot dogs, and condiments. In the cupboards, I found about a dozen bottles of Gerber's baby foods, representing virtually all varieties. There were some bananas and oranges on the kitchen counter. In general, it looked like a tidy, well-stocked kitchen. I continued to wander around. The bathroom was quite well kept. There were several combat magazines atop the toilet, which I presumed represented Russell's leisure reading.

I heard Tina hang up, and I returned to the living room. "That was my friend Gertrude from Odessa, just keeping me up to date on the latest gossip back home!" Russell was rocking Lindsay back and forth, and she appeared to be drifting off to sleep.

"Well, I'm quite impressed. This is quite a nice place," I told Tina.

"Well, it's nothing like my parents' place, but it's OK for the time being."

Tina offered me a cup of coffee, but as I was pressed for time, I declined. Despite the turmoil that had recently characterized her life, Tina appeared to have found a comfortable home for herself and her child. Furthermore, Russell seemed to enjoy looking after his girlfriend's daughter. I told Tina about the other people who were willing to help assess Lindsay's failure to thrive. She seemed anxious to get on with the evaluation. I told her I would make the necessary arrangements. I left with a positive feeling about the household and told Tina and Russell that I and the other members of the team would do our best to get to the root of Lindsay's problem.

PART IV

The Problem

Upon completing your home visit, you return to your office and arrange for Tina and Lindsay to have a social work and breast-feeding assessment in Kingman 2 days later. You call Tina with this appointment information and ask her to return the following day to your office for further evaluation.

Prior to Tina and Lindsay's return, you are called by both Joanna Fernandez and the nurse who made the breast-feeding assessment. Joanna tells you that Tina and Russell are coping extremely well with their limited income. She feels that they provide a safe and comfortable environment for Lindsay. You tell her that you had the same impression after making a home visit. The nurse tells you that Tina has appropriate technique in breast-feeding. She feeds Lindsay on demand and there is every indication that Lindsay takes to the breast very well. She is surprised that a child who feeds so well has failed to gain weight. You thank the nurse for her help and tell her you will continue to evaluate the baby.

Tina and Lindsay return to your office. Tina tells you Lindsay continues to cough, but otherwise she has been doing quite well.

Questions

1. Where would you go from here?

Discussion

1. At this point in the group discussion, it may be best to review what conclusions can be drawn from the assessment so far. Lindsay was born a healthy baby to a healthy mother. She appeared to develop growth deficiency around 3 months of age. She has been hospitalized for pneumonia and has a persistent, chronic cough. It is easy to implicate psychosocial factors in this child's failure to thrive, given that Tina is a young mother living with a somewhat peculiar young man in relative social isolation. Through the limited resources available in the community, it is apparent, however, that Tina and Russell have provided a comfortable and supportive environment for the baby.

The limited laboratory results show no evidence of obvious pulmonary disease that could account for Lindsay's chronic cough. A CBC shows anemia suggestive of chronic disease—a relatively nonspecific finding. As noted, there are a number of chronic diseases compatible with anemia and chronic cough, including pulmonary hemosiderosis and cystic fibrosis. The picture of failure to thrive, history of pneumonia, persistent cough, and anemia is certainly compatible with cystic fibrosis. A reasonable starting point for further evaluation would be testing for this condition. Some even include testing for cystic fibrosis in the initial evaluation of failure to thrive (Barness, 1992).

PART V

The Problem

You review the results of the breast-feeding evaluation and social work assessment with Tina. "See, I told you I was breast-feeding just fine," she responds.

You discuss further evaluation of Lindsay's failure to thrive and recommend evaluation for cystic fibrosis. Tina interrupts you immediately, "Cystic fibrosis! Hey, my aunt had that. She died before I was born! She was my mom's sister."

Questions

1. How is cystic fibrosis inherited?
2. Without further diagnostic testing at this point, describe a hypothesis that accounts for how Lindsay may have inherited cystic fibrosis.
3. How does one test for this condition?
4. How would you explain the need for further testing and evaluation to Tina? What would you tell her about cystic fibrosis?

See "The Rest of the Story" after the following Discussion section.

Discussion

1. Cystic fibrosis (CF) is inherited in an *autosomal recessive* fashion. The defect is on chromosome 7, in the gene that encodes the *cystic fibrosis transmembrane conductance regulator* (CFTR) protein, which regulates the transport of ions across cell membranes. Cystic fibrosis is the most common fatal autosomal recessive disease affecting Caucasians.

2. A recessive gene is expressed only when present in both members of a chromosomal pair. If there is expression of the gene for cystic fibrosis in Lindsay, she must have two copies of the defective gene, one from each parent, Tina and her former boyfriend, Ryan Voeller. As Tina is a healthy young woman, she must have only one copy of the defective gene. She must be a *carrier* of the cystic fibrosis gene or a

heterozygote. We know little about Ryan Voeller's medical problems, but according to Tina, he is in good health. As cystic fibrosis is a serious condition with many manifestations, it is likely that during her relationship with Ryan, Tina would have learned whether he has the disease. Ryan therefore is most likely a heterozygote as well. In autosomal recessive inheritance, one quarter of the offspring of heterozygotes will be homozygotes, one quarter will be normal, and one half will be heterozygotes.

We do know that Ryan had an older brother who died of a "lung problem," the nature of which is unknown to Tina. It is quite possible that this condition was a manifestation of cystic fibrosis. In other words, Ryan's brother may have been a

C = Normal CFTR gene
c = Defective CFTR gene

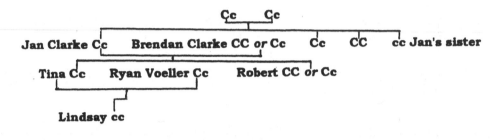

NOTE: C = normal CFTR gene; c = defective CFTR géne.

Figure 10.6   Cystic Fibrosis Pedigree for Lindsay Clarke

homozygote. Tina's mother's sister died of complications of cystic fibrosis. She was also, therefore, a homozygote.

Given this information, none of which is absolutely certain, and keeping in mind the principal of autosomal recessive inheritance, one can construct the pedigree shown in Figure 10.6.

3. Despite important discoveries in the past 10 years concerning the genetics of cystic fibrosis, widespread genetic testing remains elusive. Of the defects in the CFTR gene, 70% correspond to the mutation identified as deltaF508. There are more than 400 other mutations that account for the remainder. Genetic testing is available in many centers for potential carriers of the CF gene. The sweat test remains the mainstay of diagnosis when cystic fibrosis is suspected clinically (Veeze, 1995). The diagnosis of cystic fibrosis can be made on the basis of typical clinical features, such as pancreatitis and chronic cough, and on two separate sweat chloride results of greater than

60 mEq/L. Warwick describes a detailed point system on which the diagnosis can be made based on clinical features, family history, and laboratory results (Warwick, 1996).

Availability of the sweat test is usually quite limited. Furthermore, it should be performed in laboratories experienced in the procedure of collecting sweat and performing the analysis. Even under such conditions, the test is notoriously unreliable and may need to be repeated several times before a conclusive diagnosis can be made (Rosenstein & Langbaum, 1987). To complicate matters further, elevated sweat chloride values are found in a variety of other conditions, including celiac disease and psychosocial failure to thrive (Ruddy & Scanlin, 1987). There is little question that at this point in the management of the case, additional help is required. There are specialized clinics in larger centers with experience in testing and treatment of cystic fibrosis whose expertise should definitely be considered. Dr. Lowry may be helpful in pinpointing the appropriate resources.

4. There is no simple answer to these questions. Further testing probably needs to take place in a distant specialized center, which will be a major inconvenience to Tina and Lindsay. There is no question that testing for cystic fibrosis is justified, given the clinical picture and Lindsay's family history. There is also evidence that the earlier a diagnosis of CF is made, the better the prognosis (Danker-Roelse & te Meerman, 1995).

The possibility of a diagnosis of CF will certainly be quite disturbing for Tina and perhaps for Russell as well. The nature of this disease, its complications, and its prognosis should be carefully explained to Tina. She should be told that there is a strong chance that she is a carrier of the CF gene. Tina will undoubtedly receive more comprehensive counseling at a specialized center, but it is best to prepare her well for the ensuing further evaluation.

The Rest of the Story

You tell Tina that, given her family history and the problems Lindsay is presently having, a diagnosis of cystic fibrosis is a strong possibility. You inform her that the test cannot be reliably performed in Kingman and that she will probably have to take Lindsay to a larger center. You explain that cystic fibrosis is a serious disease and that for this reason, thorough testing is extremely important. At this point, Tina interrupts you: "Well, how serious is it?"

You tell Tina that cystic fibrosis is a genetic disease in which an important protein is made incorrectly, resulting in a variety of problems with the lungs, digestive tract, and other systems in the body. You tell her that there is presently no cure for cystic fibrosis but that a variety of treatments are available to treat complications of the disease such as frequent episodes of pneumonia.

Tina asks, "Is Lindsay going to die like my aunt Catherine?"

You inform Tina that, unfortunately, patients with cystic fibrosis do not have a normal life expectancy, but the average survival time is increasing as better treatments are developed. You tell her that many patients live well into their 30s.

At this point, Tina begins to cry and holds Lindsay tightly. You provide a comforting hand and reassure her that all will be done to ensure that Lindsay lives as long and healthy a life as possible.

"So I'm the one with the bad gene then, is that right?" Tina asks, sobbing.

You explain the genetics of cystic fibrosis and tell her that if Lindsay does indeed have the disease, both Tina and Ryan must be carriers. You also tell Tina that you suspect that Ryan's brother died of complications of cystic fibrosis.

"Where are we going to get all this testing done?" Tina asks.

At this point, you decide to find out the answer to that question, and you give Dr. Lowry a call. He tells you that he has little expertise in the testing and management of CF, and he refers you to a specialty clinic in Scottsdale, Arizona. Tina feels it would be extremely difficult to get to Scottsdale, particularly if the evaluation process takes more than a couple of days.

Doctor, if I'm going to go all the way down there, I might as well go home. I'm getting really homesick anyway. Russ hasn't found a job. He's talking about coming home. I think I'll call my parents with the news and see what they think I should do.

You tell Tina that the support of her parents would be a welcome resource at this stage, and you pledge your continued help.

Conclusion

Tina calls her parents, who are immediately distraught. They ask her to return home as soon as possible. She agrees. She stops by your office prior to leaving to thank you for all your help.

One week later, you get a call from Dr. Wood, who tells you he made arrangements for Lindsay to be seen in a CF clinic in Texas. The diagnosis has been confirmed. Genetic testing has revealed that Tina is a CF carrier. Tina and her parents are enrolled in a special counseling program. Lindsay is receiving comprehensive CF care from a multidisciplinary team. Dr. Wood plans to continue to provide routine pediatric care, and he tells you, "I hope she starts to gain weight soon." He also confesses, "You know, I should have suspected the diagnosis a while ago. When I admitted Lindsay for pneumonia, CF never crossed my mind." Dr. Wood compliments you on your clinical acumen.

References

Barness, L. H. (1992). Failure to thrive. In R. A. Hoekelman (Ed.), *Primary pediatric care* (pp. 704-707). St. Louis, MO: Mosby-Year Book.

Berwick, D. M., Levy, J. C., & Kleinerman, R. (1982). Failure to thrive: Diagnostic yield of hospitalization. *Archives of Disease in Childhood, 57*, 347-351.

Bithoney, W. G., Dubowitz, H., & Egan, H. (1992). Failure to thrive/growth deficiency. *Pediatrics in Review, 13*(12), 453-460.

Bradley, R. H., & Caldwell, B. M. (1981). Pediatric usefulness of home assessment. *Advances in Behavioral Pediatrics, 2*, 61-80.

Casey, P. H. (1983). Failure to thrive: A reconceptualization. *Journal of Developmental and Behavioral Pediatrics, 4*, 63-66.

Casey, P. H., Bradley, R., & Wortham, B. (1984). Social and nonsocial home environments of infants with nonorganic failure-to-thrive. *Pediatrics, 73*(3), 348-353.

Dankert-Roelse, J. E., & te Meerman, G. J. (1995). Long-term prognosis of patients with cystic fibrosis in relation to early detection by neonatal screening and treatment in a cystic fibrosis centre. *Thorax, 50*(7), 712-718.

Drotar, D., Malone, C., & Devost, C. (1985). Early preventive intervention in failure to thrive: Methods and early outcome. In D. Drotar (Ed.), *New directions in failure to thrive: Implications for research and practice.* New York: Plenum.

Frank, D. A., & Zeisel, S. H. (1988). Failure to thrive. *Pediatric Clinics of North America, 35*(6), 1187-1206.

Gomez, F., Galvan, R. R., Frenk, S., Muñoz, J. C., Chavez, R., & Vazquez, J. (1956). Mortality in second and third degree malnutrition. *Journal of Tropical Pediatrics, 2*, 77-83.

Kamei, R. K. (1991). Chronic cough in children. *Pediatric Clinics of North America, 38*(3), 593-605.

Leung, A.K.C., Robson, L. M., & Fagan, J. E. (1993). Assessment of the child with failure to thrive. *American Family Physician, 48*(8), 1432-1438.

MacLean, W. C., de Romana, G. L., Masse, E., et al. (1980). Nutritional management of chronic diarrhea and malnutrition: Primary reliance on oral feeding. *Journal of Pediatrics, 97*, 316-323.

Rosenstein, B. J., & Langbaum, T. S. (1987). Misdiagnosis of cystic fibrosis. *Clinical Pediatrics, 26*(2), 78-89.

Ruddy, R. M., & Scanlin, T. F. (1987). Abnormal sweat electrolytes in a case of celiac disease and a case of psychosocial failure to thrive. *Clinical Pediatrics, 26*(2), 83-89.

Schwartz, R., & Abegglen, J. A. (1996). Failure to thrive: An ambulatory approach. *Nurse Practitioner, 21*(5), 19-35.

Sills, R. H. (1978). Failure to thrive—The role of clinical and laboratory evaluations. *American Journal of Diseases of Children, 132,* 967-969.

Snow, C. W. (1989). *Infant development.* Englewood Cliffs, NJ: Prentice Hall.

Veeze, H. J. (1995). Diagnosis of cystic fibrosis. *Netherlands Journal of Medicine, 46*(6), 271-274.

Viteri, F. (1981). Primary protein-calorie malnutrition. In R. M. Suskind (Ed.), *Textbook of pediatric nutrition.* New York: Raven.

Warwick, W. J. (1996). *Guidebook for cystic fibrosis.* Minneapolis, MN: Cystic Fibrosis Center.

11. MANAGEMENT OF ASTHMA

Ms. Liane Webber

*Goal: The goal of this group discussion exercise
is to develop and evaluate the participants' understanding
of the management of asthma in a young person.*

Specific Objectives: Upon completion of this group discussion exercise, each participant should be able to accomplish the following:

1. Obtain a focused, relevant history from a patient initially presenting with typical symptoms of asthma.
2. Explain the technique of spirometry and its role in the diagnosis, assessment, and monitoring of asthma.
3. Determine the severity of asthma based on history, physical findings, and objective measures of respiratory function.
4. List the categories of present pharmacologic therapy for asthma, and provide examples and indications for each type of medication.
5. Teach a patient how to use a metered-dose inhaler, spacer device, and home peak-flow monitor.
6. Develop an individualized self-management plan that includes adjustment of medications, recording of peak flows and symptoms, and identification and avoidance of triggers by the patient.

PART I

The Patient

Social History

Liane Webber is a white, 15-year-old girl who lives with her family in the Wisconsin city of Eau Claire, where she was born and raised. She is presently enrolled in her freshman year of high school.

Liane's parents divorced 6 years ago. Her father, Peter Webber, 49, is a taxi driver in St. Paul, Minnesota. Liane's mother, Barbara Naus, works as a waitress in a diner in Eau Claire.

The patient's brother, Carl, 22, is currently enrolled in a carpentry apprenticeship program. Barbara and her children rent a small three-bedroom home that they also share with Barbara's boyfriend of 3 years, Jeff Hale. Two cats, whom Liane has smothered with affection since she was 10, complete the household.

The patient has had a difficult family life. Barbara and Peter's divorce was tough for both children, especially Carl, who dropped out of high school shortly thereafter. He has been plagued with drug and alcohol abuse and unemployment ever since. He maintains a fragile and occasionally physically abusive relationship with his girlfriend, Stella. Though he shares the same home with the patient, Carl and Liane rarely speak to each other. Liane says, "We haven't been close since we were very little. He's such a screwup. It's scary sometimes." Carl's relationship with his mother is similarly lacking in communication. On the other hand, he admires his father, whom he describes as a "free spirit." He often drives to St. Paul to spend a weekend with him, during which Carl and his father do little more than watch television together in Peter's rather shabby apartment.

Jeff Hale has not received a warm reception in the household from Carl and Liane. He neither contributes to the rent nor pays for any other household expenses, a fact Carl often brings to everyone's attention. Moreover, Mr. Hale has felt the need to exert some parental authority over Barbara's children, and this has received a cool if not sometimes openly hostile reaction. Most disturbing to Liane is the fact that Jeff and Barbara have actually talked about having a child together. In her words, "I mean. That's crazy. She wants to have a kid with this loser. She's 42 for God's sake. It just won't happen. What a stupid idea!" Although this and other disagreements characterize the relationship between Liane and her mother, they remain very close. In Barbara's words, "She's all I have left. I had Carl, but I'm losing him now. I love her more than anything."

Liane is a poor student. She came close to failing a year of middle school and is presently struggling in high school. Barbara, who has attended several parent-teacher meetings, has been told that Liane is a bright and capable girl but that she rarely hands in assignments in time, and when she does, her work is below any reasonable standard. Her poor performance on tests, Liane's mother has been told, is certainly the result of lack of preparation. Barbara has always found it difficult to motivate Liane to do her homework or to study for exams. For her part, Liane often insists, "I can't stand it sometimes. I mean I hate studying. I think I'd rather be digging a ditch or something."

The patient spends her afternoons and often her evenings at a nearby shopping mall, where she "hangs out" with a group of friends from school whom her mother describes as "kind of a bad crowd." She does not have a boyfriend. She is not involved in any extracurricular school activities, nor any other clubs or sports. She took piano lessons from age 10 to 13, but the piano she inherited from her grandmother now sits idle, gathering dust in the dining room of the family home. Liane earns a small amount of money baby-sitting the 4-year-old daughter of a young couple who live down the street.

Barbara describes her family's background as Lutheran, of Dutch and German ancestry—similar to that of her ex-husband's. Neither she nor her children is involved in any organized religious activities.

The family is presently enrolled in a government-sponsored medical assistance program that pays for doctors' visits, prescriptions, and hospital care.

Past Personal and Family Medical History

Liane suffered from frequent asthma symptoms as a young child. This was manifested as episodic attacks, usually accompanying an upper respiratory tract infection, which gradually disappeared by the time Liane was 9 years old. She has never been hospitalized for asthma or any other condition. She presently experiences mild shortness of breath and wheezing occasionally during or after gym class, for which she sometimes uses an albuterol inhaler. She has had no evaluation for asthma or any other treatment since she was very young.

Accompanied by her mother, she saw a physician 2 years ago for acne, and topical antibiotic cream was prescribed. Her acne has largely disappeared, and apart from her inhaler, she presently uses no medications.

Liane began menstruating at age 12 and has had regular periods ever since. She has never been sexually active.

Barbara Naus suffers from frequent migraine headaches and obesity. She is otherwise healthy. As noted, Carl Webber has had trouble with illicit drugs, specifically marijuana and heroin, for which he has visited and continues to visit a treatment center. He has had both gonorrhea and chlamydia in the past. He had a right second metacarpal fracture last year, acquired during a fist fight outside a local bar. He has no other past medical history.

Peter Webber's health is a bit of a mystery. Liane suspects her father is an alcoholic, but her mother insists that this is not the case. Liane knows that her father has a "heart condition" but is unsure about the details.

The entire household smokes. Liane began smoking approximately 5 months ago—usually 3 or 4 cigarettes a day with her friends from school. Her consumption has gradually increased to 15 to 20 cigarettes a day, which uses up a substantial portion of the money she earns as a baby-sitter.

The Problem

You are a family physician in a solo practice in a small city with complete access to all diagnostic facilities and specialists. Liane Webber, a 15-year-old girl, comes to your office alone, complaining of cough, wheezing, congestion, and episodic difficulty breathing. She tells you her symptoms began approximately 5 days ago and have steadily worsened. She reports no fever, sputum, otalgia, or any sore throat. She presently does not feel any chest tightness or shortness of breath (SOB). She tells you, "I think it's asthma. I think I need a new puffer. Can you give me one?"

Questions

1. What additional elements of the history would you like to obtain?

2. Describe how you would perform a focused physical examination of the patient.

3. What conditions can be confused with asthma?

4. Describe in detail what further diagnostic testing, if any, you would perform at this visit.

Discussion

1. The diagnosis of asthma is supported by the presence of the cardinal symptoms of cough, wheeze, and shortness of breath (Wiedemann & Kavuru, 1994). According to the patient profile, the patient has had little difficulty with asthma prior to this episode and therefore requires a thorough evaluation. To make an accurate diagnosis and to assess the severity of the disease, a much more detailed history is needed. In addition to the typical symptoms of asthma, it is important to gather the following information: (a) associated conditions such as rhinitis, sinusitis, nasal polyps, and atopic dermatitis; (b) age at onset and disease progression; (c) usual asthma precipitants such as exercise, medications, allergies, and so on; (d) previous and current treatments; (e) prior hospital-based care; (f) days missed from school or work; (g) nocturnal symptoms; (h) effect on lifestyle, growth, and school; (i) smoking, including exposure to passive smoke; and (j) family history of asthma or atopy (Allen & Graber, 1990). Some of this information is provided in the patient profile. For the remainder of a comprehensive initial history, refer to "The Rest of the Story," which follows this discussion section.

2. There is no mystery to what constitutes a focused physical examination of an asthmatic patient. In addition to a respiratory exam, physical evidence of associated conditions, such as nasal polyps and sinusitis, should be sought. See "The Rest of the Story."

3. It is important, in all patients presenting with a clinical picture like that above, to keep in mind conditions that can mimic asthma (Allen & Graber, 1990; Shuttari, 1995; Wiedemann & Kavuru, 1994). In adults, these include laryngeal dysfunction, mechanical obstruction of the airways, congestive heart failure, and pulmonary embolism, all of which can cause wheezing or stridor that may be confused with asthma. In children, the differential diagnosis includes foreign body obstruction, vascular rings, tracheomalacia, epiglotitis, croup, and bronchopulmonary dysplasia. There is no evidence that Liane has any of these other conditions.

4. Although the history and physical examination are certainly consistent with asthma, the clinical picture is often inaccurate, sometimes in the actual diagnosis and more often in the assessment of severity. An objective measure of lung function is valuable in confirming the diagnosis of asthma, evaluating its severity, and measuring the response to treatment. For these reasons, pulmonary function testing is widely advocated in the initial assessment of the asthmatic patient (Allen & Graber, 1990; Asthma Committee, 1996; Joint Task Force on Practice Parameters, 1995; L'Enfant & Khaltaev, 1995; Shuttari, 1995; Wiedemann & Kavuru, 1994). The usual device used in physicians' offices or testing facilities is the *spirometer.* These instruments are designed to measure respired volume or flow. Volume-recording spirometers are very outdated; they are bulky and do not normally incorporate computer technology, unlike most modern flow-sensing spirometers. This technology permits most flow spirometers automatically to calculate various measures of respiratory function, store results, determine reference values for individual patients, and so on. *Peak flow meters,* which play a valuable role in patient self-management of asthma, are more widely available in physicians' offices but provide only one mea-

sure of ventilatory function. Spirometry is the preferred method and will be described in detail.

In the technique of spirometry, the patient performs a **forced vital capacity** maneuver (FVC). The patient is asked either to sit erect or to stand, inspire fully, seal his or her lips around the mouthpiece of the spirometer, and exhale as fast and for as long as possible. Precision is improved by repeating the procedure at least twice. The measurements derived include the **forced vital capacity** (the maximal amount of expired air), the **forced vital capacity in one second** (FEV1), and the **peak expiratory flow** (PEF) or **peak flow,** the maximal rate of volume expiration. The data are graphically represented as a volume-time curve or as a *flow-volume loop.* Asthma is an obstructive lung disease, and the flow-volume loop in an acutely asthmatic patient follows a particular pattern (Pierce & Johns, 1995).

There are a number of other specialized tests that are sometimes performed in asthmatic patients, such as bronchoprovocation with methacholine or histamine. The impressive, evidence-based guidelines of the asthma committee of the Canadian Thoracic Society (Asthma Committee, 1996) include a recommendation of allergy assessment in "most asthmatics." The aim is to identify particular asthma triggers. Other important organizations (Allen & Graber, 1990; L'Enfant & Khaltaev, 1995) recommend allergy testing only on a selective basis, when triggers are not obvious. In any case, allergy testing is best done when the patient's asthma is stable. Any discussion participant who advocates allergy testing at the initial assessment should realize that the priority is to make the correct diagnosis, assess the severity of the disease, and institute an effective, immediate management plan.

The Rest of the Story

You tell Liane that before considering treatment, you would like to get more information so that you can help confirm the diagnosis of asthma and assess its severity.

Liane tells you she began to experience a runny nose about 5 days ago and that her cough began shortly thereafter. The cough has been worse at night, making it difficult for her to fall asleep. She has had three episodes of SOB, one occurring at night, over the past 4 days. She describes a feeling of "chest tightness" that accompanies her shortness of breath. She administered three or four puffs of her inhaler during each episode, which gradually brought relief in about 1 hr. Liane also tells you she can hear herself wheezing from time to time. She tells you that the cough persists, together with occasional mild shortness of breath, in between "attacks."

Liane denies symptoms of sinusitis. To the best of her knowledge, she has never had nasal polyps nor any skin disorders apart from acne. She has not felt this way in recent memory and identifies vigorous exercise as the only trigger for her asthma. According to the patient, "sometimes when we're running or playing basketball in gym class, I get a bit winded and use my puffer once. I start to feel better in about 10 or 15 minutes. That doesn't happen very often. I mean, the last time I needed a puff before last week was probably nearly a year ago. Besides, it's not nearly as bad as this. I don't think I've felt this bad since I was a little kid."

As noted in the patient profile, Liane has never been hospitalized for asthma. To the best of her knowledge, she has never received treatment in an emergency room. She does not know with which medications she has been treated in the past other than albuterol.

The patient has missed the past 3 days of school, which she describes as "one of two good things about being sick." She tells you, however, that she rarely misses school, and that asthma has had little impact on her lifestyle or attendance in recent years. She is not aware of any impact on her growth. In her words, "Hey, I'm a big girl, as you can see." You ask this young lady what the other "good thing about being sick" is, to which she replies, "Oh. I don't feel like smoking. That's the other thing. I mean, I've really cut down a lot. That has got to be good for you." Liane tells you, "Our house has five chimneys—only one made of brick!" by which she means that the entire household smokes heavily. Moreover, most of Liane's friends smoke before and after school and often between classes.

To the best of the patient's knowledge, no other family member has had asthma, eczema, or any other skin disorder.

Physical Examination (with Liane's corresponding summarized results)

General: Very pleasant, talkative, heavy-set 15-year-old girl in no apparent distress.
Vitals: P = 84/min; BP = 115/85 (no pulsus paradoxus); RR = 26/min; T = 37.2°C
HEENT: No facial tenderness
    No nasal polyps visualized
Resp: Inspection: no retractions/no accessory muscle use
Auscultation: slightly decreased breath sounds throughout
    Wheezes heard on expiration throughout

PART II

The Problem

You do not have a spirometer in your office. There is a modern flow-sensing spirometer in the office of Dr. Lars Carlsson, down the hall. Dr. Carlsson's medical assistant tells you she would be more than happy to perform pulmonary function testing on your patient. You send Liane to your colleague's office and ask her to return with a copy of her test results. She produces a piece of paper that includes the following data:

Patient: Liane Webber// DOB: 05/19/81(f)
    Height: 177 cm; race: Cauc.
    FEV1 (predicted) 3.30L
    FVC (predicted) 3.70L
    PEF (predicted) 420L/min
Results:
    flow-volume loop   FEV1 (best) = 2.31L
    best result   FVC (best) = 3.64L
                        PEF (best) = 300L/min

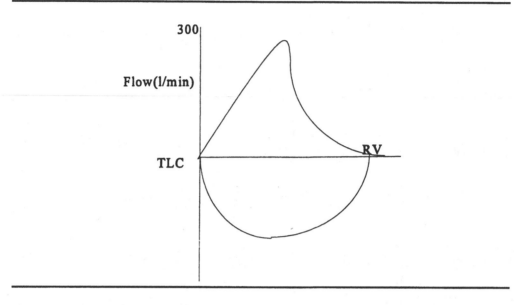

Figure 11.1 Flow Volume Loop

Questions

1. How would you interpret Liane's spirometric data?
2. Putting together the information from the history, physical examination, and spirogram, how would you assess the severity of Liane's condition?
3. Describe how you would manage this case from this point.

Discussion

1. The top part of the flow-volume loop represents expiration, whereby the lung volume decreases from total lung capacity (TLC) to residual volume (RV). The change in lung volume is the vital capacity (VC). Note that the flow rate reaches a peak and then drops off at lower lung volumes until it reaches zero at the RV. At this point, the direction of flow is reversed as the patient inspires. Asthma is an obstructive lung disease, and Liane's optimal flow-volume loop shows a typically obstructive pattern. The PEF is dimished. Upon reaching the PEF, the flow rate de-

creases more precipitously than in a normal person, giving the expiratory portion of the curve a "scooped out" appearance.

In addition to a decreased peak flow, asthmatics typically present with a decreased FEV1. The FVC, or forced vital capacity, however, is often only slightly decreased or normal. Although it is reasonable to compare the obtained FEV1 to that value predicted from age, gender, and height, further individual variation independent of these three variables makes it useful to compare FEV1 to the patient's FVC. In other words, the FEV1/FVC ratio for an individual patient is a useful parameter. The lower limit of normal for this ratio is 70% to 75%. Unfortunately, even this ratio is somewhat dependent on age. This value is not given in Liane's spirometric data but is easily calculated as 63%. Liane's peak flow is also below normal, at 71% of her predicted value. One can conclude that the patient's pulmonary function tests are consistent with asthma. You may, in addition to obtaining the pulmonary function tests described above, wish to assess Liane's response to bronchodilator therapy. This can be easily done in the office setting. Most patients with moderate asthma will demonstrate a 15% or greater improvement in FEV1 after receiving an inhaled bronchodilator.

2. The history, physical examination, and pulmonary function provide a convincing clinical picture of asthma. The next step is to assign a severity grade. Asthma can be classified as mild, moderate, or severe, depending on several variables including number of exacerbations or "attacks," exercise tolerance, nocturnal symptoms, job or school attendance, pulmonary function tests, and required medication therapy (Shuttari, 1995). The National Heart, Lung and Blood Institute/ World Health Organization (NHLBI/ WHO) guidelines (L'Enfant & Khaltaev, 1995; see also Appendix) provide a more detailed classification of asthma, based on the clinical course over a period of time, and further classify acute asthma attacks. Under this system, asthma is classified as intermittent, mild persistent, moderate persistent, and severe persistent. Individual witnessed attacks are classified as mild, moderate, or severe, depending on ability to speak, alertness, respiratory rate, accessory muscle use, decrease in peak flow,

and so on. It is difficult to apply either classification system of chronic asthma to Liane Webber. Until very recently, she had only mild, occasional, exercise-induced asthma. Over the past 5 days she has had three attacks or acute exacerbations of asthma, and one that included nocturnal symptoms. She also has persistent mild shortness of breath and cough. Judging by the past 5 days, one could say that Liane has moderate or moderate persistent asthma. In addition to the history, the pulmonary function tests are of great value in determining the severity of disease.

Mild asthma is associated with a peak flow of 80% or greater of the predicted value; moderate, with 60% to 80%; and severe, with less than 60%. Patients with mild asthma usually have no spirometric abnormalities; those with moderate asthma show an obstructive pattern with FEV1 greater than 60% of the predicted value. Patients with severe asthma have an abnormal spirogram and an FEV1 often less than 60% of that predicted. Based on Liane's pulmonary function, therefore, she has moderate asthma.

3. There are an overwhelming number of comprehensive, well-researched guidelines for the management of asthma. The NHLBI/WHO (L'Enfant & Khaltaev, 1995) describes a *stepwise* approach to therapy in which the number and frequency of use of medications increases as the severity grade of asthma worsens. The asthma committee of the Canadian Thoracic Society has rejected the stepwise approach in favor of an **asthma continuum** (Asthma Committee, 1996), which is described as a "more dynamic therapeutic approach" that does not promote "an overly rigorous stratification of levels of asthma care." One can interpret this as the

adjustment of drug therapy to achieve good control, with less reliance on the severity grade. Whether this distinction has any practical value is uncertain. What is common in the management recommendations of most important organizations is the extensive involvement of the patient in the management of his or her own disease. As part of the management plan, for example, patients are expected to make adjustments to their medication based on self-monitoring of their PEF. This sort of self-management of asthma requires a great deal of patient education. In this regard, the National Asthma Education Program (1992) is a superb resource for both doctors and their patients with asthma that provides excellent information and worksheets on self-monitoring of peak flow and so on.

How would one begin to manage Liane's asthma? Management has three main components (Canadian Lung Association, 1994). **Patient education and self-management** have already been mentioned. **Environmental control,** which includes such measures as the avoidance of known triggers, is crucial. Finally, unlike the diabetic or hypertensive who can in some mild cases manage his or her own disease through nonpharmacologic means, the patient with asthma usually requires some form of **pharmacologic therapy** at the outset. The goals of therapy are to relieve symptoms, maintain normal activity, prevent exacerbations, and normalize tests of pulmonary function (Wiedermann & Kavuru, 1994).

Pharmacologic therapy is most likely to have an immediate impact on Liane's well-being. A more detailed discussion of the various drug treatments, their mechanism of action, side effects, and so on can be found elsewhere ("Drugs for Asthma,"

1995). The approach to drug therapy has changed in recent years. Asthma is now viewed as a chronic inflammatory disease, and anti-inflammatories, therefore, are the fundamental forms of therapy (British Thoracic Society, 1990). Corticosteroids, either in oral or inhaled form, are the most widely used anti-inflammatories and include *beclomethasone, budesonide, and flunisolide* (inhalers) and *prednisone* and *methlyprenisolone* (oral). They are effective in reducing airway swelling, mucus production, microvascular leakage, and increasing responsiveness of smooth-muscle beta receptors (L'Enfant & Khaltaev, 1995). *Cromolyn* and *nedocromil* are anti-inflammatory medications that are primarily used in the prevention of symptoms of mild to moderate asthma (Joint Task Force on Practice Parameters, 1995). They are both available in inhaled form.

Inhaled beta-2 agonists are the safest and most effective treatment for acute episodes of asthma. They include relatively nonselective and (the preferred) highly selective beta-2 agonists such as *albuterol.* They can be given orally or by inhalation and are available in short-acting and sustained-release forms (e.g., *salmeterol*).

Theophylline, when used as maintenance therapy, can reduce the frequency and severity of symptoms in the patient with chronic asthma (Joint Task Force on Practice Parameters, 1995). It is associated with a number of side effects and should be used with caution. Other medications that sometimes play a role in the management of asthma include anticholinergics and antihistamines. Their use is not conventional treatment for the patient initially presenting with asthma and should not be considered at this point in Liane's case.

As noted, it is fair to characterize the patient's asthma as "moderate" in severity. Precise recommendations as to drug therapy in such patients are variable. A reasonable approach is to prescribe an inhaled corticosteroid at a dose equivalent to 100μg to 400μg of beclomethasone dipropionate twice daily. An inhaled beta-2 agonist such as albuterol (100μg to 200μg) should be used only on an "as needed" basis. When used in conjunction with mild exercise-induced asthma, Liane should administer this medication 20 to 30 min *prior* to the start of exercise as a prophylactic measure (Wiedermann & Kavuru, 1994).

It is probably best to hold off on prophylactic agents such as cromolyn or theophylline until the remaining components of the management plan have been implemented and their effects assessed. One must also consider the question of whether to supplement the inhaled corticosteroids with steroids in oral form (usually prednisone). This is a controversial issue. Oral corticosteroids are known, when used early in an asthma exacerbation, to reduce emergency department visits and hospitalizations (Allen & Graber, 1990). The Asthma Committee of the Canadian Thoracic Society recommends the use of oral steroids only in cases of severe asthma (Asthma Committee, 1996). Not only are the precise indications for the use of oral corticosteroids uncertain, but recommendations about dosage vary greatly. Some recommend 0.5 to 1.0mg/kg of prednisone per day for a period of 1 to 2 weeks (Asthma Committee, 1996), others a universal dose of 40mg/day for just 5 days in adults (Allen & Graber, 1990). Liane is 15 years old, and although we do not know her precise weight, we do know she is a tall, heavy-set girl. It is easy to see that these two recommendations for prednisone dosage, when applied to Liane, would result in vastly different total dosages over the entire treatment period. Participants will probably already have been exposed to quite different clinical practices with respect to the use of oral steroids in asthma, and this issue may be a contentious one. The side effects of short courses of oral steroids are minimal.

The goals of education and self-management are to allow the patient to use medications correctly, to identify and avoid triggers, and to monitor disease status and take appropriate action. The preferred route of administration of many asthma medications is through a metered-dose inhaler (MDI) or "puffer." Unfortunately, roughly 30% of adults and 50% of children do not use their metered dose inhalers properly (Pierce & Johns, 1995). It is therefore important to review Liane's technique.

A "spacer" is a device that holds the inhaler medication in a chamber long enough for it to be inhaled slowly. It overcomes the problem of coordination of medication release and inspiration that often accompanies MDI use. Some advocate the use of spacers only in young children and those who demonstrate an inability to use an inhaler alone. Liane, who has some familiarity with the use of an inhaler, probably does not require a spacer. The National Asthma Education Program (1992) has excellent patient worksheets on the correct use of spacers and inhalers. There is no substitute, however, for a good demonstration. As inhalers and spacers are commonly prescribed and their ineffective use is a serious problem, family physicians should themselves be skilled in their use for demonstration purposes. At this point in the group discussion, a brief practical session in the use of inhalers and spacers would be appropriate.

When using an MDI alone, the cap is removed and the inhaler shaken. The user exhales slowly. The MDI is brought either in the mouth or 5cm from the open mouth. The release mechanism is pressed while the user inspires slowly and as deeply as possible. The breath is held for about 10 s prior to a slow expiration. The technique of use of a spacer is quite similar, except that the inhaler is first attached to a spacer, which in turn has a mouthpiece. As noted, the inhalation phase need not be coordinated with release of medication, as it remains in the chamber for several seconds.

In general, when a patient takes both beta-2 agonists and corticosteroids in inhaled form, the beta-2 agonist is inhaled first. It is recommended that after use of an inhaled corticosteroid, especially without a spacer, the patient rinse his or her mouth thoroughly to prevent oral candidiasis (Shuttari, 1995).

Asthmatic patients should have the ability to monitor their disease objectively through home peak flow monitoring. Small, inexpensive peak flow monitors are widely available, reasonably accurate, and easy to use with some basic teaching. Decreasing peak flow is a sensitive sign of airway obstruction that often appears prior to the onset of symptoms or presence of physical findings such as wheezing. Home monitoring, therefore, serves as a valuable gauge of the severity of asthma. It can be used to determine if the present medication regimen is working well, if a severe attack is imminent, and even to identify triggers. The technique of peak flow meter use is virtually identical to spirometry. In other words, the patient performs the forced expiratory maneuver in the erect position

three times and records the best result. Peak flow should be taken at least twice daily, morning and evening, for 2 weeks during the initial management period. It is normally lowest early in the morning and by evening increases by approximately 20% in the asthmatic patient who uses beta-2 agonists. Indeed, this characteristic peak flow *variability* is one criterion by which asthma can be diagnosed. Peak flow readings should also be taken before and after beta-2 agonist use to assess the response to therapy. During the first 2 weeks of self-monitoring, the patient should identify a "personal best" peak flow. As the predicted value is a function of age, height, and gender and does not account for further individual variation, the "personal best" value should be substituted for it as a basis for comparison.

The peak flow **zone system** (National Asthma Education Program, 1992) should be used by patients to make decisions about self-management. In the **green zone,** the peak flow is 80% to 100% of the patient's personal best, which means that no asthma symptoms are present and that medications should be taken as usual. The **yellow zone,** where peak flow is 50% to 80% of personal best, signals caution and a possible need for increased pharmacologic control. The **red zone** (peak flow less than 50%) signals that the patient should take immediate action. All this information should be kept in an asthma diary (National Asthma Education Program, 1992; see also Appendix), where peak flows are recorded together with any corresponding symptoms. Since Liane has yet to determine her personal best peak flow, she can in the interim use her predicted peak flow value of 420L/min for calculations in the *zone system*. The action plan that corresponds to the zone system should be individualized, but some possible recommendations are given below. Most important, the plan should be explained clearly to the patient. As noted, in the green zone, no intervention is required. In the yellow zone, the patient should take two extra puffs of beta-2 agonist and recheck peak flow in 20 to 30 min. If still in the yellow zone, the treatment can be repeated with two to four puffs. If peak flow still does not improve, the dosage of inhaled steroids should be doubled, and Liane's physician should be contacted. In the red zone, two to six puffs of beta-2 agonist should be taken immediately. Lack of improvement should be reported to the physician immediately. Oral steroids at a dose of 30mg of prednisone should be taken simultaneously.

Adolescents often have poor compliance with an asthma treatment plan. Liane neither benefits from the extremely close supervision provided by a parent to a young child nor the maturity and personal understanding that usually comes with adulthood. It would help if her mother were made thoroughly familiar with the action plan and were also involved in other aspects of self-management. She could, for example, encourage the patient to maintain good peak flow records and help identify triggers.

Home peak flow monitoring, of course, is not the only way to identify worsening asthma. Symptoms such as chronic cough, especially at night; shortness of breath; and chest tightness are all warning signs of deterioration. Liane should not hesitate to contact her physician if her symptoms worsen, at least for the next couple of weeks.

A **trigger** is an environmental or other stimulus that either precipitates an attack of asthma or makes existing asthma symptoms worse. Common triggers include pollens, molds, dust mites, animal danders, infections, exercise, and cold weather. The identification and avoidance of triggers is a key component of asthma management. At this point, Liane's history reveals four potential triggers. She herself has already identified vigorous exercise such as running as a stimulus that sometimes brings on mild asthma symptoms. As a child, asthma exacerbations accompanied an upper respiratory tract infection or "cold." This is the situation at present. Liane began having symptoms of rhinorrhea 5 days ago, and her asthma symptoms followed shortly thereafter. It is unlikely, however, that this was the first cold she has had since she was a young child. In other words, Liane has probably had several upper respiratory tract infections in recent years that were not associated with exacerbations of asthma. What has changed recently that has made her feel so lousy? Tobacco smoke, inhaled either firsthand or passively, is widely recognized as a trigger of asthma (Asthma Committee, 1996; L'Enfant & Khaltaev, 1995; Joint Task Force on Practice Parameters, 1995; National Asthma Education Program, 1992; Shuttari, 1995; Troisi, Speizer, Rosner, Trichopoulos, & Willett, 1995). Liane began smoking about 5 months ago, and it is probable that the severity of her asthma at present is directly related. Furthermore, there is evidence that children of lower socioeconomic status whose mothers smoke are more likely to develop asthma (Martinez, Cline, & Burrow, 1992). This factor may have played a major role in the patient's early childhood asthma. Smoking cessation and avoidance of secondhand smoke should be a top priority. It is a good sign that Liane has expressed some desire to quit, but this is often a difficult process, and will be discussed in detail in Chapter 12. For the time being, the patient should at least be made aware that her asthma is made worse by cigarette smoking and that help in smoking cessation is available.

The final potential trigger is likely a sensitive issue for Liane. She is the owner of two cats, which could be the source of allergens associated with asthma. The Asthma Committee of the Canadian Thoracic Society (Asthma Committee, 1996) has concluded that, "The reduction of exposure to cat allergen cannot be achieved without removing the pet from the home." Such a hard-line position would probably not be acceptable to Liane. As an alternative, some effort could be made to confirm the presence of the cats as a trigger. This could involve allergy testing. More simply, Liane could be asked if she ever experiences allergic symptoms such as watery, itchy eyes in addition to asthma symptoms such as shortness of breath when she is close to her or someone else's pets. Simple measures such as keeping the cats out of her bedroom and washing them weekly (National Asthma Education Program, 1992) may be effective in reducing exposure to allergens. These ideas should be presented to Liane as suggestions if and when she accepts her cats as possible asthma triggers rather than as strict recommendations that should be acted upon, such as smoking cessation.

For a discussion of the implementation of an initial management plan, see "The Rest of the Story," which follows.

The Rest of the Story

You review the spirometric data with the patient and tell Liane that it, together with her history and physical examination, are consistent with moderate asthma with persistent symptoms. You prescribe for her a new albuterol inhaler, which she is to use at a dose of 2 puffs only as needed. You also prescribe beclomethasone inhaler, 100μg bid, and prednisone, 40mg/day for 5 days, as well as a home peak flow monitor. You explain the role of each medication and advise Liane to rinse her mouth thoroughly after using her steroid inhaler. Liane tells you she is comfortable with the use of inhalers, but you insist that it would be of some benefit for you to demonstrate the proper use and review her technique.

Upon completion of your demonstration with a placebo inhaler, Liane shows you that she is able to use an inhaler effectively. You tell her that she must be very involved in the management of her condition and describe to her the role and technique of home peak flow monitoring. You ask her to take peak flow readings twice daily and before and after albuterol use, and you explain the importance of identifying her personal best peak flow. You give her several sheets on which she can record peak flow and asthma symptoms. You explain the *zone system* and asthma action plan. You tell her that symptoms such as cough at night and chest tightness are warning signs of worsening asthma and that she should not hesitate to contact you if her symptoms or peak flow do not improve with repeated doses of her albuterol inhaler. You tell Liane that if she has no objection, you will call her mother and explain the action plan to her as well.

You discuss asthma triggers at length with the patient. Liane expresses a genuine desire to quit smoking and tells you she has tried several times in the past couple of months without success. In her words, "I'm always edgy without a cigarette. I mean, unless I'm sick, I feel like smoking all the time." You inform the patient that smoking and asthma are related and that you are willing to help her quit. She seems very receptive to your offer.

You tell Liane that to prevent asthma symptoms during vigorous exercise, she should use her albuterol inhaler prior to gym class. You bring up the role her cats may play in her asthma. Liane tells you,

> Well, I know what you're saying. But I've had those cats for a long time. They don't make my eyes watery or anything. Anyway, I can't imagine getting rid of them. I don't want to get tested for cat allergy or anything because if I'm allergic my mom will make me get rid of them. I'll keep them out of my bedroom from now on, and they could stand a bath once in a while.

You tell the patient that you understand that she is very attached to her pets and that any effort to reduce exposure to cat allergens may be beneficial.

Liane appears to understand the management plan very well. She tells you, "I hope I won't have to do a lot of math for that asthma diary. I have trouble with that kind of stuff." You tell the patient that completing her diary should not prove difficult, and you complete her predicted, green-, yellow-, and red-zone boundaries for peak flow on her diary form. You ask her to return in 2 weeks with her asthma diary and emphasize once again that you are available for help in the interim.

You call Barbara Naus later that day and explain the management plan. She is very grateful for your call and assures you that she will do all she can to ensure that Liane is compliant.

PART III

The Problem

Liane returns and immediately tells you she feels much better. Her symptoms have gradually improved such that she has had no attacks for the past 10 days and only occasional mild symptoms for the past week. She completed the course of prednisone and continues to take her beclomethasone inhaler as prescribed. She has not used her albuterol inhaler for approximately 1 week. She has not missed a single day of school and has been participating in her other usual activities for the past 10 days. Unfortunately, this includes tobacco use—Liane has been smoking about one pack of cigarettes per day over the past few days.

The patient presently reports no shortness of breath, cough, fever, rhinorrhea, chest tightness, wheezing, or other symptoms. She has been performing self-monitoring of peak flow. Her diary for the past 2 weeks is summarized in Figure 11.2.

Questions

1. Describe how you would manage the case from this point.

420L/min	My predicted peak flow	
440L/min	My personal best peak flow	
> 340L/min	My Green (OK) Zone (80% to 100% of personal best)	
> 210L/min	My Yellow (Caution) Zone (50% to 80% of personal best)	
< 210L/min	My Red (Danger) Zone (less than 50% of personal best)	

Day	One a.m./p.m.	Two a.m./p.m.	Three a.m./p.m.	Four a.m./p.m.	Five a.m./p.m.	Six a.m./p.m.	Seven a.m./p.m.
Peak Flow	p.m.340 night pre 240 night post 340	320/360 a.m. pre 320 a.m. post 330	340/400	240/400 a.m. pre 240 a.m. post 240 a.m. post 340	340/400	340/300 p.m. pre 300 p.m. post 340	340/340 a.m. pre 340 a.m. post 400
No asthma symptoms						No symptoms but used puffer due to low peak flow	
Mild asthma symptoms	Mild symptoms at night	Mild symptoms in a.m.					Mild symptoms in a.m.
Moderate asthma symptoms				Moderate symptoms in a.m.			
Serious asthma symptoms							
Medicine used	albuterol, 2 puffs at night	albuterol, 2 puffs in a.m.		albuterol, 4 puffs in a.m.		albuterol, 2 puffs in a.m.	albuterol, 2 puffs in a.m.
Urgent visit to doctor							

Day	Eight a.m./p.m.	Nine a.m./p.m.	Ten a.m./p.m.	Eleven a.m./p.m.	Twelve a.m./p.m.	Thirteen a.m./p.m.	Fourteen a.m./p.m.
Peak flow (L/min)	320/360	320/400	340/400	320/440	340/300	340/330	440/420
No asthma symptoms							
Mild asthma		Mild symptoms in a.m.			Mild symptoms in p.m.		
Moderate asthma symptoms							
Serious asthma symptoms							
Medicine used		No puffer used		No puffer used	No puffer used	No puffer used	
Urgent visit to doctor							

Figure 11.2   My Weekly Asthma Symptom and Peak Flow Diary

Discussion

1. Liane is doing quite well. She is more or less asymptomatic. Although her peak flow measurements have greatly improved, there is still evidence of occasionally compromised respiratory function. After an exacerbation of asthma, pulmonary function may take several weeks to improve. Corticosteroids should be continued during this period, both to promote recovery and to prevent relapse of moderate or severe asthma (Joint Task Force on Practice Parameters, 1995; L'Enfant & Khaltaev, 1995). It is recommended that once reasonable control of asthma has been achieved, the dose of steroids be reduced to the minimum needed (British Thoracic Society, 1990). Liane should continue on the same or a lower dose of beclomethasone inhaler until her asthma can be reassessed at a later date. As she has good control with inhaled steroid, there is no need to consider other anti-inflammatory medications or long-acting inhaled beta-2 agonists in her present situation. Liane should, of course, continue to use her albuterol inhaler as needed. The patient's pulmonary function could be objectively assessed at present with a repeat spirogram or with a simple office recording of peak flow.

In school-aged children, 80% to 85% of asthma exacerbations are associated with common viral infections (Johnston et al., 1995). Such infections usually cannot be prevented. There is, however, value in administering influenza and pneumococcal vaccine to asthmatics (L'Enfant & Khaltaev, 1995). Liane should receive these immunizations either at this visit or in the near future.

Management of asthma is an ongoing process founded upon a therapeutic partnership between the patient and physician. The issue of tobacco avoidance remains an extremely important one, especially as Liane has resumed smoking heavily. She should be asked to return for help in quitting, not only to prevent the adverse effects of tobacco smoke on her asthma but also as a way of improving her general health now and in the future.

Conclusion

You tell Liane that you are pleased that her symptoms and peak flows have improved. You explain to her that it is best for her to continue her beclomethasone inhaler for at least a few more weeks until her asthma can be reassessed. You ask her to continue the same dose of 100μg bid. You re-emphasize the importance of smoking cessation and once again offer your help. Liane responds, "Yeah, doing it on my own isn't easy. I want to come back and talk about it. I've got a test next week that I really have to pass. I just can't quit right now. I'm too edgy."

You measure Liane's best peak flow in the office as 360L/min. You administer both influenza and pneumococcal vaccines.

You wish Liane the best of luck on her test and tell her you understand that it is difficult to stop smoking during periods of stress. She tells you, "Oh, I'm not stressed out or anything. I just need the cigarettes to get me through next week."

You ask Liane to return in 2 weeks for reassessment of her asthma and to discuss smoking cessation. She agrees.

References

Allen, R. J., & Graber, M. A. (1990). Asthma. In M. A. Graber, R. J. Allen, & B. T. Levy (Eds.), *University of Iowa family practice handbook. Chapter 3: Pulmonary medicine.* Iowa City: University of Iowa. (http://indy.radiology.uiowa.edu/Providers/ClinRef/FPHandbook/03.html; accessed October 20, 1996)

Asthma Committee, Canadian Thoracic Society. (1996). Canadian Asthma Consensus Conference summary of recommendations. *Canadian Respiratory Journal, 3*(2), 89-100.

British Thoracic Society, Research Unit of the Royal College of Physicians of London, King's Fund Centre, National Asthma Campaign. (1990). Guidelines for management of asthma in adults (Statement). *British Medical Journal, 301*, 651-653.

Canadian Lung Association. (1994). *Asthma management.* (http://www.lung.ca/asthma/manage/index.html; accessed October 17, 1996)

Drugs for asthma. (1995). In M. Abramowicz (Ed.), *Drugs of choice from the Medical Letter.* New Rochelle, NY: Medical Letter, Inc.

Johnston, S. L., Pattermore, P. K., Sanderson, G., Smith, S., Lampe, F., Josephs, L., Symington, P., O'Toole, S., Myint, S. H., Tyrrell, D. A., & Holgate, S. T. (1995). Community study of role of viral infections in exacerbations of asthma in 9-11 year old children. *British Medical Journal, 310*, 1225-1228.

Joint Task Force on Practice Parameters, representing the American Academy of Allergy, Asthma, and Immunology, the American College of Allergy, Asthma and Immunology, and the Joint Council of Allergy, Asthma and Immunology. (1995, November). Practice parameters for the diagnosis and treatment of asthma. *Journal of Allergy and Clinical Immunology, 96*(5, Pt. 2), 707-870.

L'Enfant, C., & Khaltev, N. (1995, December). *Asthma: A practical guide for public health officials and health care professionals* (NIH Publication No. 96-3659A). Bethesda, MD: National Heart, Lung and Blood Institute. (http://www.ginasthma.com/gina/PRACTICAL/PRACTICAL.HTML; accessed October 2, 1996)

Martinez, F. D., Cline, M., & Burrow, B. (1992). Increased incidence of asthma in children of smoking mothers. *Pediatrics, 89*(1), 21-26.

National Asthma Education Program, Office of Prevention, Education and Control, National Heart, Lung and Blood Institute. (1992). *Teach your patients about asthma: A clinician's guide* (Publication No. [NIH] 92-2737). Bethesda, MD: Author.

Pierce, R., & Johns, D. P. (1995). *Spirometry: The measurement and interpretation of ventilatory function in clinical practice.* Melbourne, Australia: National Asthma Campaign.

Shuttari, M. G. (1995). Asthma: Diagnosis and management. *American Family Physician, 52*, 2225-2235.

Troisi, R. J., Speizer, F. E., Rosner, B., Trichopoulos, D., & Willett, W. C. (1995). Cigarette smoking and incidence of chronic bronchitis and asthma in women. *Chest, 108*(6), 1557-1561.

Wiedemann, H. P., & Kavuru, M. D. (1994). *Diagnosis and management of asthma.* Caddo, OK: Professionals Communications.

Appendix
Classify Severity of Asthma

	Clinical Features Before Treatment	*Medication Required to Maintain Control*
STEP 4 (Severe persistent)	Continuous symptoms, frequent exacerbations, frequent night-time asthma symptoms, physical activities limited by asthma symptoms, PEF or FEV1 60% predicted; variability > 30%	Multiple daily long-term preventive medications: high doses inhaled corticosteroid, long-acting bronchodilator, and oral corticosteroid long term
STEP 3 (Moderate persistent)	Symptoms daily, exacerbations affect activity and sleep, night-time asthma symptoms > 1 time per week, daily use of inhaled short-acting beta-2 agonist, PEF or FEV1 60%; variability > 30%	Daily long-term preventive medications: inhaled corticosteroid and long-acting bronchodilator (especially for night-time symptoms)
STEP 2 (Mild persistent)	Symptoms 1 time per week but 2 times per month, PEF or FEV1 80% predicted; variability 20-30%	One daily long-term preventive medication: possibly add a long-acting bronchodilator to anti-inflammatory medication (especially for night-time symptoms)
STEP 1 (Intermittent)	Intermittent symptoms 80% predicted; variability	Intermittent quick-relief medication taken as needed only: inhaled short-acting beta-2 agonist. Intensity of treatment depends on severity of exacerbation: Oral corticosteroids may be required.

SOURCE: L'Enfant & Khaltaev (1995).
NOTE: If even one of the items listed in the Clinical Features Before Treatment column is present, the patient falls into the category in that row.

Worksheet No. 16

My Weekly Asthma Symptom and Peak Flow Diary

_____ My predicted peak flow
_____ My personal best peak flow
_____ My Green (OK) Zone (80% to 100% of personal best)
_____ My Yellow (Caution) Zone (50% to 80% of personal best)
_____ My Red (Danger) Zone (below 50% of personal best)

Date   a.m. p.m. a.m. p.m. a.m. p.m. a.m. p.m. a.m. p.m. a.m. p.m. a.m. p.m.

<u>Peak Flow Reading</u>

    No asthma symptoms
    Mild asthma symptoms
    Moderate asthma symptoms
    Serious asthma symptoms
    Medicine used to stop
    Urgent visit to the doctor

1. Take your peak flow reading every morning (a.m.) when you wake up and every night (p.m.) at bedtime. Try to take your peak flow readings at the same time each day. If you take an inhaled beta-2 agonist medicine, take your peak flow reading before taking that medicine. Write down the highest reading of three tries in the box that says peak flow reading.
2. Look at the box in the upper left of this sheet to see whether your number is in the green, yellow, or red zone.
3. In the space below the date and time, put an X in the box that matches the symptoms you have when you record your peak flow reading.
4. Look at your asthma control plan for what to do when your number is in one of the zones and you have asthma symptoms.
5. Put an X in the box beside "Medicine used to stop" if you took extra asthma medicine to stop your symptoms.
6. If you made any visit to your doctor's office, emergency room, or hospital for treatment of an asthma episode, put an X in the box marked "Urgent visit to the doctor." Tell your doctor if you went to the emergency room or hospital.

"No asthma symptoms" = No symptoms (wheeze, cough, chest tightness, or shortness of breath) even with normal physical activity. "Mild asthma symptoms" = Symptoms during physical activity but not at rest: They do not keep you from sleeping or being active. "Moderate asthma symptoms" = Symptoms while at rest: Symptoms may keep you from sleeping or being active. "Serious asthma symptoms" = Serious symptoms at rest (wheeze may be absent): Symptoms cause problems walking or talking; muscles in neck or between ribs are pulled in when breathing.

SOURCE: National Asthma Education Program (1992).

12. SMOKING CESSATION

Ms. Liane Webber

*Goal: The goal of this exercise is to evaluate and develop
the participants' understanding of how
physicians can help their patients quit smoking.*

Specific Objectives: Upon completion of this group discussion exercise, each participant should be able to accomplish the following:

1. Obtain a comprehensive tobacco use history from a patient who smokes.
2. Describe the most common concerns expressed about smoking cessation by patients.
3. Address, in an effective manner, the concerns of a young female smoker relating to postcessation weight gain.
4. Assist a smoker in a cessation attempt by providing suggestions on how and when to quit, how to cope with withdrawal symptoms, how to deal with individual threats to abstinence, and how to cope with relapse when it occurs.
5. Describe the role of carbon monoxide monitoring in smoking cessation.

PART I

The Patient

Social History

Liane Webber is a white, 15-year-old girl who lives with her family in the Wisconsin city of Eau Claire where she was born and raised. She is presently enrolled in her freshman year of high school.

Liane's parents divorced 6 years ago. Her father, Peter Webber, 49, is a taxi driver in St. Paul, Minnesota. Liane's mother, Barbara Naus, works as a waitress in a diner in Eau Claire. The patient's brother, Carl, 22, is currently enrolled in a carpentry apprenticeship program. Barbara and her children rent a small three-bedroom home they also share with Barbara's boyfriend of 3 years, Jeff Hale. Two cats, whom Liane has smothered with affection since she was 10, complete the household.

The patient has had a difficult family life. Barbara and Peter's divorce was difficult for both children, especially Carl, who dropped out of high school shortly thereafter. He has been plagued with drug and alcohol abuse and unemployment ever since. He maintains a fragile and occasionally physically abusive relationship with his girlfriend, Stella. Although he shares the same home with the patient, Carl and Liane rarely speak to each other. Liane says, "We haven't been close since we were very little. He's such a screwup. It's scary sometimes." Carl's relationship with his mother is similarly lacking in communication. On the other hand, he admires his father, whom he describes as a "free spirit." He often drives to St. Paul to spend a weekend with him, during which Carl and his father do little more than watch television together in Peter's rather shabby apartment.

Jeff Hale has not received a warm reception in the household from Carl and Liane. He neither contributes to the rent nor pays for any other household expenses, a fact Carl often brings to everyone's attention. Moreover, Mr. Hale has felt the need to exert some parental authority over Barbara's children, and this has received a cool if not sometimes openly hostile reaction. Most disturbing to Liane is the fact that Jeff and Barbara have actually talked about having a child together. In her words, "I mean. That's crazy. She wants to have a kid with this loser. She's 42 for God's sake. It just won't happen. What a stupid idea!" Although this and other disagreements characterize the relationship between Liane and her mother, they remain very close. In Barbara's words, "She's all I have left. I had Carl, but I'm losing him now. I love her more than anything."

Liane is a poor student. She has come close to failing a year of middle school and is presently struggling in high school. Barbara, who has attended several parent-teacher meetings, has been told that Liane is a bright and capable girl but that she rarely hands in assignments on time, and when she does, her work is below any reasonable standard. Her poor performance on tests, Liane's mother has been told, is certainly the result of inadequate preparation. Barbara has always found it difficult to motivate Liane to do her homework or to study for exams. For her part, Liane often insists, "I can't stand it sometimes. I mean, I hate studying. I think I'd rather be digging a ditch or something."

The patient spends her afternoons and often her evenings at a nearby shopping mall, where she "hangs out" with a group of friends from school whom her mother describes as "kind of a bad crowd." She does not have a boyfriend. She is not involved in any extracurricular school activities or any other clubs or sports. She took piano lessons from age 10 to 13, but the piano she inherited from her grandmother now sits idle, gathering dust in the dining room of the family home. Liane earns a small amount of money baby-sitting the 4-year-old daughter of a young couple who live down the street.

Barbara describes her family's background as Lutheran, of Dutch and German ancestry—similar to that of her ex-husband's. Neither she nor her children are involved in any organized religious activities.

The family is presently enrolled in a government-sponsored medical assistance program that pays for doctors' visits, prescriptions, and hospital care.

Past Personal and Family Medical History

Liane suffered from frequent asthma symptoms as a young child. This was manifested as episodic attacks, usually accompanying an upper respiratory tract infection, which gradually disappeared by the time Liane was 9 years old. She has never been hospitalized for asthma or any other condition.

Until recently, Liane had been experiencing only occasional, mild shortness of breath and wheezing after vigorous exercise. A few weeks ago, she presented to her family physician with a moderate asthma exacerbation, which she has been told was likely triggered by an upper respiratory tract infection as well as cigarette smoking—an activity the patient began about 5 months ago. Liane has been monitoring her symptoms and peak flow and recording this information in an asthma diary. She presently uses a beclomethasone inhaler, 100µg bid, as well as a albuterol inhaler, 2 puffs on a prn basis.

Accompanied by her mother, she saw a physician 2 years ago for acne, and topical antibiotic cream was prescribed. Her acne has largely disappeared.

Liane began menstruating at age 12 and has had regular periods ever since. She has never been sexually active.

Barbara Naus suffers from frequent migraine headaches and obesity. She is otherwise healthy. As noted, Carl Webber has had trouble with illicit drugs, specifically marijuana and heroin, for which he has visited and continues to visit a treatment center. He has had both gonorrhea and chlamydia in the past. He had a right second metacarpal fracture last year, acquired during a fist fight outside a local bar. He has no other past medical history.

Peter Webber's health is a bit of a mystery. Liane suspects her father is an alcoholic, but her mother insists that this is not the case. Liane knows that her father has a "heart condition" but is unsure about the details.

The Problem

You are a family physician in a solo practice in a small city with complete access to all diagnostic facilities and specialists. You last saw Liane 2 weeks ago for reassessment of an asthma exacerbation. You emphasized the importance of smoking cessation at that time and asked her to return to discuss this matter further. The patient told you that she had an important test coming up and that for this reason it was not an appropriate time to consider quitting smoking.

Liane returns today and tells you she has been feeling quite well. She has had no recent asthma attacks and has been completely asymptomatic for the past 10 days. She has recorded normal peak flow values for the past 2 weeks. She continues to use her beclomethasone inhaler as prescribed but has had no need for albuterol.

You recommend that Liane discontinue use of her beclomethasone inhaler. When asked about her test, Liane tells you, "Well, I passed, but just barely! Anyway, I think I'm ready to at least talk about quitting smoking."

Questions

1. How would you obtain a comprehensive tobacco use history from the patient?
2. After reviewing "The Rest of the Story" that follows the second discussion section, how would you describe Liane's pattern of tobacco use?
3. How would you address Liane's concerns about smoking cessation?

Discussion

Helping Liane to quit smoking is likely to be a long and difficult process whose course will be greatly influenced by the patient's home environment, peer influences, ability to cope with adverse situations, and self-image. There are few recommendations in the literature that pertain specifically to smoking cessation among adolescents. Some authorities, however, recommend that the same interventions used to help adults quit smoking be applied to adolescent patients (Agency for Health Care Policy and Research [AHCPR], 1996). *Participants are encouraged to be creative in their approach to this problem and to individualize their suggestions for smoking cessation whenever possible to meet Liane Webber's specific needs and concerns.*

1. Assessment of tobacco use by all adolescent patients and institution of a cessation plan are recommended by the American Medical Association ("Guidelines for Adolescent," 1995). The enormous negative impact of cigarette smoking on the health of North Americans has led to the development of a number of comprehensive guidelines on smoking cessation (AHCPR, 1996; American Academy of Family Physicians [AAFP], 1993; Canadian Council on Smoking and Health, 1992; Glynn & Manley, 1993). Most guidelines divide the physician's role in smoking cessation into three or more components that commonly include **ask, ad-**

vise, and **assist.** The "three As" can be expanded to include **arrange, anticipate,** and **advocate.** The precise meaning of this terminology will be explained as needed throughout this discussion. At present, the issue is how to obtain a comprehensive tobacco history. This pertains to the **ask** component, which involves much more than simply determining if a patient smokes (Canadian Council on Smoking and Health, 1992). A comprehensive history includes when smoking began and for what reasons. In addition, it is important to know if the patient has tried to quit in the past. The success of past quit attempts and the perceived reasons for relapse should be determined. The patient's reasons for wanting to quit now should be explored.

Patients often express serious concerns about smoking cessation that commonly include weight gain, withdrawal symptoms, and the influence of other smokers. These issues should be addressed.

Smoking more than 20 to 25 cigarettes per day and having a cigarette within 30 min of waking up in the morning are two useful indicators of nicotine dependence (Fagerstrom & Melin, 1985).The presence of these patterns of tobacco consumption should be determined.

Finally, as the success of physician guidance in smoking cessation is largely dependent on the patient's desire to quit, it is useful to ask Liane how interested she is in stopping smoking on a scale of 1 to 10. See

"The Rest of the Story" following this section for a comprehensive tobacco use history.

2. Liane Webber's pattern of tobacco use is typical of that of many young people. Five stages of youth tobacco use have been described (Thomas & Thomas, 1995). The first stage is **anticipation,** or preparation, during which young children often become curious about smoking. This is followed by **initiation,** or the consumption of a first cigarette. Next is **experimentation,** during which children explore tobacco use and their reactions to it. In the fourth stage, **habituation,** they smoke regularly with peers. Finally, in stage five, children follow a pattern of **adult smoking** and regularly smoke alone. According to this categorization, Liane is already in the final stage.

Another way to examine Liane's tobacco consumption pattern is to consider her risks for tobacco use and her reasons for starting smoking. Children whose parents smoke are much more likely to become smokers than the children of nonsmokers. Children who belong to lower socioeconomic classes are much more likely to smoke than those of higher socioeconomic status. The patient was clearly at risk for these two reasons (Committee on Adolescence, 1987). Liane's actual specific reason for initiation deserves considerable attention. A study by Klesges and Klesges (1988) revealed that 39% of female smokers in a university population reported using smoking as a weight loss strategy. Furthermore, overweight females were much more likely to begin smoking to lose weight. Liane's reason for starting smoking (given in "The Rest of the Story") is, therefore, not uncommon among many young female smokers.

Not only is Liane's pattern of tobacco use common, her reasons for wanting to quit are typical of adolescent smokers. In a survey of 77 adolescents at a youth detention center in Washington (Dozois, Farrow, & Miser, 1995), the most common reasons cited for wanting to quit smoking were health related. Liane, through the guidance of her family physician, has come to understand that her asthma is made worse by cigarettes and has mentioned this as a motivation to quit, together with fears of long-term addiction and lung cancer.

3. Presently available evidence indicates that the weight loss achieved by smoking is modest or nonexistent in many cases (Klesges, Meyers, Klesges, & LaVasque, 1989). Indeed, Liane has discovered that smoking is an ineffective weight loss strategy. There is support, however, for Liane's concern about postcessation weight gain, and it is best to be open and honest about this issue. Most smokers who quit gain less than 4.5kg (Agency for Health Care Policy and Research, 1996), which has a negligible impact on health in relation to the adverse effects of continued tobacco use. For many adolescent girls and young women, however, weight gain is less of a health matter than a question of attractiveness and social acceptability. This is Liane's predominant concern.

All smokers should be **advised** to quit, and the advice given should be personalized. Young females concerned about weight, like Liane, should be told that smoking cessation is often associated with weight gain but that in most cases the amount of weight gained is modest. Liane should be told that cigarette smoking itself is unattractive in many ways, as it causes bad breath, stained teeth and fingers, and smelly clothes. As this information may not be enough to allay concerns about weight gain, it is important to consider different strategies to tackle the problem.

The smoking cessation guidelines of the Canadian Council on Smoking and Health (1992) advocates a pro-active approach to weight gain, through which exercise and dietary modification are recommended at the same time as the cessation effort. The difficulty is that postcessation weight gain is not only due to the commonly observed increase in caloric intake upon quitting but also metabolic adjustments that take place in the absence of cigarettes (Klesges & Shumaker, 1992). In a study by Pirie et al. (1992), a behavioral weight control program that included caloric restriction, when combined with an effective smoking cessation program, was ineffective in preventing postcessation weight gain. Consistent with such evidence, the Agency for Health Care Policy and Research (AHCPR, 1996) does not recommend a simultaneous weight control and smoking cessation effort. It advocates that clini-

cians emphasize that smoking cessation should be the immediate priority, the problem to be tackled first. Weight gain can be dealt with once the cessation effort has been successful. Strict dieting during the quit attempt may be counterproductive, as the added anxiety over weight may lead to relapse in smoking. Nicotine gum has been shown to delay the onset but not the amount of weight gain (Gross, Stitzer, & Maldonado, 1989).

As rational as the AHCPR's approach to weight and smoking cessation appears, the idea of postcessation weight gain as a problem of much less importance than smoking cessation may be a difficult one for Liane to accept, particularly as she actually began smoking as a weight-control measure. This is one opportunity for discussion participants to contribute creative solutions to help Liane. She could, for example, be discouraged from stepping on a scale until she has quit smoking completely.

The Rest of the Story

You tell Liane that before discussing quitting smoking, you would like to get a detailed history of her tobacco use.

Liane tells you she began smoking about 5 months ago, soon after beginning high school. She tells you,

I usually stay away from bathroom scales, but one day after gym class, a whole bunch of girls decided to weigh themselves on the scale in the locker room. I know I've always been heavy, but man was I shocked—211 pounds! It was so depressing! My friend Tracy noticed how upset I was. Tracy's a little rail—weighs like 90 pounds dripping wet, and she gets a lot of attention from the boys at school. I started thinking, this is high school. It's time I started meeting guys. There are dances and proms all the time. No guy will come near me at this size. Besides, it's disgusting to be so huge! I asked Tracy what was her secret for staying so thin. She said, "It comes in a little cardboard box" and handed me my first cigarette. At first it was gross—made me cough a lot, but I got used to it. Before long, Tracy, Jen, and I were smoking outside school and between classes. They got tired of me bumming cigarettes off of them, so I started buying my own. It's not hard. Just walk into a store—no one asks you for ID or anything. There are machines everywhere too.

You ask Liane about her family's reaction, if any, to her smoking. She responds,

Well, the whole house smokes, but we all try to be secret about it for some reason. My mom has always tried not to smoke around me because of my asthma. She noticed a pack of Virginia Slims in my jean jacket pocket a couple of months ago and started lecturing me on how bad smoking is and how I should stop right away. I told her I knew all about that and that she was a fine one to talk. I told her I didn't plan to be a smoker forever. Ever since then she's been nagging me to quit. Once she suggested that we both quit together. I took her up on that offer, but she kept saying she wasn't ready. Anyway, Jeff smokes too. He likes to smoke on the porch. I think I'd kick him in the head if *he* ever started lecturing me about quitting. My brother smokes cigarettes and other things. He's not around the house a lot, and I'm sure he doesn't care if I'm a smoker. I haven't seen my father for 6 months, and he doesn't know about my smoking.

Liane tells you that for the past 2 weeks she has been smoking 20 cigarettes, or one pack, per day and that she has her first while waiting for her school bus, approximately 1 hr after awakening. She tells you she tried to quit "cold turkey" 2 months ago. In her words,

It didn't go very well. I was under a lot of pressure to pass tests and stuff. I got so edgy without a cigarette. I lasted about a day and was back to smoking a pack. I've tried cutting down a lot. Well, I told you when I was sick I cut down. I was smoking only three or four cigarettes there for awhile, but every time I cut down I bounce back up to a whole pack.

You ask Liane why she is interested in quitting now. She tells you,

Lots of reasons. Like you said, smoking makes my asthma worse, and I don't want to feel the way I did 3 weeks ago. Also, I don't want to wind up like my mom. I think it's easier to quit when you're young—when you're not so addicted to it. My mom's been smoking for like 30 years, and she's tried all kinds of things and can't quit. I'm afraid she's going to wind up with lung cancer or something if she keeps it up.

You ask Liane if she has any fears or concerns about quitting. She responds,

Well. I think I've learned that Tracy is just a natural twig. I don't think I've lost a pound with cigarettes. I am worried about gaining weight when I stop, though. I've heard people gain a lot of weight. I can't afford for that to happen. I can't imagine being even bigger. That's my big worry. I'm pretty tall, and I can hide those 200-plus pounds pretty well, but if I got bigger, people would notice how huge I was.

When asked how motivated she is to quit smoking on a scale of 1 to 10, Liane tells you, "Well, I would say 8 or 9. I really want to stop. I just need help."

PART II

The Problem

You tell Liane that you are very pleased that she is so interested in quitting and tell her you will provide any assistance you can. You tell her that smoking is associated with modest weight gain that does not constitute a major health concern. You emphasize that although she may feel that the added weight would be unattractive, continued smoking, for a number of reasons, has a negative impact on attractiveness and desirability. Liane tells you, "I really don't want to gain weight, but I'm not too hung up on it or anything." You inform the patient that smoking cessation should be the priority and that you would be happy to help her lose any excess weight once the cessation effort has been successful. Liane tells you that she believes your approach to weight gain "makes sense" and agrees not to be too concerned about weight in the short term. At this point Liane asks you, "Well, I'm not going to have to stop cold turkey, am I? I mean, I can gradually cut down, right?"

Questions

1. How would you answer Liane's question?
2. What should be the next step in management of this case?
3. Would you recommend nicotine replacement?
4. Discuss the role of objective measures of tobacco consumption.
5. When would you like to see Liane for follow-up?

Discussion

1. Reducing consumption of tobacco is neither a substitute for cessation nor an effective means of eventually quitting. Most patients are unable to reduce their consumption of cigarettes to zero. Furthermore, smokers often compensate for the reduced number of cigarettes by extracting 3 to 4 times more chemicals from each cigarette (AAFP, 1993). Stopping cold turkey, therefore, is the most effective way to quit.

2. A thorough tobacco use history has been obtained. Liane's main concern about smoking cessation has been considered. She has indicated a strong desire to quit. The next step is to decide on an actual day for cessation, a "quit date." Preferably, a date within the next 2 weeks should be chosen. Liane implied earlier that anxiety over a test would hinder a cessation effort. A quit date should be chosen, therefore, to minimize interference from such obstacles. Helping to select a quit date is one way in which Liane's physician can **assist** her with smoking cessation. The initial cessation effort requires some preparation. Liane should inform her family and tobacco-using friends about her plan to quit and request their support. She should prepare her environment by removing cigarettes from her immediate vicinity. Prior to the quit date, it is recommended that the

patient avoid smoking in places where she spends a lot of time (e.g., the mall, at home, etc.) (AHCPR, 1996).

Liane has identified weight gain as her primary concern about smoking cessation. Cessation, however, is often associated with other challenges, such as nicotine withdrawal symptoms, stress that may lead to relapse (which apparently was the case with Liane's one previous quit attempt), and the presence of other smokers. These problems should be *anticipated* and discussed at this visit. Indeed, withdrawal symptoms and the presence of other smokers are two of the most common concerns expressed about cessation ("Guidelines for Adolescent," 1995). Common withdrawal symptoms include severe urges to smoke, irritability, difficulty concentrating, difficulty sleeping, increased appetite, and headaches. Liane may have experienced some of these symptoms during her previous quit attempt. She should be told that such symptoms are at their worst for the first 3 to 4 days, after which they abate considerably. Cravings for cigarettes normally last only a few minutes. The National Cancer Institute's smoking cessation guidelines (Glynn & Manley, 1993) include specific recommendations on how to cope with the urge to smoke. These include several important strategies, among which is, first, reviewing the circumstances under which a particular urge took place (time, activity, thoughts, etc.). Another involves quickly reviewing why one has decided to stop smoking during an urge. The ex-smoker should learn to anticipate and avoid specific identified triggers. For example, the urge to smoke immediately after a meal can be avoided by immediately rising from the dinner table and washing the

dishes. Other ways to deal with urges include changing one's daily routine and normal habits and patterns, using positive thoughts to reinforce the desire to abstain, and using deep breathing exercises. These suggestions can be briefly reviewed with Liane at this visit.

Enlisting the support and understanding of close friends and family members is helpful in avoiding exposure to other smokers. However, there are likely to be situations in which the presence of other smokers cannot be avoided. Liane should make a conscious effort to avoid such situations. She should stay away from the smoking sections of restaurants, for example.

Liane can be provided with self-help materials such as the *I'm in Charge Now . . . What's My Secret?* (for women) booklet available from the American Cancer Society (1993). There is no evidence that provision of such self-help materials without personalized counseling is an effective smoking cessation aid (AHCPR, 1996). Providing such a booklet to Liane may, however, help reinforce some of the advice given her by her physician.

Liane can be asked to sign a "stop smoking contract," which confirms the patient's desire to quit smoking and makes note of the quit date. Whether making smoking cessation a written contractual obligation influences the success of the effort is uncertain. An example of a stop smoking contract is available from the National Cancer Institute (see Appendix).

3. There is no question that nicotine replacement is an effective cessation aid that helps relieve withdrawal symptoms in patients dependent on this drug (Miller, Golish, & Cox, 1992). The AHCPR (1996)

recommends liberal use of nicotine replacement, including administration to adolescents with evidence of dependence. Liane smokes roughly a pack of cigarettes per day and has her first cigarette relatively early in the morning. She is therefore likely to benefit from nicotine replacement. It is available in patch, gum, and a recently approved nasal spray form. Of these, the patch is easiest to use and is associated with few compliance problems.

Nicotine patches are available in different strengths and are usually each applied for either 24- or 16-hr periods. Most patch systems deliver a steady dose of nicotine for several weeks that is gradually tapered. Most courses are 8 weeks long. Specific instructions should accompany the prescription of nicotine patches. The patient should not smoke while using the patch. He or she should place a new patch on a relatively bare area of skin between the neck and waist daily. Patients should start using the patch as soon as they awaken on their quit day. The patch should be prescribed with caution in pregnant and lactating woman and those with cardiovascular illnesses. It causes local skin irritation in up to 50% of users that is usually self-limiting. This is the side effect that Liane is most likely to encounter.

4. There are objective, biochemical methods of determining tobacco consumption. Patients are sometimes, for a variety of reasons, unreliable in reporting their smoking status. Biochemical measures, therefore, can provide a picture of the effectiveness of a smoking cessation program either for one or a group of individuals. Furthermore, the mere existence of such measures may encourage more accurate self-reporting. The scrutiny provided by such tests may also provide added pressure to abstain from smoking. Biochemical markers include measures of serum thiocyanate, nicotine, and cotinine (a metabolite of nicotine), as well as carbon monoxide (CO) in expired air (Jarvis, Tunstall-Pedoe, Feyerabend, Vesey, & Saloojee, 1987). The serum tests are quite expensive and difficult to obtain. Furthermore, for obvious reasons, serum nicotine or cotinine cannot be used as a measure of cigarette consumption in patients on nicotine replacement.

Carbon monoxide monitors are relatively inexpensive devices that can be used to confirm nonsmoking claims or quantify cigarette consumption (Jarvis, Belcher, Vesey, & Hutchison, 1986). The amount of carbon monoxide in expired air is, however, influenced by time of day, exposure to passive smoke, exposure to atmospheric pollution, physical exercise, and other factors. Indeed, it is not as reliable a measure as serum cotinine in patients not using nicotine replacement. Carbon monoxide in expired air does drop quickly after a patient quits smoking, and the feedback to patients of dropping CO levels is a tangible way for them to appreciate their cessation effort that may contribute to its success (Jamrozik et al., 1984). This is probably the best use of carbon monoxide monitoring with Liane, rather than repeated verification of cessation status, which seems somewhat authoritarian. A CO reading could be taken at this visit and then again soon after the quit date (Canadian Council on Smoking and Health, 1992).

5. Follow-up contact with the patient, either in person or by telephone, should take place within a week of the quit date, as it is this early period that patients often find most difficult.

See "The Rest of the Story," which follows.

The Rest of the Story

You tell Liane that gradually cutting down cigarette consumption, although it may seem easier than abrupt cessation, is not an effective way to stop smoking. She responds, "Oh. Well, I didn't know I had to stop so suddenly. When I quit last time, I gradually cut down and stopped, but that didn't last too long." Liane is willing to set a quit date on which she agrees to stop smoking completely. She does not anticipate any exams or other stressors that would interfere with a quit attempt in the near future. You and the patient agree on a quit date 1 week from now. You provide Liane with information on how to prepare her environment prior to cessation. You discuss some of the difficulties smokers sometimes encounter upon quitting, such as withdrawal symptoms and the presence of other smokers, together with strategies to deal with these problems.

You inform the patient about the role of nicotine replacement in smoking cessation and tell her that she may benefit from the nicotine patch. Liane agrees, and you prescribe a 24-hr patch system that begins with 21mg/day of nicotine and is tapered to 7mg/day over an 8-week period. You provide specific instructions on how to use the patch.

There is a carbon monoxide monitor in the office of your colleague, Dr. Lars Carlsson, down the hall, to which you send Liane for an expired CO reading. A value of 11 ppm is recorded. You tell Liane that her CO level will decrease once she quits.

You provide Liane with several self-help booklets on smoking cessation. You ask her to return 2 days after her quit day but tell her you are available to help should she have any problems or concerns prior to that date.

PART III

The Problem

Liane returns as scheduled. It has been 2 days since she had her last cigarette. She has been using nicotine replacement as prescribed.

When asked how she feels, Liane responds, "Well, I've been a little edgy. I guess I'm holding up. I have been feeling some pretty powerful urges though. It's funny, I'm starting to cough a lot too. I would have thought quitting smoking *wouldn't* make me cough. Why is that?"

Questions

1. How would you respond to Liane's question?
2. What is your agenda for this visit?
3. When would you like to see Liane again?

Discussion

1. Roughly 20% of ex-smokers will experience increased cough upon cessation (AAFP, 1993). This is due to increased phlegm production and recovery of the

mucociliary expulsion mechanism after the damage inflicted by cigarette smoke. The cough, therefore, is a healthy sign of recovering lungs. It usually lasts only a short time. Liane should be reassured with this information.

2. Smoking cessation is a difficult task, and Liane should be commended for her effort. This visit is an opportunity to provide her with as much support as possible and to identify, *anticipate,* and provide solutions to problems. The focus of this visit should be on preventing relapse in smoking. The AHCPR (1996) has identified several relapse prevention strategies. The benefits of smoking cessation and the importance of remaining abstinent should be reviewed with the patient. Problems encountered in maintaining abstinence and possible solutions should be discussed. Liane and her physician should make an effort to anticipate any threats to abstinence that may come up in the near future. This visit is also an ideal time to obtain another CO reading to demonstrate to Liane that her respiratory function is improving. See "The Rest of the Story," which follows.

3. There is a positive correlation between the success of an individualized smoking cessation program and both the number of counseling sessions and the number of weeks over which care is provided (AHCPR, 1996). The AHCPR recommends that clinicians should meet with quitting smokers a minimum of four times. Liane should be told that your help with smoking cessation will be a long-term effort. She should be seen once again in a relatively short period of time of perhaps 1 to 2 weeks.

The Rest of the Story

You explain to Liane that the increased cough she is having is actually a sign of the recovery of her lungs from the effects of cigarette smoke and that it should disappear shortly. You ask the patient how she prepared for cessation and whether she has had any problems. She responds,

> I talked to my mom and Jeff. They were both really supportive. They haven't smoked anywhere near me at all. I've tried to keep away from my friends who are smokers. I told them I'm trying to quit. They were pretty supportive and wished me the best of luck. It's too bad they just can't stop smoking. I haven't felt stressed out at all—just a little edgy. I do get a lot of urges though, usually after eating, so I started doing the things you talked about. I've been taking a lot of walks. I've also been taking a lot of hot showers to get rid of that edgy feeling. I feel relaxed with the hot water running.

You congratulate Liane on her cessation effort. You tell her that taking walks and showers are good ways to deal with urges. You review the benefits of smoking cessation and the importance of remaining abstinent. Liane reports no withdrawal symptoms apart from "edginess" and the urge to smoke. She has had no difficulties in using nicotine patches.

You ask Liane if she foresees any specific challenges to her cessation effort in the near future. She responds, "I haven't got any tests coming up or anything. I think I'll be OK for awhile. I just hope I can keep this up." You remind Liane that withdrawal symptoms such as urges do not last forever. You tell her to think about her cessation effort one day at a time and that every new day that she abstains represents a significant accomplishment.

A measurement of expired CO returns as 7 ppm. You tell Liane that this is already a sign of improving lung function.

Liane appears confident and optimistic. She thanks you for your help. You ask her to return in 1 week and tell her you are available in the meantime for help.

PART IV

The Problem

Liane returns as scheduled and says, "Bad news, Doctor. I started smoking again. I smoked nearly a pack yesterday. I'm sorry. I know how much you've tried to help me."

Questions

1. What information would you like to know about Liane's relapse?
2. Describe your management of the case from this point.

Discussion

1. It is important to know when, where, and under what circumstances Liane began smoking again. Other important information includes the source of the cigarette that led to relapse, the coping mechanisms the patient employed, if any, to avoid relapse, and whether Liane has been using her nicotine patch properly (AAFP, 1993; Glynn & Manley, 1993). See "The Rest of the Story" following this section.

2. Relapse is extremely common, and Liane should be told this. On the average, it takes four to five quit attempts before cessation is permanent (Canadian Council on Smoking and Health, 1992). It is best to view relapse as a part of the quitting process and not as a failure. Liane should not feel "sorry" about having resumed smoking. She should be told that you are prepared to help her through the whole cessation process and not only through one quit attempt. It is important to determine the patient's willingness to make another quit attempt, and a new quit date should be set. Discussion participants should volunteer creative solutions for how Liane should deal with circumstances like those she described that led to relapse.

Primary care physicians also have the option of referring refractory cases of tobacco use to specialized intensive programs to treat nicotine dependence (Hurt et al., 1992). This option could be considered at some point if Liane's physician feels such treatment is needed and the patient is willing to enroll in such a program.

The Rest of the Story

When asked what led her to smoke again, Liane tells you,

Well. My mom and I were having an argument 5 days ago. She and Jeff are going away on vacation. She wants me to look after the house, like totally. I mean she wants me to do everything—vacuuming, raking leaves, the whole works. Carl doesn't have to anything, because my mom says "he's going through a hard time." Like I'm not! I don't mind doing the chores. I mean, it will keep my mind away from smoking. I just didn't like her attitude. My brother is such a bum. I mean he really should do his share. Anyway, I snatched a cigarette and a lighter out of my mother's purse and stormed out of the house to smoke. It was just instinct. I was mad. I had done that so many times before. I wasn't thinking. I lit it without even thinking. Before I knew it, I had smoked two cigarettes. Later that day, I bought a pack, and that's how I got where I am. I didn't even think about using some of my ways to cope with urges. I just got flustered and reached for a cigarette.

Liane indicates that she has been using her nicotine patch properly. She has not used it since the day after her relapse, as she kept in mind that she cannot smoke and use the patch simultaneously.

Conclusion

You assure Liane that relapse is an extremely common part of the smoking cessation process and that it should not be viewed as a failure. You tell her that often several attempts are needed to quit for good. You also offer your continuing help.

As easy access to cigarettes and a verbal confrontation led to relapse, you suggest to Liane ways in which access to cigarettes be limited. Her mother, for example, could make sure her cigarettes are not accessible by keeping them on her person or in a location unknown to Liane. You review ways to deal with stress and "feeling flustered." Rather than going outside to smoke, Liane could take a walk in the fresh air.

Liane tells you she is willing to make another quit attempt and that she is very grateful for your willingness to help. You set a quit date 1 week from now and ask Liane to return 2 days after that quit date. You instruct her to use the nicotine patch as previously, and you review ways to cope with withdrawal symptoms as well as how to prepare her environment once again for the cessation effort.

References

Agency for Health Care Policy and Research. (1996). *Smoking cessation clinical practice guideline number 18* (Publication No. 96-0693). Rockville, MD: U.S. Department of Health and Human Services, Public Health Service.

American Academy of Family Physicians. (1993). *AAFP stop smoking program.* Kansas City, MO: Author.

American Cancer Society. (1993). *I'm in charge now . . . What's my secret?* Atlanta, GA: Author.

Canadian Council on Smoking and Health. (1992). *Guide your patients to a smoke free future.* Ottawa: Author.

Committee on Adolescence, American Academy of Pediatrics. (1987). Tobacco use by children and adolescents. *Pediatrics, 79,* 479-481.

Dozois, D. N., Farrow, J. A., & Miser, A. (1995). Smoking patterns and cessation motivations during adolescence. *International Journal of Addictions, 11,* 1485-1498.

Fagerstrom, K. O., & Melin, B. (1985). Nicotine chewing gum in smoking cessation: Efficiency, nicotine dependence, therapy duration, and clinical recommendations. In J. Grabowski & S. M. Hall (Eds.), *Pharmacological adjuncts in the treatment of tobacco dependence* (National Institute of Drug Abuse Research Monograph No. 53, pp. 102-109). Bethesda, MD: National Institutes of Health.

Glynn, T. J., & Manley, M. W. (1993). *How to help your patients stop smoking—A National Cancer Institute manual for physicians* (NIH Publication No. 93-3064). Rockville, MD: U.S. Department of Health and Human Services, Public Health Service/National Institutes of Health.

Gross, J., Stitzer, M. L., & Maldonado, J. (1989). Nicotine replacement: Effects of postcessation weight gain. *Journal of Consulting and Clinical Psychology, 57,* 87-92.

Guidelines for adolescent preventive service (GAPS). (1995). Chicago, IL: American Medical Association.

Hurt, R. D., Dale, L. C., McClain, F. L., Eberman, K. M., Offord, K. P., Bruce, B. K., & Lauger, G. G. (1992). A comprehensive model for the treatment of nicotine dependence in a medical setting. *Medical Clinics of North America, 76*(2), 495-514.

Jamrozik, K., Vessey, M., Fowler, G., Wald, N., Parker, G., & Van Vunakis, H. (1984). Controlled trial of three different antismoking interventions in general practice. *British Medical Journal, 288,* 1499-1502.

Jarvis, M. J., Belcher, M., Vesey, C., & Hutchison, D.C.S. (1986). Low cost carbon monoxide monitors in smoking cessation. *Thorax, 41,* 886-887.

Jarvis, M. J., Tunstall-Pedoe, H., Feyerabend, C., Vesey, C., & Saloojee, Y. (1987). Comparison of tests used to distinguish smokers from nonsmokers. *American Journal of Public Health, 77*(11), 1435-1438.

Klesges, R. C., & Klesges, L. M. (1988). Cigarette smoking as a dieting strategy in a university population. *International Journal of Eating Disorders, 7,* 413-419.

Klesges, R. C., Meyers, A. W., & Klesges, L. M., & LaVasque, M. E. (1989). Smoking, body weight, and their effects of smoking behavior: A comprehensive review of the literature. *Psychology Bulletin, 106*(2), 203-230.

Klesges, R. C., & Shumaker, S. A. (Eds.). (1992). Proceedings of the National Working Conference on Smoking and Body Weight. *Health Psychology, 11*(Suppl.), 1-22.

Miller, G. H., Golish, J. A., & Cox, C. E. (1992). A physician's guide to smoking cessation. *Journal of Family Practice, 34*(6), 759-766.

Pirie, P. L., McBride, C. M., Hellerstedt, W., Jeffery, R. W., Hatsukami, D., Allen, S., & Lando, H. (1992). Smoking cessation in women concerned about weight. *American Journal of Public Health, 82,* 1238-1243.

Thomas, R. E., & Thomas, A. P. (1995). Preventing children from smoking. *Canadian Family Physician, 41,* 1517-1523.

Appendix

I agree to stop smoking on _____

(date)

I understand that stopping smoking is the single best thing I can do for my health and that my health professional has strongly encouraged me to quit.

_____   _____

Patient's Signature   Professional's Signature

_____

Today's Date

QUIT FOR GOOD RX

SOURCE: Glynn and Manley (1993).

13. MANAGEMENT OF
EARLY HIV INFECTION

Mr. Adam Moore

*Goal: The goal of this group discussion exercise
is to assess and develop participants' ability to evaluate
and treat early HIV infection in an adult patient.*

Specific Objectives: Upon completion of this group discussion exercise, each participant should be able to accomplish the following:

1. Provide a patient who requests a test for the HIV virus with accurate and comprehensive pre- and posttest counseling.
2. Conduct a thorough review of systems and physical examination in a patient recently diagnosed with HIV infection that takes into consideration the broad impact of this disease.
3. Recognize the enormous psychosocial impact of a positive HIV result and respond to the patient's reaction in a way that takes into consideration his or her individual needs in terms of counseling, support groups, and so on.
4. Provide a patient with early HIV infection with a health maintenance and monitoring program that includes timely administration of vaccines, immune function monitoring, and starting antiretroviral therapy.
5. Recognize the burden of suffering of opportunistic infections such as tuberculosis and institute strategies to lessen their impact.

PART I

The Patient

Social History

Adam Moore is a single, white, 31-year-old man who lives and works in New York City. Born in Quincy, Massachusetts, Adam is the only child of Mrs. Phyllis Moore of Brookline, Massachusetts and her late husband Harvey, who died in 1974. Adam grew up in the Boston area, where he completed high school in 1983. His mother, a factory worker, had high hopes for Adam and managed to save several thousand dollars for a college education that he never pursued. An aspiring photographer, Adam convinced his mother to give him the money she had saved so that he could purchase photographic equipment. Hence began a brief and unsuccessful career in commercial photography. Adam became somewhat of a drifter for several years after high school, earning small amounts of money taking freelance pictures. In October 1986, his uninsured cameras and lenses were stolen from a youth hostel in Boulder, Colorado. Frustrated by his lack of success and misfortune, he gave up photography and settled in New York, where he found work as a delivery man for a catering company.

It was in New York in 1988 that Adam met Peter Metz, an openly gay 35-year-old public servant. Adam had been sexually attracted to men since he was 12 or 13 years old, but it was Peter who, in the patient's words, "pulled me out of the closet and into the real world." The two began an intimate relationship that lasted 3 years, during which time they lived in Peter's comfortable Queens apartment. In Metz, the impoverished Adam found not only a partner but a means of financial support. This, unfortunately, led to the decay of the couple's relationship. In Adam's words, "He said he was tired of me sponging off of him. He had a job, a car, and an apartment. I had nothing except a lousy job. What was I supposed to do?" Metz asked Adam to leave the apartment in September 1991. Adam does accept some responsibility for the failure of the relationship. "Well, I guess I could have gone out and gotten a better job. I also spent Peter's money like water. On top of all that, I wasn't exactly monogamous. He was."

The failure of his relationship with Metz began a terrible downhill spiral for Adam Moore. He moved into a decrepit hotel in Brooklyn. He began experimenting with drugs, including marijuana and crack cocaine. He lost his job with the catering company after several months of poor performance characterized by tardiness and unreliability, and he applied successfully for welfare. Adam began frequenting several New York area gay bars, and the year after losing Metz was characterized by a great deal of sexual promiscuity.

It was in the autumn of 1992 that Adam started to turn his life around. He enrolled in a drug rehabilitation program and emerged "clean." He found a job as a salesclerk in a camera store. He began to heal what had for several years been a very strained relationship with his mother. In his words,

> I love my mother. My being gay is not easy for her. She wanted me to be this married professional with a beautiful wife and two beautiful kids. That will never happen. She has to accept that—but I also have to be much nicer to her. I can still be a good son. That's what I have to start being.

The improvement in relations with Phyllis could not have come at a better time. In January 1993, she was diagnosed with breast cancer and underwent surgery. She has since done fairly well, but the experience has been an extremely difficult one for her and her son. Adam visited his mother frequently in 1993 and told her he was through with drugs forever.

Today, Adam continues to work at the camera store. He shares a modest but clean three-bedroom apartment in Queens with a young couple and their 2-year-old son. He is presently not involved in an intimate relationship. The patient has few friends. His only social activities are occasional dinners with other employees from work. He does not enjoy sports, music, or other pastimes. Much of his free time is spent in front of his black-and-white television or reading magazines.

The patient describes himself as an "Irish-American Catholic," but he has never belonged to an organized religion and considers himself "pretty much an atheist." While involved with Peter Metz, Adam belonged to a number of gay rights organizations and movements, but he has since withdrawn his participation entirely. His roommates describe the patient as "very withdrawn" but pleasant.

Past Personal and Family Medical History

From a medical standpoint, Adam's childhood and adolescence were quite unremarkable. He was never hospitalized and suffered no major childhood diseases. In 1990, he was struck by a car while crossing a busy intersection. He was taken to hospital by ambulance, but apart from a few contusions and small lacerations, he was fine and was discharged the same day. His illicit drug abuse in the early 1990s brought him into contact with the health care system several times, including two trips to the emergency room for symptoms of cocaine withdrawal. He received some counseling from an addictions specialist in 1991 but without much success. As mentioned earlier, Adam enrolled in a rehabilitation program that was successful in ending his drug abuse. He remains clean. He neither smokes nor consumes alcohol. The patient presently uses no medications. He is presently enrolled in a government medical assistance program.

Adam received all routine childhood immunizations. He has never been vaccinated against hemophilus influenzae, hepatitis B, or tuberculosis (BCG). He had a tetanus booster shot in 1990 after his accident. He has no known exposure to tuberculosis.

Harvey Moore, who was plagued by alcoholism and depression much of his life, shot himself in the head in 1974 at the age of 36. He had been separated from Phyllis for 5 years, having left the family when Adam was just 4 years old.

Phyllis Moore, 56, was a heavy smoker until she was diagnosed with breast cancer, at which point she quit with the help of her family physician. She is an obese woman, carrying nearly 130kg on her 167cm frame. She has no history of other health problems.

The Problem

You are a family physician working in a publicly funded primary care center in the heart of a large city. Adam Moore, a single, 31-year-old man, comes to your office and says, "I'm here for an AIDS test, Doctor."

Questions

1. Describe how you would proceed with the interview from this point.

Discussion

1. A diagnosis of AIDS or HIV infection has a profound impact on a patient's medical, social, psychological, and even financial well-being. AIDS has received more attention in the past 15 years, both by the lay public and the medical community,

than any other illness. For these reasons, testing for HIV infection is an extremely serious matter, which must be accompanied by appropriate counseling. Such counseling is among the most important roles of the primary care physician in the management of HIV disease (Miller & Lipman, 1996). A number of detailed, authoritative guidelines designed for primary care physicians are available. These include those distributed by the American Medical Association (AMA Division of Health Sciences, 1993, 1994), the Agency for Health Care Policy and Research (AHCPR; Early HIV Infection Guideline Panel, 1994), and the College of Family Physicians of Canada (CFPC; National Working Group on Comprehensive Care, 1993). Interestingly, as pointed out by Wagner (1994), the guidelines issued by the AHCPR do not include pretest procedures, although they point out that pretest counseling is important. In this regard, the AMA provides the most comprehensive guidelines pertaining to pretest management. These guidelines are divided into four categories: **providing information about the HIV test, HIV education, conducting risk assessment, and counseling about risk reduction.**

A discussion of HIV testing should begin with asking why the patient wants the test. This should be followed by an explanation of the meaning of a positive or negative test. Issues of confidentiality need to be addressed, such as state reporting requirements and different types of testing (e.g., anonymous). The way in which the test is done (in two stages, enzyme-linked immunosorbent assay [ELISA] followed by confirmatory Western Blot) should be

explained. It is imperative for the physician to explain the "window period" during which HIV infection may have taken place but antibodies to the virus have yet to appear, giving a negative test result. This is usually 6 to 12 weeks. The benefits of testing (such as helping to prevent passing the infection to others) as well as disadvantages (e.g., effect on employment and insurance if test is positive) should be addressed.

According to the AMA (1993), HIV education should include information about the modes of transmission of HIV, the course of HIV disease, and presently available therapies. Risk assessment means taking a thorough history of past and present sexual behavior and drug use. Although this is a very sensitive issue, questions relating to specific high-risk sexual behaviors such as anal-genital activity should be posed. It is important to keep in mind that all drug use, whether intravenous or not, increases the risk of HIV infection because it impairs judgment and subsequent sexual practices.

Risk reduction counseling includes recommendations for reducing high-risk sexual behavior such as using condoms, limiting the number of sexual partners, and avoiding sexual activities that can cause cuts or tears in the lining of the rectum, penis, or vagina. Sharing used needles or syringes should be avoided.

All pretest counseling sessions should include an assessment of the patient's coping skills and social supports. Finally, once the session has resulted in an exchange of information satisfactory to both the physician and patient, formal informed consent should be obtained.

The Rest of the Story

You engage the patient in a comprehensive pretest counseling session. Adam tells you that he wants an HIV test because he found out that a man whom he met shortly after breaking up with Peter Metz, and with whom he had unprotected anal-genital intercourse on a number of occasions, recently died of AIDS in a New York hospital.

> I read about it in the newspaper. Terence Ruhlmann . . . dead at age 34. I figured it was AIDS, but I went down to one of the bars and asked around. Everyone said it was AIDS. Anyway, I got to thinking, there must be dozens of other guys I had sex with who are dead now. That's why I want to be tested.

Adam is uncertain about how many sexual contacts he has had, but believes the number to be over 100. He has never had heterosexual intercourse. His use of condoms in the early 1990s was sporadic at best.

Adam denies sexual intercourse of any kind in the past 3 years. He admits to a long history of crack cocaine abuse but considers himself rehabilitated and clean since January 1993. Adam denies ever using drugs intravenously.

You tell Adam that he has the option of undergoing anonymous testing, whereby only he will have access to his result. Otherwise, his HIV status will be a confidential matter between you and the patient. The state of New York does not require reporting of positive results to public authorities. You describe the benefits of testing. First and foremost, if his result is positive, a careful monitoring program can be implemented, together with a number of presently available therapies to improve both the length and quality of Adam's life. Furthermore, knowledge of positive HIV status can help Adam to protect others from infection. You inform Adam that, unfortunately, a positive HIV result can have a profound negative impact on personal relationships, finances, employment, and insurance.

You describe the conventional test for HIV as a two-step process, with the Western Blot normally used to confirm a positive ELISA. You explain the window period to Adam. You tell him that a positive result means that he is infected and can pass the infection on to others. He is also told that there is a small "false positive" rate and that sometimes the result returns as "indeterminate," necessitating repeat testing. A negative result almost certainly means he is not infected but does not mean that he is immune to HIV. You go on to describe AIDS as a viral illness caused by the HIV virus, which attacks the body's immune system, gradually weakening it so that resistance to infection is compromised. It is spread through exchange of blood, body organs, semen, and vaginal secretions. You tell Adam that there is presently no cure for AIDS.

You briefly review risk reduction strategies such as avoidance of unprotected sex and sharing needles. Adam tells you, "I have no intention of doing anything like that, for sure."

Your interview concludes with an exploration of Adam's social supports. He confesses that he has no close friends in New York. He loves his mother very much and has always relied on her for support. When asked how he would react if he is HIV positive, Adam tells you,

Well. I don't know. I mean, I don't think it would be the end of the world. I wouldn't off myself or anything. I think life would just go on, and I would make the most of the years I would have left. I think I might move in with my mom—we could look after each other.

In the case of a negative result, Adam tells you,

I'd be awfully relieved, of course. I don't think much else would change in my life. Any future relationships I have are going to involve safe sex. I'm not a junkie anymore. I've got a clear head on my shoulders.

Adam tells you he has no further questions or concerns at the present time. He is not interested in anonymous testing. He signs a form indicating his informed consent for the HIV test. You arrange a posttest appointment in 2 weeks and make it clear to Adam that you will disclose the result in person only. Before leaving, Adam tells you, "OK. For the next 2 weeks, I'm just going to go on with life as usual. I'm not going to worry about it now. I'll deal with the result when it comes." You tell him that sounds like a good plan and that you look forward to seeing him soon.

PART II

The Problem

Adam Moore's HIV test result returns as positive and he comes back as scheduled for his posttest appointment.

Questions

1. How would you disclose the test result to Adam?
2. Beyond disclosure, what else would you do at this visit?

Discussion

1. The AMA (1993) favors a direct and immediate disclosure of HIV status in a posttest session. "Your tests show you have the virus" is an acceptable way of conveying a positive result. Regardless of the patient's own suspicions and the thoroughness of pretest counseling, this is never an easy moment for either the physician or patient. The next step is to allow and encourage the patient to express his or her feelings and understanding of the result.

2. The patient should be told once again how to prevent passing the infection to others. Adam should not donate blood, semen, or organ tissues. He should practice only "safer sex." A review of avoidance of high-risk practices at the posttest visit has been shown to reduce future incidence of sexually transmitted disease (Zenilman, Erickson, Fox, Reichart, & Hook, 1992). He should not share razors, toothbrushes, needles, or syringes with others. Furthermore, he should inform other health pro-

fessionals with whom he comes in contact about his HIV seropositivity. Adam should be encouraged to inform any past sexual contacts about his HIV status so that they may consider HIV testing. This is an area in which the physician should offer help.

Adam is a relatively poor, isolated young man who has lived a troubled life. His lack of social supports is a major concern, given his HIV result. In this case, the physician should ask Adam about his interest in HIV support groups, individual counseling, and other support services. Adam's physician should take an active role in coordinating these other levels of care. There is a positive association between AIDS and suicide (Gibson & Saunders, 1994). Adam should be closely monitored throughout his HIV care for depressive symptoms and suicide risk.

Finally, the posttest session should mark the beginning of comprehensive management of early HIV infection. Upon completion of this visit, Adam should be told to return in a relatively short period of time for a full medical evaluation, appropriate laboratory testing, and reassessment of his coping abilities.

PART III

The Problem

You tell Adam that his test result is positive and ask him how he feels about that. He says nothing for several seconds, and finally responds in an annoyed fashion, "Well, how do you think I feel? I mean. God damn it! I should have known. No one could have wreaked havoc the way I did and gotten away with it. I guess I just have to deal with this."

You ask Adam if he fully understands the meaning of the result. He says,

Yeah. I know what it's all about. I'm HIV positive. I don't have AIDS. I can transmit this to others . . . through sex and stuff, that I don't do anyway. I guess I just have to stay healthy. I'm not planning on sleeping around or shooting drugs. I've given up that forever.

You tell Adam about other ways of infecting others, including donation of body fluids and tissue. You ask him about how he feels about informing other concerned parties about the result.

Well, I don't mind telling anyone I have to. I've never donated blood or anything, so I'm not worried about that. Man, but I was high on crack back when I was sleeping around. I don't know if I can go around tracking people down to tell them that I've got it. I wouldn't know where to start.

You ask Adam if he feels there are any specific individuals who should know about his positive result.

Yeah, Peter for one. I have to tell him. I mean, I cheated on him a lot. God, I hope he hasn't got it. I haven't talked to him for 5 years. He's not my biggest fan. I don't think I'll bother telling the family I live with. I don't eat with them. I don't share brushes, forks, or anything. I've got my own bathroom in the apartment. I mean I hardly see those people. There is one person who should never know. It would kill her for sure—my mother.

Adam appears agitated and angry throughout the interview. You ask Adam if he is interested in a support group or specialized individual counseling. "Yeah. I'd like to talk to other people who have got it. I mean no offense, but talking to you about this is really kind of bullshit. 'How do I feel about the result?' What a ridiculous question."

You emphasize the importance of close follow-up for Adam that will include a thorough medical evaluation and staging of his illness. You tell him you would like to see him again in 1 week, at which point you could discuss participation in a support group further, as well as how he is coping. You tell Adam that if he has any questions or concerns prior to this appointment, he should feel free to contact you. Adam rises from his chair with a look of contempt on his face. "Whatever, Doc," he says, as he storms out of your office.

Questions

1. How would you assess Adam's reaction to his test result?

Discussion

1. Initial reactions to a positive HIV test result are extremely varied and unpredictable (Gibson & Saunders, 1994). Adam reacts with anger, which is certainly not unusual. It is important for the physician to allow him to express this emotion without criticism (Fallowfield & Lipkin, 1993) to prevent an even more hostile reaction and a seriously compromised doctor-patient relationship. although Adam's reaction may be difficult to handle, the physician must still try to meet the agenda of the posttest session, especially making sure the patient returns for further evaluation. A follow-up phone call, after Adam has had time to digest the meaning of the diagnosis he has received and cool off, may be helpful in reaffirming some points of the posttest session. It has also been suggested that a tape recording of such encounters, in which bad news has been delivered, be made available to the patient so that information can be reviewed in a less distressed state (Fallowfield & Lipkin, 1993).

PART IV

The Problem

Adam returns as scheduled for his follow-up appointment. You have not spoken to him in the interim. He appears calm and relaxed. "First of all, Doctor," he says, "I want to apologize for my behavior last week. So many things were going through my mind, I didn't know what to think or say."

You tell Adam that, under the circumstances, his reaction was completely understandable, and you are pleased he has returned. You ask him how he has been during the past week.

At first, it was rough. I just went home and cried. I called my mother several times. She sensed that something was wrong. I just told her I missed her and was feeling lonely. I was also really afraid. I'm not sure what life is going to be like from now on. Three days ago, I got up enough courage to call Peter. That was an amazing conversation. I told him I have HIV and that he should get tested. He was so kind and compassionate. I mean, I treated the guy like crap, and here he was feeling bad for me. He even offered to help me in any way he could. He was so sincere. He said I shouldn't worry about him, and that he had tested negative recently. I was so relieved. I told him I was through with drugs and that I have a good job. He said that was wonderful, and that we should be friends. I felt better after talking to him. The last couple of days have been good.

Adam seems enthusiastic about getting on with the medical evaluation and joining a support group.

Questions

1. Describe what elements of the medical history and physical examination you would incorporate into an initial evaluation.
2. What laboratory tests would you request?
3. What immunizations, if any, would you consider at this point for Adam?

Discussion

1. Adam's present attitude is certainly a positive development. Nevertheless, it is best to review the content of the posttest session, especially to make sure he has a thorough understanding of what it means to be HIV positive.

The CFPC (National Working Group, 1993) has a simple but comprehensive approach to the patient who is first diagnosed with HIV infection. HIV disease can affect virtually every system of the body, and an initial evaluation should take this into account. This includes a baseline history, in which general health status, past medical history, drug and sexual history, risks of infectious complications (e.g., immunizations, travel history, exposure to TB), and psychosocial history are assessed. Much of this information has already been gathered. The next step is a thorough review of systems, followed by a baseline physical examination, baseline lab tests, and, finally, administration of appropriate immunizations and tests for tuberculosis.

The initial review of systems and physical examination should be quite exhaustive, both to pick up signs and symptoms of early disease and to serve as a control for future assessments (see "The Rest of the Story," which follows).

2. The baseline laboratory investigations, in addition to serving as markers for future abnormalities, may also pick up signs of immune compromise when no physical signs or symptoms exist.

A CBC and differential are required. A decreased hemoglobin level is a nonspecific indicator of HIV disease progression (Clement & Hollander, 1995). This lab test is also of value because *zidovidine* (ZDV, formerly AZT), a common therapeutic medication used in HIV patients, can suppress neutrophil count and cause macrocytosis. The baseline MCV and neutrophil count can serve as markers for future adverse effects of such therapy. Similarly, a baseline B-12 and folate level are suggested, as uncorrected deficiencies of these in the setting of ZDV administration would likely exacerbate macrocytosis.

Appropriate swabs for STDs, along with tests for syphilis, hepatitis B, hepatitis C, and toxoplasmosis, are required to rule out exposure to or infection by the corresponding pathogens.

Tuberculosis is a major opportunistic infection in HIV patients. All authorities (AMA Division of Health Sciences, 1994; Canadian Task Force on the Periodic Health Examination, 1994; Early HIV Infection Guideline Panel, 1994; National Working Group, 1993; U.S. Preventive Services Task Force, 1996) recommend PPD skin testing. The AHCPR (Early HIV Infection Guideline Panel, 1994) recommends *simultaneous* anergy screening using two of three antigens (candida, mumps, tetanus toxoid). Alternatively, an anergy panel can be administered only in the case of a negative skin test result for TB. The CFPC (National Working Group, 1993) recommends a baseline CXR in all patients initially diagnosed with HIV, regardless of PPD status.

The CD4 (also known as T4 or T-Helper) cell count is the standard marker used to assess the degree of immune system dysfunction in an HIV positive patient (Bally, 1993). A baseline value is universally recommended.

Routine tests of renal and hepatic function are important, as many pharmacotherapies can affect these parameters. Furthermore, certain opportunistic infections or neoplasms can penetrate the liver. Interestingly, the AMA (1994) also recommends obtaining an assay for glucose-6 phosphate dehydrogenase (G-6PD) deficiency. G-6PD deficiency is a common glycogen storage disease characterized by hypoglycemia, hepatomegaly, and bleeding diathesis (Beaudet, 1994). It is usually detected early in life. No rationale is given in the AMA guidelines for this recommendation.

3. An annual vaccination against influenza is recommended, as well as a one-time pneumococcal vaccine. Vaccination against hepatitis B is recommended to those with no evidence of immunity. Adam has had a tetanus booster (Td) in the past 10 years and does not require one now. The CFPC (1993) recommends administration of inactivated polio vaccine (IPV) every 10 years. Vaccination against hemophilus influenzae b (Hib) is considered optional. As Adam has received the routine childhood immunizations, these need not be readministered. All live vaccines, with the exception of MMR (National Working Group, 1993), are contraindicated in HIV positive patients.

The Rest of the Story

Initial suggested medical evaluation (corresponding results for Adam Moore summarized)

Review of systems:

General: no recent fatigue, fever, sweats, or any loss of appetite or weight
Skin/mucous membranes: Patient has noticed no abnormalities
Respiratory: No nasal or sinus congestion or pain. No cough, sputum, shortness of breath, or chest pain

Gastrointestinal: No dys- or hypogeusia, dysphagia, odynophagia, nausea, vomiting, abdominal or rectal pain, diarrhea, or jaundice

Genitourinary: No dysuria or penile discharge

Neurologic: No seizures, weakness, tingling or pain in extremities, change in balance, or visual changes

Psychiatric: Adam describes his mood as "still down in the dumps, but getting better." He tells you he is learning to accept his illness and wants to get on with his life while trying to stay as healthy as possible. When asked about his libido or sex drive, Adam says, "Haven't had any sex drive recently at all. It's not something that's on my mind." Patient reports no change in memory, concentration, or any sleep disturbance. He denies any suicidal thoughts or plans.

Physical examination:

General: Quiet, pleasant young man

  Wt. = 72.5kg; height = 1.75m; T = 37.2°C; BP = 117/60mmHg

Head and neck: No oral lesions

  No sinus tenderness

  No visual field defects, retinal hemorrhages, or any visible exudate on funduscopic examination

Lymph nodes: No cervical, supraclavicular, axillary, or inguinal lymphadenopathy noted

Skin: No rashes, ulcers, or lesions

Chest and cardiovascular: Examination unremarkable

Abdominal and rectal: No hepatosplenomegaly; no abdominal tenderness; no rectal or anal lesions

Genitourinary: No genital lesions; no penile discharge

Neurologic: Normal strength in all four limbs

  Normal sensation over all four limbs

Mental status: Formal mental status examination not carried out at this visit. Patient describes mood as slightly depressed. Has appropriate affect. Appears to have no obvious impairment of cognition or judgment.

PART V

The Problem

After examining Adam, you tell him that he appears very healthy. You administer vaccinations against influenza, polio, and pneumococcus, as well as a PPD test (5 TU). You send him to the lab for blood tests and a CXR and arrange follow-up in 4 days. Once again, you ask him to call you in the interim should he have any questions or concerns. Adam agrees to this plan and returns as scheduled. He tells you that he is feeling very well.

Questions

1. After reviewing the results of Adam's lab tests in "The Rest of the Story" immediately following, how would you proceed?

The Rest of the Story

Suggested laboratory tests and corresponding results (all values in standard SI units when not specified)

CXR-PA + Lat: Read as "within normal limits, demonstrating no evidence of pulmonary disease" by radiologist

CBC:

Hb 142

Hematocrit 48.0%

MCH 2.01 (normal)

MCHC 21.2 (normal)

MCV 90.3

Total leukocytes 8.3

Lymphocytes 3.0

Mononuclear cells 0.4

Granulocytes 4.9

Platelets 310

Reticulocytes 0.008 (normal)

BUN 7.0Mm

Creatinine 50μmol/L

B-12 210 (normal)

Folate (plasma) 6.8 (normal)

ALT 0.16 (normal)

AST 0.34 (normal)

Alkaline phosphatase 1.62 (normal)

Penile swabs chlamydia and gonorrhea: Both negative

VDRL: Negative

HBsAg: Negative

Anti-HBs: Negative

Anti-HCV: Negative

Toxoplasmosis titre: negative

PPD: 7mm

CD4: 390 cells/cubic Mm (This is the absolute CD4 count. Some clinicians prefer to use the percentage of CD4 cells as a more stable measure, as the absolute count varies with time of day, the particular laboratory, age, and gender [AMA, 1994])

Discussion

1. The laboratory results reveal two significant abnormalities. First, although Adam is an asymptomatic HIV patient, his CD4 count, which is below the lower limit

of normal (500 cells/cubic Mm), reveals mild immune dysfunction. Second, Adam's PPD test is positive (over 5mm of induration is considered positive in HIV patients). He has been infected with TB but has no signs of active disease.

The decreased CD4 count raises the question of whether to initiate antiretroviral therapy. This is usually ZDV. The value of early administration of ZDV to asymptomatic, HIV patients with evidence of immune system compromise is a controversial issue. Early studies showed that ZDV delayed the onset of opportunistic infections and prolonged survival in patients with HIV (Fischl, Richman, & Grieco, 1987). The "Concorde Study," which questioned the benefit of such therapy, is among the evidence against early administration of ZDV (Albouker & Swart, 1993). The AHCPR and other authorities recommend "offering" ZDV to patients like Adam. Adam should be told that the value of this medication is an unresolved matter. He should also know about the side effects of ZDV, which, early in the course of treatment, commonly include insomnia, headache, nausea, vomiting, myalgia, and dyspepsia. These usually resolve within 12 weeks. Late side effects include hepatic dysfunction, bone marrow suppression, anemia, neutropenia, and myopathy (Early HIV Infection Guideline Panel, 1994; National Working Group, 1993). ZDV is usually started at 600mg/day, given in divided doses.

HIV positive patients with a positive PPD test have a 10% annual risk of developing active TB, compared with just a 10% lifetime risk in PPD-positive, HIV negative patients (Early HIV Infection Guideline Panel, 1994). Preventive therapy with isoniazid (INH) is recommended (AMA, 1994; Early HIV Infection Guideline Panel, 1994; National Working Group, 1993). Adam should take either 300mg per day of INH or 900mg twice a week for a full year. Pyridoxine (50 to 100mg/day) is given concomitantly to prevent INH-induced peripheral neuritis. Adam shows no evidence of exposure to or infection by hepatitis B. This is a good opportunity to administer the hepatitis B vaccine (usually given in three doses).

PART VI

The Problem

You tell Adam that he is infected with tuberculosis and has a considerable risk of developing active disease. You also tell him that his CD4 count, a marker of the health of his immune system, is decreased. You describe prevention of TB with INH and the possible benefit of ZDV, as well as its adverse effects. Adam shares your concerns about tuberculosis and agrees to start INH prophylaxis. He also decides to start therapy with ZDV. You administer the first of three doses of the hepatitis B vaccine.

Questions

1. When would you like to follow up with Adam?

Discussion

1. ZDV therapy requires close monitoring, both for adverse symptoms and hematologic dysfunction. A follow-up visit within a short period of time would also allow the physician to continue monitoring Adam's mood, social circumstances, and ability to cope. The AMA recommends follow-up in 2 weeks for those started on ZDV, at which point a CBC and differential should be repeated.

Conclusion

Adam schedules a follow-up appointment in 2 weeks. He visits the lab for a CBC and differential test the day before his appointment. Upon his arrival, you have the result, which is normal. You ask him how he has been doing. He responds,

> Not so good. Well, I should say, I'm doing OK. I've been attending the support group you suggested, and it's great. I mean, we share all kinds of experiences. I get so much useful info, even about things like housing and insurance. The problem is my mother. She visited the doctor last week for terrible headaches. Her cancer has come back in a big way. It has spread all over—even to her head. She's in a terrible state . . . crying all the time. I have to go to Boston now. I quit my job. I have to be with her now for sure. I want to thank you for all your help.

Adam tells you that he has been doing quite well on the ZDV. He says that he was nauseated for the first couple of days and vomited once or twice but has since been fine; he reports no other side effects.

You tell Adam that his lab test is normal and that you are sorry that his mother is in such a condition. You explore Adam's mood and how he is coping with the difficult circumstances that have enveloped him. Adam tells you his mood has been good. He has been sleeping and eating well. He still "feels a little down" but is not considering harming himself in any way. He tells you he actually feels a bit hopeful for the future. "My mom and I are going to pull through this together," he tells you.

You provide Adam with the names of several primary care physicians in the Boston area with experience in managing HIV positive patients, together with information about social services and support groups that are available. Adam agrees to find a new physician and to follow up in 2 weeks to receive the second dose of the hepatitis B vaccine. You also tell him that he should have a repeat CD4 test within 3 months. You inform Adam that when a formal request is made by his new physician, you will forward all his old records, including his lab tests. Once again, you emphasize that you are available to help him in any way you can during this challenging point in his life, and you wish him all the best.

References

Aboulker, J. P., & Swart, A. M. (1993). Preliminary analysis of the Concorde trial [Letter to editor]. *Lancet, 341,* 889.

American Medical Association Division of Health Sciences. (1993). *HIV blood test counseling: Physician guidelines* (2nd ed.). Chicago: American Medical Association.

American Medical Association Division of Health Sciences. (1994). *HIV early intervention: Physician guidelines* (2nd ed.). Chicago: American Medical Association.

Bally, G. (1993). Caring for patients with HIV infection. *Canadian Family Physician, 39,* 2175-2182.

Beaudet, A. L. (1994). The glycogen storage diseases. In J. D. Wilson, E. Braunwald, K. J. Isselbacher, R. G. Petersdorf, J. B. Martin, A. S. Fauci, & R. K. Root (Eds.), *Harrison's principles of internal medicine.* New York: McGraw-Hill.

Canadian Task Force on the Periodic Health Examination. (1994). *The Canadian guide to clinical preventive health care.* Ottawa: Minister of Supply and Services.

Clement, M., & Hollander, H. (1995). Initial evaluation of and health care maintenance for the HIV-infected adult. In M. A. Sande & P. A. Volberding (Eds.), *The medical management of AIDS.* Philadelphia: W. B. Saunders.

Early HIV Infection Guideline Panel. (1994). *Evaluation and management of early HIV infection* (AHCPR Publication No. 94-0572). Rockville, MD: Agency for Health Care Policy and Research.

Fallowfield, L. J., & Lipkin, M. (1993). Delivering sad or bad news. *Lancet, 341,* 476-478.

Fischl, M. A., Richman, D. D., & Grieco, M. H. (1987). The efficacy of azidothymidine (AZT) in the treatment of patients with AIDS and AIDS related complex: A double-blind placebo-controlled trial. *New England Journal of Medicine, 317,* 185-191.

Gibson, G., & Saunders, D. (1994). HIV disease: Psychosocial issues for patients and doctors. *Canadian Family Physician, 40,* 1422-1426.

Miller, R., & Lipman, M. (1996). HIV pre-test discussion: Not just for specialists. *British Medical Journal, 313,* 130.

National Working Group on Comprehensive Care for Persons With HIV Disease. (1993). *A comprehensive guide for the care of persons with HIV disease.* Mississauga, Ontario: College of Family Physicians of Canada.

U.S. Preventive Services Task Force. (1996). *Guide to clinical preventive services* (2nd ed.). Baltimore, MD: Williams and Wilkins.

Wagner, R. A. (1994). Pretest counseling, informed consent and HIV testing [letter]. *American Family Physician, 50,* 48.

Zenilman, J. M., Erickson, B., Fox, R., Reichart, C. A., & Hook, E. W. (1992). Effect of HIV posttest counseling on STD incidence. *Journal of the American Medical Association, 267,* 843-845.

14. MENOPAUSE

Ms. Esmerelda Gutierez

*Goal: The goal of this group discussion exercise is to develop
and evaluate the participants' knowledge of the signs
and symptoms of the climacteric as well as the management
of this developmental phase in a healthy woman.*

Specific Objectives: Upon completion of this group discussion exercise, each participant should be able to accomplish the following:

1. Describe the wide spectrum of signs and symptoms that can accompany the climacteric.
2. Counsel a patient effectively about the risks and benefits of hormone replacement therapy.
3. Describe health promotion strategies complementary to hormone replacement therapy, including diet, exercise, and drug therapies.
4. Describe the various hormone replacement regimens currently available, and customize a prescription for an individual patient's needs.

PART I

The Patient

Social History

Esmerelda Gutierez is a 51-year-old office manager who lives and works in Ft. Lauderdale, Florida. Born in Santiago, Cuba, she came to the United States as a teenager with her father, Rudolfo; her mother, Rosa; and her younger sister, Alicia, in 1961. The Gutierez family settled in Miami, where Esmerelda completed high school. An aspiring singer, she later attended 1 year of music school and went on to perform in a number of Miami-area night clubs. Having achieved only very limited success after 2 years, Esmerelda took a secretarial course at a vocational college and landed a job with a local bank.

The patient met Diego Perron, a Miami attorney, in 1964. The two were married 2 years later. Diego was 38 at the time; Esmerelda was just 21. The patient describes her marriage as brief and unhappy, characterized by frequent verbal and physical abuse as well as numerous extramarital indiscretions by her husband. Despite all this, the couple did have one child, Julianna, born in 1967. They separated in 1968 and divorced in 1970.

Diego had no interest in helping to raise Julianna and no desire to contribute financially to the well-being of his ex-wife or daughter. Consequently, Esmerelda and Julianna moved in with Rudolfo and Rosa. Esmerelda continued to work at the bank as a secretary while Julianna was under the loving care of her adoring grandmother. The patient left the bank in 1977 for a higher-paying secretarial position in an insurance company in Ft. Lauderdale. Despite a still modest income, Esmerelda's careful management of money allowed her to purchase a small house in 1980. A hardworking and faithful employee, the patient was eventually promoted to office manager in 1988. She continues to work in that capacity, overseeing the processing of automobile insurance claims.

Rudolfo Gutierez, now 80 years old and a retired employee of a shipping company, and Rosa, 73, live together in a senior citizens residence in Miami. The patient's sister, Alicia, is a married housewife with four children and lives in Port Jefferson, New York. Julianna, a physical therapist, has been married for 2 years and lives in Sarasota, Florida. She has no children.

Esmerelda is a soft-spoken, ever-smiling woman whom her coworkers describe as "Mrs. Sunshine" because of her pleasant demeanor. She has a number of very close friends, many of whom she has known since high school. Julianna and Esmerelda are very close and are in touch with each other at least once a week. The patient's parents also keep in touch, especially as they are in need of some help with transportation and shopping for food, which Esmerelda happily provides. Alicia ran away from home when she was 17. Since that time she has had only sporadic contact with her parents, but she does manage to speak with Esmerelda once or twice a year.

The patient describes herself as "born Catholic" and a "true believer," but she rarely attends church. She enjoys having dinner with friends, watching television, and reading. Esmerelda and a coworker have recently enrolled in golf lessons that they are both enjoying immensely.

Past Personal and Family Medical History

The patient was a healthy child who grew up to be a healthy young woman. Indeed, she has no memory of any childhood hospitalizations or illnesses. Esmerelda began menstruating at age 13. She gave birth to Julianna at age 22. This represents her first and only pregnancy, and it was completely uncomplicated, except that "Julianna showed up a couple of weeks early." There is no other significant medical or surgical history.

Esmerelda began smoking soon after separation from her husband and continues to this day. Her consumption of cigarettes varies, or as she puts it, "depends on my stress level." Normally the patient smokes one pack of cigarettes per day. She has tried unsuccessfully to quit on her own on a number of occasions. She drinks about two to three glasses of wine per week, usually with dinner and rarely without company. The patient consumes approximately five to six cups of coffee a day at work. Esmerelda presently uses no medications except for one ginseng tablet per day, which she purchases at a health food store.

The patient's father is in very poor health. He has been admitted to the hospital three times in the past year for exacerbations of congestive heart failure. He suffered his first myocardial infarction in 1971. This was followed by another in 1992. He has extremely poor exercise tolerance and is more or less confined to his apartment. In addition, Rudolfo's cognitive function has deteriorated markedly in recent years. He frequently seems disoriented and confused, and he becomes frustrated and tearful with minor aggravations. His family physician has told the Guttierez family that Rudolfo suffers from senile dementia.

By comparison, Rosa is in good health. She has had no heart problems. Her only health concern has been basal cell carcinoma on her face, which was treated successfully in 1990. She is an active but somewhat frail woman who spends much of her time looking after her husband.

Esmerelda's daughter Julianna is in good health but smokes very heavily. To the best of the patient's knowledge, her sister is in good health.

The Problem

You are a family physician in a large metropolitan area with easy access to all diagnostic facilities and specialists. Esmerelda Gutierez, a divorced, 51-year-old woman, comes to see you and tells you she is "going through the change of life." More precisely, she reports that her previously "clockwork" menstrual periods have been very irregular for the past 8 months. She believes she has had only three menses during this time period, each with very scant bleeding. Esmerelda has been troubled by "hot flashes" occurring approximately four or five times a week, usually at night. She describes these as a feeling of warmth over her chest followed by profuse sweating. Esmerelda usually feels nauseated during these flashes. On one occasion, she actually vomited as a result. The flashes are brief, lasting approximately 1 min. The patient tells you, "They don't last long, but they're awful. I wake up at night completely soaked sometimes, and I have trouble falling back asleep. I'm a person who really needs her sleep."

Esmerelda reports no urinary frequency, nocturia, incontinence, or dysuria. She reports no vaginal dryness, itching, or irritation. There is no history of dizziness, headaches, dry mouth, or palpitations. When asked to describe her mood over the past 8 months, the patient, replies, "Well, I guess I've been as happy as usual. I mean, I worry about my parents. My father's pretty sick and my mother fusses over him so much she's driving herself crazy—but this isn't anything new."

The patient denies feeling depressed, irritable, or anxious. She tells you her appetite has been good and that actually she is afraid she may have gained some weight recently. She remains active, continuing to spend time with her friends and family. She has not missed any work, although she tells you, "After sleeping poorly because of night sweats, it's hard to drag myself to work in the morning." The patient denies any other sleep disturbance, including early morning awakening.

When asked what finally precipitated her visit, Esmerelda says,

Well, I know the menopause is a natural part of life—something I have to deal with. I guess I'm here for two reasons. First, I'm tired of the hot flashes and night sweats. Second, I've heard a lot about hormones to protect my bones—both good and bad things. I'd like to learn as much about that as possible.

Questions

1. Is Esmerelda menopausal?
2. What important information is missing from the history given?
3. What can you offer to relieve Esmerelda's hot flashes?
4. What would you tell Esmerelda about hormone replacement therapy and complementary health promotion strategies?

Discussion

1. The classic definition of menopause is the "cessation of menses for more than one year" (Dzerzko, 1995). Esmerelda Gutierez is, therefore, not yet "menopausal." Some, however, use the word *menopause* to refer to the spectrum of physiological changes and symptoms that happen at this time (Drife, 1993). A better term to describe Esmerelda's situation is *climacteric,* which refers to the entire transition from the reproductive to the postreproductive phase in a healthy woman (Hammond, 1996).

2. The climacteric is associated in many women with profound changes in sexual health (McCoy & Davidson, 1985). Many experience sexual dissatisfaction, often characterized by a loss of libido. Furthermore, physiological changes to the genitourinary tract, such as vaginal dryness and postcoital bleeding, can present as dyspareunia and consequent decrease in frequency of sexual activity. A history from a woman presenting with menopausal symptoms should certainly include an inquiry into her sexual well-being. Questions relating to sex, when posed tactfully and appropriately, should not be embarassing or offensive to either the physician or patient. Interestingly, physicians are often more uncomfortable with questions about sex than their patients (Kentsmith, 1979). The history provided makes no mention of Esmerelda's relationships from a romantic point of view. Is she presently involved in an intimate relationship? Is she presently sexually active? If involved but not sexually active, why not? If Esmerelda is having sex, is she satisfied? If dissatisfied, is it the result of pain, irritation, bleeding, lack of desire, or some other reason? All these issues should be addressed, and the preceding questions provide a good framework for such a discussion with the patient. Open-ended questions such as "Is there anything else you would like to tell me?" are also suitable, as they encourage the patient to express concerns she may otherwise withhold (Bates, 1991).

See "The Rest of the Story" following this discussion section for Esmerelda's response to questions of sexual health.

3. It is perhaps best to discuss therapy for hot flashes with Esmerelda in the context of overall management of the climacteric. The hot flashes, however, are her primary concern, and at this point in the consultation, she would benefit from knowing that effective management strategies are available. Hot flashes and associated night sweats, considered a symptom of "vasomotor instability" (Dzerzko, 1995), are of hypothalamic origin. They gradually disappear, but 25% of women report hot flashes of more than 5 years' duration. Hormone replacement therapy provides substantial relief of hot flashes in 90% of women (Drife, 1993). Clonidine,

an alpha-adrenergic agonist, has been shown to be of benefit in some patients (Clayden, Bell, & Pollard, 1974). Other pharmacotherapies, including propanolol and *bellergal* (belladonna, ergotamine tartrate, and phenobarbital), have been shown to provide only minimal relief and are not commonly used. It is important for Esmerelda to understand that pharmacotherapy does not provide an instant cure for hot flashes but, rather, effective symptomatic relief. Caffeine, alcohol, and spicy foods may increase the frequency or severity of hot flashes, and their avoidance is a worthwhile strategy for Esmerelda to pursue (Hammond, 1996). Wearing loose, layered clothing also is beneficial to some patients. Presenting these approaches to the management of hot flashes provides a good introduction to a general discussion of hormone replacement therapy and health promotion during the climacteric.

4. Patient education is by far the most important component of management in the case of Esmerelda Gutierez, for several reasons. The decision to receive hormone replacement therapy is not an easy one for many women. It involves a long-term commitment and can itself be associated with unpleasant side effects. Many women, quite correctly, view the climacteric as a natural phase. Some also believe that hormone replacement therapy interferes with the "natural process." Surveys have shown that most people are extremely poorly informed about the menopause. Many women receive their information on this matter from the lay press rather than from their physicians (Andrews, 1996). Esmerelda has revealed few preconceived ideas about the benefits and risks of hormone replacement therapy. A good place to begin a discussion on this subject would be to ask her what she knows about hormone re-

placement therapy and health before and after the menopause (see "The Rest of the Story" at the end of this section). This can be followed by an informative review of hormone replacement therapy and complementary health promotion strategies, based on what is currently available in the literature and without judging or disputing Esmerelda's own views. Such an approach, where the doctor does not immediately prescribe a management plan, is compatible with a good doctor-patient relationship. Esmerelda should be encouraged to make her own decision about therapy, using the information she has received from her physician and others, if she so chooses.

A discussion of the benefits and risks of hormone replacement therapy should be kept simple and concise, without quoting figures or studies, which are likely to be of less interest to the patient than "the bottom line."

First, Esmerelda should be told that there is abundant evidence that estrogen replacement therapy is protective against heart disease and strokes (Wild, 1996). She should also know these are the number one killers of women. Second, she should be told that she is correct about the effect of hormone replacement on bones. Continuous, long-term estrogen replacement does protect women from the rapid loss of bone mass in the postmenopausal period and reduces the incidence of vertebral and hip fractures, which in turn are associated with significant morbidity and mortality (Lindsay, 1996).

Hormone replacement therapy preserves muscle strength in postmenopausal women, which in the untreated patient decreases quickly after menopause (Phillips, Rook, Siddle, Bruce, & Woledge, 1993). This has obvious implications relating to mobility, balance, level of activity, and frequency of falls.

The effects of the menopause on cognitive function and mood are not completely clear at this point in time. There is evidence that hormone replacement therapy enhances mood (Sherwin, 1996). There is little evidence, however, contrary to popular belief, that the menopausal period is associated with an increase in depressive symptoms (Hammond, 1996). Estrogen replacement therapy is believed to enhance "verbal" memory in healthy postmenopausal women (Kampen & Sherwin, 1994). There is also evidence in the literature that hormone replacement is protective against Alzheimer's disease (Henderson, Paganini-Hill, Emanuel, Dunn, & Buckwalter, 1994).

As discussed earlier, estrogen replacement is effective in relieving hot flashes. Other symptoms, including those resulting from genitourinary atrophy such as vaginal dryness and irritation, respond to oral estrogen. Genitourinary atrophy can also result in frequent urinary tract infections. In addition, sexual dysfunction, characterized by loss of libido, is greatly improved with hormone replacement (Dzerzko, 1995).

Esmerelda's symptoms at the present time are hot flashes and subsequent night sweats. She should be told of all the benefits of hormone replacement therapy, including relief of symptoms with which she does not present. After all, symptoms of genitourinary atrophy often develop much later than hot flashes (Griffing & Allen, 1994), and changes in sexual well-being could also occur later. Estrogen replacement would, in this context, therefore, represent a preventive measure. Some physicians may choose to provide a more personalized review of the benefits of estrogen replacement. Esmerelda has been a smoker for many years and does have a family history of heart disease. These put her at increased risk of cardiovascular disease. Furthermore, though no physical description of the patient is given, she does have a "frail" mother and may certainly have inherited her physique. This, together with her smoking, put her at increased risk for osteoporosis. These personal considerations may help the patient make a decision about hormone replacement therapy. In addition, measurement of bone mass to identify patients at risk of osteoporosis is used by some physicians to help patients decide about hormone replacement (Dzerzko, 1995). Widespread screening for osteoporosis with bone densitometry, however, is not recommended (Canadian Task Force on the Periodic Health Examination, 1994; U.S. Preventive Services Task Force, 1996).

The risks of estrogen replacement therapy have been the focus of a great deal of attention. Estrogen is known to cause endometrial hyperplasia and to increase the risk of endometrial cancer two- to threefold (Griffing & Allen, 1994). For this reason, in women who have an intact uterus, progesterone is added to the hormone replacement regimen. The risk of endometrial cancer in women for whom both hormones are prescribed is actually lower than the same risk in those receiving no therapy (Gambrell, 1982).

The association between estrogen replacement therapy and breast cancer is still unclear, despite the publication of nearly 40 observational studies on the subject. At this point in time, most experts believe that the risk of developing breast cancer as a result of hormone replacement therapy is slight and that the benefits of therapy, particularly its cardio- and osteoprotective effects, outweigh this potential risk (Griffing & Allen, 1994; Speroff, 1996).

Health promotion during the climacteric should not consist of hormone replacement therapy alone. Complementary approaches to health promotion include good nutrition and supplements, exercise, and stress management (Menopause Consensus Committee, 1994). A healthy, well-balanced diet should, as for all patients, be recommended for women who present with menopausal symptoms. Excessive caffeine intake is a risk factor for osteoporosis (Dzerzko, 1995). Esmerelda should definitely moderate her consumption of coffee. Calcium and vitamin D are known to be osteoprotective. Total daily calcium intake should be 1,500 to 2,000mg per day, which is normally achieved through diet plus supplementation. One multiple vitamin tablet per day usually provides an adequate 400 IU of vitamin D per day (Prior, 1995).

Exercise in the form of walking, swimming, aerobics, hiking, and so on is both cardio- and osteoprotective and improves strength, balance, and sense of well-being (Menopause Consensus Committee, 1994; Prior, 1995). Esmerelda's interest in golf is a positive development in this respect. Such leisure activities represent, without doubt, an effective form of stress management. She should be encouraged to pursue this and other recreational activities.

Esmerelda should be told that her smoking is a major health concern. Smoking cessation, as for any patient, should be an important health promotion strategy. The patient's visit to ask about hot flashes and hormone replacement therapy provides an ideal introduction for a follow-up visit specifically to discuss smoking cessation. It is probably best not to overwhelm Esmerelda with smoking cessation strategies at this point, as she already has a good deal of information to digest. One possible approach is to end the consultation by asking Esmerelda how interested she is in quitting smoking. A positive response can be followed by an offer of help with smoking cessation.

The Rest of the Story

You ask the patient if she is involved in an intimate or romantic relationship and if she is sexually active. She responds,

> Oh, no. I was involved with someone several years ago. He was with the Navy and is now retired. I spoke to him a few months ago, and we even talked about getting back together, but it was just talk. He was the last person I had sex with.

You ask Esmerelda how she would describe her sex drive or desire.

> Oh . . . I don't know. I haven't noticed any change. I don't have any more or any less desire to have sex right now. It's not something I'm worried about. It's not a high priority. I enjoy my friends, family, and work. If I meet someone and we hit it off, then great, but I'm not in the hunt, if you know what I mean!

You ask the patient what she knows about hormone replacement therapy and other health promotion strategies. Esmerelda responds as follows:

Well . . . let me see. I know that I can take estrogen to protect my bones. I think that's important. You hear about a lot of old women who break their bones easily. My mother is a frail little lady. I'm afraid she'll fall and break her hip some day. So as far as I know, that's why I should take estrogen—but I also know that taking it for a long time can cause breast cancer. So I guess one has to balance the two.

You ask Esmerelda, "Do you know of any other benefits or risks of hormone replacement therapy?"

"No, I can't say I do."

"How about other strategies for healthy living during this part of life?"

"Well, I know that some women take calcium to protect their bones. Beyond that I don't know of any."

PART II

The Problem

Esmerelda thanks you for the information you have provided. She tells you, "This is a lot to think about. I'm not going to decide about all this right now. Is it OK if I think about what you've told me and come back next week?"

You tell Esmerelda that, indeed, deciding about therapy during this phase of life should be done carefully, and taking some time to do so is not only acceptable but advisable. You agree to meet Esmerelda in 1 week's time.

The patient returns and tells you,

Well, I've made up my mind. I never even knew about the risk of heart disease before you told me. I certainly don't want to wind up like my father. All things considered, I think I would like to start hormone replacement. Getting some relief from the hot flashes would be very welcome right now! I will definitely continue exercising and eating properly. I'm also going to add calcium and vitamin D tablets to my daily routine. As far as the smoking goes, well, I don't know if I'm quite ready for it. I want to quit for good, and I know I'll need help. I will definitely get in touch with you when I am ready.

Questions

1. What would you do now?

Discussion

1. Esmerelda requires an initial evaluation prior to starting hormone replacement therapy. This must definitely include both pelvic and breast examinations, as well as a Pap smear if she is due for one. Some authorities recommend a baseline fasting cholesterol and triglyceride level (Menopause Consensus Committee, 1994). Recommendations for mammographic evaluation vary (Canadian Task Force, 1994; Menopause Consensus Committee, 1994; U.S. Preventive Services,

1996). This visit is also a good time to incorporate other components of the periodic health examination, including assessment of blood pressure, height, and weight (U.S. Preventive Services, 1996). Endometrial sampling should not be carried out routinely on all patients prior to receiving hormone replacement therapy. The indications for an endometrial biopsy are highly irregular bleeding patterns or risk factors for endometrial cancer (Menopause Consensus Committee, 1994).

PART III

The Problem

Esmerelda's physical examination and lab results are unremarkable.

Questions

1. What is the next step?

Discussion

1. Upon completion of the initial evaluation, Esmerelda should be informed about the options she has for hormone replacement therapy. As noted earlier, together with estrogen (usually 0.625mg conjugated estrogen per day), Esmerelda should receive progesterone (usually 5 to 10mg/day), as she has an intact uterus. Hormone replacement can be administered "cyclically" or "continuously." One cyclical regimen involves taking oral estrogen for days 1 through 25 of each month and progesterone from days 12 through 25. Another is administration of oral estrogen every day of each month, with progesterone given for the first 2 weeks. A minimum of 12 days of progesterone is needed for endometrial protection (Griffing & Allen, 1994).

A continuous oral hormone replacement regimen consists of taking estrogen (usually 0.625mg) each day of the month together with a lower dose of progesterone (usually 2.5mg per day). The cyclical regimens are associated with menstrual bleeding that can be distressing to some women. This can be avoided by using the continuous regimen, although scant bleeding may still occur irregularly during the first year of therapy.

In addition to oral therapy, transdermal preparations of estrogen are available in the form of patches. In Canada, a combined estrogen-progesterone transdermal regimen is available (Novartis Pharmaceuticals, 1995). Although patches have proved effective in relieving menopausal symptoms and preventing osteoporosis, the cardioprotective value of transdermal preparations is uncertain, as they do not appear have the same beneficial impact of serum lipids as oral preparations (Chetkowski et al., 1986).

Side effects of hormone replacement therapy include mastalgia, which is very common but usually resolves in 3 months (Dzerzko, 1995). Mastalgia can be avoided or diminished by using a lower dose of estrogen or a continuous replacement regimen. Some women also complain of bloating, headaches, nausea, and menorrhagia. In addition, transdermal preparations are known to cause skin irritation (Chetkowski et al., 1986).

Esmerelda should be seen 3 months after beginning hormone replacement therapy (Menopause Consensus Committee, 1994). Her physician should ask about side effects. Blood pressure should be repeated. The importance of smoking cessation should be re-emphasized.

Conclusion

Esmerelda Gutierez decides to begin a cyclical oral hormone replacement regimen. She returns 3 months later and tells you she feels pretty well.

She has had two regular menses and reports no mastalgia or other complaints. Her blood pressure is normal. You tell her that you are pleased that things are going well, but her smoking remains a concern. She agrees and arranges follow-up 3 weeks later to discuss strategies for smoking cessation.

References

Andrews, W. C. (1996). Menopause and hormone replacement: An introduction. *Obstetrics and Gynecology, 87,* 1S.

Bates, B. (1991). *A guide to physical examination and history taking.* Philadelphia, PA: J. B. Lippincott.

Canadian Task Force on the Periodic Health Examination. (1994). *The Canadian guide to clinical preventive health care.* Ottawa: Minister of Supply and Services Canada.

Chetkowski, R. J., Meldrum, D. R., Steingold, K. A., Randle, D., Lu, J. K., Eggena, P., Hershman, J. M., Alkjaersig, N. K., Fletcher, A. P., & Judd, H. L. (1986). Biologic effects of transdermal estradiol. *New England Journal of Medicine, 314,* 1615-1620.

Clayden, J. R., Bell, J. W., & Pollard, P. (1974). Menopausal flushing, double blind trial of nonhormonal medication. *British Medical Journal, 1,* 409-412.

Drife, J. O. (1993, September). The menopause. *Medicine North America,* pp. 632-636.

Dzerzko, C. M. (1995, October). Indications for HRT in older women. *Canadian Journal of Diagnosis,* pp. 40-59.

Gambrell, R. D., Jr. (1982). The menopause: Benefits and risks of estrogen-progesterone replacement therapy. *Fertility and Sterility, 37,* 457-474.

Griffing, G. T., & Allen, S. H. (1994). Estrogen replacement therapy at menopause: How benefits outweigh risks. *Postgraduate Medicine, 96,* 131-140.

Hammond, C. B. (1996). Menopause and hormone replacement therapy: An overview. *Obstetrics and Gynecology, 87,* 2S-15S.

Henderson, V. W., Paganini-Hill, A., Emanuel, C. K., Dunn, M. E., & Buckwalter, J. G. (1994). Estrogen replacement therapy in older women. *Archives of Neurology, 51,* 896-900.

Kampen, D. L., & Sherwin, B. B. (1994). Estrogen use and verbal memory in healthy postmenopausal women. *Obstetrics and Gynecology, 83,* 979-983.

Kentsmith, D. K. (1979). *Treating sexual problems in medical practice.* New York: Arco.

Lindsay, R. (1996). The menopause and osteoporosis. *Obstetrics and Gynecology, 87,* 16S-19S.

McCoy, N. L., & Davidson, J. M. (1985). A longitudinal study of the effects of the menopause on sexuality. *Maturitas, 7,* 203-210.

Menopause Consensus Commitee. (1994). Canadian Menopause Consensus Conference. *Journal of the Society of Obstetrics and Gynecology Canada, 16,* 1-39.

Novartis Pharmaceuticals. (1995). *Estracomb product monograph* [Package insert]. Dorval, Quebec: Author.

Phillips, S. K., Rook, K. M., Siddle, N. C., Bruce, S. A., & Woledge, R. C. (1993). Musculoskeletal weakness in women occurs at an earlier age than in men, but strength is preserved by hormonal replacement therapy. *Clinical Science, 84,* 95-98.

Prior, J. C. (1995). Menopause. In J. Gray (Ed.), *Therapeutic choices*. Ottawa, Ontario: Canadian Pharmaceutical Association.

Sherwin, B. B. (1996). Hormones, mood and cognitive functioning in postmenopausal women. *Obstetrics and Gynecology, 87,* 20S-26S.

Speroff, L. (1996). Postmenopausal hormone therapy and breast cancer. *Obstetrics and Gynecology, 87,* 44S-53S.

U.S. Preventive Services Task Force. (1996). *Guide to clinical preventive services*. Baltimore, MD: Willliams and Wilkins.

Wild, R. A. (1996). Estrogen: Effects on the cardiovascular tree. *Obstetrics and Gynecology, 87,* 27S-35S.

15. ACUTE LOW BACK PAIN

Mr. Thomas Ishigawa

*Goal: The goal of this exercise is to evaluate and develop
the participants' understanding of the assessment and management
of back pain of less than 3 months' duration in an adult patient.*

Specific Objectives: Upon completion of the group discussion exercise, each participant should be able to do the following:

1. Take a focused history and perform a focused physical examination of an adult patient who presents with back pain of acute onset.
2. Identify the most common causes of acute back pain as well as less common and more insidious conditions that can present as back pain.
3. Prescribe a suitable regimen of activity, medications, and other treatment upon initial assessment of low back pain.
4. Assess the psychosocial impact of low back pain upon a previously active adult and be able to counsel the patient effectively.
5. Order diagnostic tests, including radiographs and bloodwork, only when appropriate.
6. Refer patients for surgical evaluation appropriately. ·

PART I

The Patient

Social History

Tom Ishigawa is a 46-year-old, married, Japanese-Canadian high school chemistry teacher who lives in Burnaby, British Columbia.

Originally from Abbotsford, BC, the patient is the eldest of three children born to Yasuo Ishigawa and his wife Nobi, who immigrated to Canada from Japan in 1948. Tom spent his early life in Vancouver, where he completed high school. He later attended the University of Victoria, where he obtained a bachelor's degree in biology. Tom went on to complete his teacher's training at the University of British Columbia, where he received a B.Ed. certificate in 1973. He has been a teacher in the metropolitan Vancouver area for 23 years and has been working in his present position since 1982.

Tom married Alison West, whom he met in college, in 1976. The Ishigawas have three children: Christina, 17 years old; Daniel, 15; and Trevor, 11. Alison works part-time as a real estate agent in Burnaby, where the family also owns a large three-bedroom home. Both Tom and Alison are very active in community affairs. They participate in the local parent-teacher association (PTA). In addition, Alison has been involved in several committees organized by their city council.

Yasuo, 73, and Nobi, 70, live in a beautiful bungalow on Vancouver Island, approximately 200km from Tom's home. They make a trip to the city roughly once a month. Tom and his family in turn are frequent visitors to the island, especially during the summer months.

The patient has two younger siblings. His younger sister, Jennifer, 43, is a married housewife with two children and lives in nearby Port Coquitlam, BC. Tom's brother, Walter, 38, a computer consultant, is single and lives and works in San Diego, CA.

The patient inherited the Shinto faith from his parents but considers himself "not religious in the least." Neither he nor his wife ascribe to any organized religion.

Tom Ishigawa has a number of close friends, most of whom are fellow teachers and with whom he gets together about once a week outside of work. He is an avid golfer and loves to play basketball at the local YMCA about twice a week. Tom and Alison maintain a superb vegetable garden in their backyard. Much of the couple's remaining spare time is spent attending the numerous activities of their children, including Trevor's hockey games, Daniel's basketball games, and Christina's piano recitals.

Tom describes his marriage and family life as "hectic but happy." Indeed, he and Alison have had no major marital difficulties and refer to themselves as "enthusiastic parents" who have raised three healthy, normal kids.

Past Personal and Family Medical History

Tom Ishigawa was a healthy child. In 1961, at the age of 11, he had his tonsils and adenoids removed after repeated throat and ear infections. In 1965, he injured his knee during a soccer match. He is uncertain as to the precise diagnosis, but he did require rest and some form of gradual physical rehabilitation for several weeks. Tom has had no other major illnesses, significant injuries, or surgery. He has never smoked tobacco but confesses that he was a "big fan of marijuana" in his college days. He gave this up when he met Alison, who had no tolerance for that indulgence. He describes himself as a "social drinker" who consumes three to four beers a weekend, usually with friends. The patient normally uses no medications.

Tom's wife and children are in excellent health. His mother, Nobi, suffers from osteoporosis and fractured her left hip in 1993. She subsequently underwent hip replacement surgery and now ambulates reasonably well. Yasuo describes himself as "healthy as a horse" but does suffer from chronic open-angle glaucoma, which, despite several laser treatments, continues to progress. He is unable to drive. His ability to read is compromised. To the best of the patient's knowledge, his parents have no other serious problems. Tom's brother and sister are in good health.

The Problem

You are a family physician practicing in a wealthy suburb of Vancouver, British Columbia, with easy access to all diagnostic facilities and specialists.

Tom Ishigawa comes to your office complaining of back pain that began approximately 3 weeks ago. He describes this pain as sharp, more or less constant, and worst in the right lowermost area of his back and right buttock but also radiating down the back of his right thigh. He awoke with the pain 3 weeks ago, and it has been getting steadily worse. Tom has noted that the pain increases significantly when he bends over and when he sits for prolonged periods of time, usually 30 min or more. The pain also increases considerably when he lifts heavy objects, over 20kg. The patient has not noted any increase in pain with coughing, sneezing, straining, or walking. He has noted no pain in his right calf, heel, or toes, or any paresthesias or numbness of these areas.

The patient cannot recall any particular incident involving lifting, twisting, falling, or other injury immediately preceding the onset of pain. During the first week after onset, Tom tried to cope with his problem by using generous doses of ibuprofen and Tylenol. He was able to participate in his usual sports activities, although with considerable discomfort. For the past 2 weeks, the medication has been completely ineffective. Tom has applied an ice pack to his right lower back with minimal relief. He has stopped playing basketball and canceled several rounds of golf. Alison has been insisting for some time that her husband seek medical attention, but for nearly 3 weeks, Tom felt that was completely unnecessary. He held the belief that the pain would spontaneously resolve.

During the past 3 days, Tom's back pain has gotten even worse. He has not gone to work. Sitting for more than 10 to 15 min has become unbearable, and the patient has spent much of his time lying in bed, the position that offers him the most comfort. Finally able to overcome her husband's stubbornness, Alison convinced Tom to see a doctor.

The patient reports no recent fever, chills, or weight loss. He reports no increased urinary frequency, incontinence, or difficulty voiding. There has been no change in bowel habits. There is no history of weakness in the lower legs. The patient reports no abdominal pain. There is also no history of recent joint stiffness.

When asked about his mood recently, Tom states that he is "depressed and frustrated." His inability to be active has affected him considerably. He tells you, "I just lie there watching soap operas . . . I feel so useless . . . like an old man. I can't believe I just can't kick this thing and get on with my life." When asked why he was so convinced that he would be able to overcome his problem on his own, Tom tells you he has had this same pain at least twice in the past year, but of much less severity and duration, and with no limitation of activities. In his words, "I just ignored it, and it went away in a couple of days." You ask Tom what he hopes to accomplish during this visit, to which he responds, "Just want to know what precisely is wrong and what can get me back to work as fast as possible."

Questions

1. How would you describe Tom as a person and Tom as a patient from what you know so far?

2. Describe how you would perform a physical examination of the patient, given the history presented.

3. How would you initially manage this patient?

Discussion

1. This question will likely introduce a wide variety of responses to the group discussion. Some general observations may include that Tom Ishigawa is an active person with diverse interests. He has had few health problems in the past. Furthermore, the history reveals a definite reluctance to seek the help of a physician. The patient appears to expect a quick recovery and return to usual activities. This may present an interesting challenge. Tom clearly has high expectations, and his reaction to the failure to meet these expectations should be anticipated. At the same time, Mr. Ishigawa is a well-educated and well-motivated patient, who is likely to respond favorably to the physician's recommendations and also become an active partner in the management plan.

2. There are many potentially serious conditions that can present as back pain. These include possible fracture, tumor, or infection, or possible cauda equina syndrome, in which nerve roots below L1 are severely compressed and characterized by bowel/bladder symptoms and saddle anesthesia. Tom's history does not include any trauma, constitutional symptoms, or neurologic problems suggestive of any of these conditions or "red flags." The physical examination of any patient presenting with back pain should be guided by the medical history. Tom is, in many ways, a typical back pain patient, and an appropriate physical examination in this case should include four principal components (Bigos et al., 1994): (a) general observation of the patient, including his or her appearance, mood, affect, and gait; (b) a regional back exam, including inspection and palpation of the lumbar spine; (c) neurologic screening, including testing for muscle strength, circumferential measurements of the calf and thigh bilaterally, testing of the deep tendon reflexes of the lower limbs, and a sensory exam using light touch of the feet; and, finally, (d) testing for sciatic nerve tension using the straight leg raising or sitting knee extension test.

The maneuvers described above have been found to be the most valuable by the Agency for Health Care Policy and Research (AHCPR) (Bigos et al., 1994). Some authorities also recommend evaluation of the range of motion of the lumbar spine (Hall, 1992; Hresko, 1992). The AHCPR states that this sort of testing is unnecessary, as there is a wide variation in range of motion in patients both with and without back pain.

See "The Rest of the Story" for a description of the recommended physical examination together with Tom Ishigawa's corresponding summarized results.

3. The focus of an appropriate history and physical examination in the back pain patient is the identification of red flags, or dangerous conditions; the understanding of activity limitations; and understanding of the patient's outlook and expectations. Less emphasis should be placed on arriving at a specific diagnosis. A careful review of Tom's history and exam, however, reveals that he does have evidence of a lumbar disk herniation, specifically of the

L5-S1 disk. The patient's pain is aggravated by sitting. He gets relief when his spine is relaxed or "unloaded" (e.g., standing or lying down). Both these characteristics are common in disk herniations. The vast majority of patients with disk herniations will have a positive ipsilateral straight leg raise test (Deyo, Loeser, & Bigos, 1990). Crossover pain, elicited by raising the asymptomatic leg, is far more specific for nerve root irritation. Furthermore, the exam reveals slight but significant atrophy of the gastrocnemius muscle supplied by the S1 root. The diminished ankle jerk and numbness of the lateral aspect of the right foot is also suggestive of S1 nerve root compression.

A first consideration in the management of this patient is whether or not to order any diagnostic tests, particularly imaging studies. This area remains controversial. The AHCPR believes that radiographs and other imaging studies are unnecessary in the patient presenting acutely with back pain of less than 4 weeks duration unless a red flag has been identified through the history and physical examination. Thus, even in Tom's case, where a herniated disk is suspected, imaging studies are not immediately needed. The C.M.E. joint committee of the American Association of Neurological Surgeons and Congress of Neurological Surgeons, on the other hand, recommends a plain film of the lumbosacral spine in all patients with a suspected herniated disk (Gilmer, Papadopoulos, & Tuite, 1993). The rationale for this is to rule out spondylolisthesis, osteomyelitis, and metastatic disease. There is nothing suggestive in Tom's history of metastatic disease. The patient reports no fever, nor is there any history of local infection or soft tissue swelling consistent with osteomyelitis. Spondylolisthesis refers to the anterior

shifting of the vertebral column upon a lower vertebra. It is more common in children than adults. Spondylolisthesis can be identified on plain radiographs and, when associated with pain, warrants an orthopedic referral (Hresko, 1992).

As the routine use of imaging studies in patients presenting acutely with back pain is controversial, discussion participants who insist on ordering such studies in this case should be able to rationalize their decision in precise terms.

Most authorities are agreed that the initial management of a patient presenting acutely with back pain, and without severe neurologic compromise, should be "conservative." Unfortunately, there are different interpretations of conservative management. Initial care should consist of three main elements (Bigos et al., 1994): **(a) patient education and reassurance, (b) patient comfort, and (c) recommendations for activity alterations.**

Patient education should be individualized. Tom should be told that he can expect to recover from his symptoms and that the majority of patients presenting with back pain are able to return to a reasonable level of activity within 4 weeks (Conochie, Marshall, & Bigos, 1996). He should also be informed that his symptoms cause you to suspect a herniated disk. Tom would benefit from the knowledge that this is not an "old man's" problem and that many disk herniations occur in healthy, often active adults. The patient definitely needs to be told that there is no sign of a dangerous cause of back pain. As this is the case, there is no need at the present time for further testing or referral to a specialist.

Comfort measures include nonprescription and prescription medications. Among over-the-counter drugs, acetaminophen has been found to be safe and effective.

NSAIDS, such as the ibuprofen Tom uses, are also effective. Unfortunately, the patient has been using both of these and not getting substantial relief. The use of more powerful analgesics is discouraged by the AHCPR, as they have been shown to have no greater benefit than NSAIDS or acetaminophen. Discussion participants who recommend the use of opiates or muscle relaxants for a short period of time cannot be faulted, as the issue of the patient's comfort is a matter of the individual physician's style, experience, and his or her perception of the patient's needs.

Using heat or cold modalities has been shown to be of questionable benefit. Tom gets some relief from an ice pack and should be encouraged to continue this at his discretion.

Controversy exists about activity alteration **recommendations** upon initial presentation of a patient with back pain. Some advocate strict bed rest on a firm mattress (Vlok & Hendrix, 1991). This supposedly minimizes intradiskal pressure. Others believe that specific back exercises are valu-

able in the first days of treatment (Wheeler, 1995). A study of public service employees with back pain in Helsinki, Finland revealed that ordinary activity is superior to bed rest or back exercises in promoting recovery (Malmivarra et al., 1995).

Other recommendations for activity are universally accepted. Tom should avoid postures that aggravate his symptoms, such as sitting. He should avoid lifting heavy objects, twisting, and reaching. A previously active person like Tom should be encouraged to pursue some aerobic conditioning such as walking or swimming. These should not aggravate his symptoms and may help maintain his fitness and improve his sense of well-being. Such an exercise regimen is likely to be enthusiastically embraced by Mr. Ishigawa.

Having incorporated the elements of patient education, comfort, and alteration of activity into an agreeable management plan, Tom and his physician should probably agree to meet once again in 1 week to monitor his progress.

The Rest of the Story

Suggested Physical Examination and Corresponding Results

Gen: Well-groomed, pleasant, fit-looking East Asian male (ht.= 1.68m; wt. = 68.5kg); walks with normal gait

MSK: Regional back exam

Inspection: No deformity, normal lumbar curve, no scoliosis

Palpation: Moderate tenderness to palpation of right paraspinal muscles at the L4 and L5 level

Neurologic screening: Evaluation of muscle strength—no difficulty toe walking, heel walking, or squatting and rising (see note below)

Circumferential measurements: Left thigh 55.0cm

Right thigh 56.0cm

Left calf 37.5cm

Right calf 35.0 cm

Reflexes: Left knee 2+ (normal)

Right knee 2+

Left ankle 2+

Right ankle 1+ (diminished)

Sensory exam: Patient reports very slight numbness upon light touch to lateral aspect of right foot

Straight Leg Raising Test

Right leg: Patient reports pain shooting down right leg into right calf upon raising leg to approximately 45 degrees

Dorsiflexion of the ankle of the raised leg makes this pain slightly worse

Left leg: Patient reports pain shooting down right leg into right calf upon raising leg to approximately 60 degrees

Dorsiflexion of the ankle of the raised leg makes this pain slightly worse.

Note: Toe walking evaluates the calf muscles that are innervated predominantly by the S1 nerve root. Heel walking tests the ankle and toe dorsiflexors, supplied mostly by the L5 nerve root. Rising from a squat requires the use of the quadriceps muscles, supplied mostly by the L4 nerve root. Direct testing of these nerve roots can be accomplished by asking the patient, for example, to dorsiflex each foot against the examiner's hand (L5). The sequence of toe walking, heel walking, and squatting and rising, although not very highly sensitive, is a reasonable way to evaluate muscle strength in a busy practitioner's office.

PART II

The Problem

You and Tom agree on an initial management plan and to meet in 1 week's time. The patient returns and tells you immediately that there has been little improvement in his symptoms. He is still unable to sit for more than 15 to 20 min. Bending over remains uncomfortable. He went to work one day after his last visit, but his postural limitations made the day unbearable and he was forced to leave early.

Tom has been swimming at the YMCA for roughly 20 min daily. He thanks you for this recommendation, as it "gets me out of the house and doesn't make my pain worse." The patient continues to notice no increased pain with coughing, straining, or walking. There is still no history of limb weakness, bowel or bladder symptoms, or any significant numbness or paresthesias in the lower extremities. Tom continues to report no constitutional symptoms.

Tom tells you, "I guess things are a little better, but I was hoping to be shooting baskets by now."

You perform a repeat physical examination that is unchanged, except that the patient's face bears a more sombre expression. While you inspect his lumbar spine, Tom asks, "You know, Doctor, I was thinking about visiting a chiropractor. What do you think about that?"

Questions

1. How would you respond to Mr. Ishigawa's question?
2. How would you manage this problem now?

Discussion

1. Many physicians have strong views about chiropractors and the value of the services they provide. Undoubtedly, the best response to Tom's question would be a rational and unbiased one. Manipulation of the spine is regarded as a legitimate means of speeding recovery in patients with back pain of less than 3 weeks duration and no evidence of nerve root entrapment. However, manipulation may make any entrapment worse (Jenner & Barry, 1995). As Tom's pain has persisted for 4 weeks and is accompanied by signs of entrapment, he should be told that for these reasons, a visit to a chiropractor would probably not be in his best interests.

2. Tom's pain has persisted for 4 weeks. He has evidence suggesting an L5-S1 disk herniation. The AHCPR has a well-defined algorithm in cases such as these. At this time, diagnostic imaging is recommended to clearly identify pathology in the lumbar spine that is the cause of the patient's symptoms and that may be amenable to surgical correction. An orthopedic surgeon or radiologist can be consulted about the best diagnostic modality. In the interim, conservative measures should continue.

PART III

The Problem

You discuss Tom Ishigawa's case with R. J. de Montgrain, M.D., F.R.C.S.C., a prominent orthopedic surgeon with a great deal of experience in treating back problems. He recommends a CT scan to delineate any disk pathology. The test is performed 2 days later. It reveals a herniated nucleus pulposus of the L5-S1 disk without significant stenosis.

You call Tom at his request with the results and arrange a follow-up appointment the next day. He is feeling no better.

Questions

1. How would you proceed?

Discussion

1. There are many possible management strategies. Discussion group members are expected to generate a variety of responses. One sound suggestion is that the orthopedic surgeon consulted about the choice of diagnostic imaging should be involved at this point in the management plan. Surgery is certainly an option but should be considered in light of the surgeon's expectations of a positive outcome as well as the patient's interest in such an invasive procedure. There is certainly evidence that nonoperative treatment of herniated disks produces positive results (Saal & Saal, 1989; Saal, Saal, & Herzog, 1990).

Conclusion

Upon reviewing Tom's CT scan and discussing his case with you, Dr. de Montgrain recommends a conservative management plan consisting of continued comfort measures and aggressive physical rehabilitation (Saal & Saal, 1989). Tom, who definitely has no interest in back surgery at this point, is enthusiastic about this plan, especially as it allows him to expand the range of his physical activity.

You see Tom after 4 weeks of exercise training. He feels much better. He has been able to work for the past 2 weeks. He can sit for prolonged periods with minimal discomfort. He has been playing golf. He uses only small amounts of plain Tylenol (one to two tablets roughly once a day) for pain control. Tom tells you, "I feel better day by day. . . . I think I'll be a 100% in a couple of weeks."

You tell the patient that you are delighted by his progress and that as long as he continues to improve, there is no need for further follow-up. You make it clear to Tom, however, that should a problem arise, you are available to help in any way you can.

References

Bigos, S. J., Bowyer, O. R., Braen, G. R., Brown, K. C., Deyo, R. A., Haldeman, S., Hart, J. L., Johnson, E. W., Keller, R. B., Kido, D. K., Liang, M. H., Nelson, R. M., Nordin, M., Owen, B. D., Pope, M. H., Schwarz, R. K., Susman, J. L., Triano, J. J., Tripp, L., Turk, D., Watts, C., & Weinstein, J. (1994). *Acute low back problems in adults* (Clinical practice guideline No. 14, AHCPR Pub. No. 95-0643). Rockville, MD: U.S. Department of Health and Human Services, Public Health Service.

Conochie, L. B., Marshall, K. G., & Bigos, S. J. (1996). The new thinking on low-back pain. *Patient Care, 7,* 30-52.

Deyo, R. A., Loeser, J. D., & Bigos, S. J. (1990). Herniated lumbar intervertebral disk. *Annals of Internal Medicine, 112,* 598-603.

Gilmer, H. S., Papadopoulos, S. M., & Tuite, G. F. (1993). Lumbar disk disease: Pathophysiology, management and prevention. *American Family Physician, 47,* 1141-1152.

Hall, H. (1992, December 15). A simple approach to back-pain management. *Patient Care,* pp. 77-98.

Hresko, T. M. (1992). Thoracic and lumbosacral spine. In G. G. Steinberg (Ed.), *Ramamurti's orthopaedics in primary care* (pp. 132-158). Baltimore, MD: Williams and Wilkins.

Jenner, J. R., & Barry, M. (1995). Low back pain. *British Medical Journal, 310,* 929-933.

Malmivarra, A., Hakkinen, U., Aro, T., Heinrichs, M.-L., Koskenniemi, L., Kuosma, E., Lappi, S., Paloheimo, R., Servo, C., Vaaranen, V., & Hernberg, S. (1995). The treatment of acute low back pain—Bed rest, exercises, or ordinary activity? *New England Journal of Medicine, 332,* 351-355.

Saal, J. A., & Saal, J. S. (1989). Nonoperative treatment of herniated lumbar intervertebral disc with radiculopathy—An outcome study. *Spine, 14,* 431-437.

Saal, J. A., Saal, J. S., & Herzog, R. J. (1990). The natural history of lumbar intervertebral disc extrusions treated nonoperatively. *Spine, 15,* 683-686.

Vlok, G. J., & Hendrix, M. R. (1991). The lumbar disc: Evaluating the causes of pain. *Orthopaedics, 14,* 419-425.

Wheeler, A. H. (1995). Diagnosis and management of low back pain and sciatica. *American Family Physician, 52,* 1333-1341.

◆ Index

Acute low back pain, 237-245
    activity, level of, 242
    chiropractic service, 244
    disk herniation, 240-241
    exercise objectives, 237
    management of, 240-242, 244-245
    patient history, 237-239
    pharmacologic therapy, 241-241
    physical examination, 240, 242-243
Agency for Health Care Policy and Research
    (AHCPR), 8, 10, 15, 17, 114, 199, 200, 206,
    242, 244
AIDS. *See* HIV infection
American Academy of Pediatrics (AAP), 143
American Association of Clinical Endocrinologists
    (AACE), 75, 80
American College of Cardiology/American Heart
    Association Task Force, 113, 114
American Diabetes Association (ADA), 74, 75, 78, 79
American Heart Association, 101, 113, 114
    Step 1 Diet, 101
    Step 2 Diet, 101, 103, 104
American Psychiatric Association (APA), 7, 14
American Sleep Disorders Association:
    International Classification, 34
    Standards of Practice Committee, 37
Anxiety, 3
Asthma, 176-194
    classification, graded, 183, 193-194
    diagnosis, 179
    exercise objectives, 176
    management of, 183-184, 188-189, 191
    patient history, 176-178
    pharmacologic therapy, 184-185
    physical examination, 179, 180-181
    screening procedures, 179-180, 181-182, 182
        (figure)
    self-management, 185-187
    spirometric data, 182-183
    symptom/peak flow diary, 190
    triggers, 187-188, 189

Back pain. *See* Acute low back pain
Behavioral therapy, 16
Biopsychosocial model, ix
Bipolar disorder, 8
Brief dynamic psychotherapy, 16
British Diabetic Association, 74

Cancer, 3, 4
Cardiovascular disease, 4, 96-97
Case management, ix, x
Case studies, vii
    acute low back pain, 237-245
    asthma, 176-194
    diabetes, type {2}, 72-93
    dizziness and falls, 46-54
    failure to thrive, 153-175
    gastroesophageal reflux disease, 123-137
    headache, 55-71
    heart failure, 109-122
    HIV infection, 211-225
    hyperlipidemia, 94-108
    infantile diarrhea, 138-152
    insomnia, 27-45
    menopause, 226-236
    smoking cessation, 195-210
    weight loss, involuntary, 1-26
Cigarettes. *See* Smoking cessation
Circadian rhythm disturbances, 34, 39
Clarke, Lindsay, 153-175
Climacteric. *See* Menopause
Cystic fibrosis. *See* Failure to thrive

Dementia, 3, 5, 9-10
    Mini-Mental Status Examination, 10, 26
    See also Geriatric patients
Depression, 3, 4, 5
    categorization of, 8
    diagnosis of, 7-9, 13-15, 25
    Geriatric Depression Scale, 8, 10, 11 (figure), 24

insomnia and, 31, 32 (figure)
pharmacologic therapy, 18-19, 20 (figure), 21
prevalence of in elderly, 7
relapse, 22
risk factors for, 8, 14
treatment modalities, 15-17
See also Weight loss, involuntary
Diabetes, Type II, 72-93
　·exercise objectives, 72
follow-up care, early, 81-83
glucose log, 90-91, 92
glycemic control, inadequate, 87-89
guidelines, initial evaluation, 75
insulin therapy, 88-89, 90
management of, 77-78, 88-89
nonpharmacologic therapy, assessment of, 83-84
ongoing care, 85-86
patient history, 72-74
pharmacologic therapy, 84-85
physical examination, 75-77
risk factors, 74
screening recommendations, 74-75, 77
therapeutic modalities, 78-80
Diagnostic and Statistical Manual of Mental Disorders (DSM-IIIR, DSM-IV), 7, 14
Diarrhea. *See* Infantile diarrhea
Dizziness and falls, 46-54
exercise objectives, 46
Get-up and Go Test, 51
patient history, 46-48
physical examination, components of, 51, 52-53
risk factors, dizziness, 50-51
risk factors, falls, 50
threshold model for falls, 49-50
Drumdonald, Joseph, 1-26
Dysphagia, 5
Dysthemia, 8, 9

Edstrom, Roger, 123-137
Elderly patients. *See* Geriatric patients

Failure to thrive, 153-175
cough, chronic, 166, 167-168
cystic fibrosis, 170, 171-173, 172 (figure)
defined, 156, 159, 162
developmental factors, 165
exercise objectives, 153
growth charts, 156, 157, 158, 160, 161
home visit, 168-169
infection/malnutrition cycle, 164
medical factors, 163-164
nutritional factors, 162-163
patient history, 153-155
physical examination, 166-167
psychosocial factors, 164-165

Falls. *See* Dizziness and falls
Family-centered medicine:
biopsychosocial model, ix
insomnia evaluation/treatment, 30

Gastroesophageal reflux disease (GERD), 123-137
complications of, 128, 134
data sheet, 137
diagnostic procedures, 132
exercise objectives, 123
factors in, 127-128
FM/SW TABLE, 128
heartburn, 125
management of, 130-131, 132-133
nonpharmacologic therapies, 128-129
patient history, 123-124, 126
pharmacologic therapies, 130, 134, 135-136
physical examination, 126, 127
surgical treatment, 130
symptom severity, 125-126
Gastrointestinal disease, 4
Geriatric Depression Scale, 8, 10, 11 (figure), 24
Geriatric patients:
antidepressants and, 21
dementia in, 3, 5, 9-10
depression in, 5, 7-9, 13-14
threshold model for falls, 49-50
weight loss, factors in, 3-4, 5
See also Geriatric Depression Scale
Get-up and Go Test, 51
Growth deficiency. *See* Failure to thrive
Gutierez, Esmerelda, 226-236

Headache, 55-71
calendar of, 67, 71
classification, 61-62
danger signals, 57-58
exercise objective, 55
history taking, 58-59
International Headache Society (IHS), 61, 69-70
medications, 64-66, 67
migraine, 58, 61-66
neurological screening, 59, 60-61
nonpharmacologic therapies, 63-64
oral contraceptives, 63
patient history, 55-56
physical examination, 59, 60
Heart failure, 109-122
diagnostic evaluation, 112-115
exercise objectives, 109
functional classification, 115-116
management of, 116-117, 118
patient history, 109-111
pharmacologic therapy, 117-118, 120, 121

HIV infection, early management of, 211-225
    evaluation, comprehensive baseline, 219, 220-221
    exercise objectives, 211
    laboratory investigation, baseline, 219-220, 222-223
    patient history, 211-213, 215
    pharmacologic therapy, 223-224
    pre-test counseling guidelines, 214
    risk reduction, 214, 216-217
    suicide, 217
    test result disclosure, 216, 218
    vaccinations, 220
Hodge, William, 72-93
Hormone replacement therapy. *See* Menopause
Hypercholesterolemia. *See* Hyperlipidemia
Hyperlipidemia, 94-108
    cardiovascular disease, risk factors, 96-97
    clinical evaluation, 98-100
    exercise objectives, 94
    genetic factors, 99
    hypercholesterolemia, 97-98
    patient history, 94-96
    pharmacologic therapy, 105-107
    therapeutic approaches, 100-102, 103, 104

Ianonne, Enza, 46-54
Infantile diarrhea, 138-152
    BRAT diet, 146
    dehydration, symptoms of, 140-141, 141 (figure)
    etiology, 143-144
    exercise objectives, 138
    giardia lamblia, 149-150
    management of, 141, 144-146, 148
    patient history, 138-140
    physical examination, 142
    practice guideline, 140
    rehydration, oral, 142-143, 144-145
    screening recommendations, 147-148
Insomnia, 27-45
    classification systems, 34
    defined, 30
    evaluation of, 30-32
    exercise objectives, 27
    medications, 37-38
    nonpharmacologic therapies, 38-39
    patient history, 27-29
    polysomnography, 36-37
    qualification algorithm, 33-34
    sleep restriction, 38-43, 41-43 (figures)
International Headache Society (IHS), 61, 69-70
Interpersonal psychotherapy, 16
Ishigawa, Thomas, 237-245

Lipid disorders. *See* Hyperlipidemia

Major depressive disorder, 8
Management. *See* Case management; specific condition
Medical practice. *See* Family-centered medicine; Primary care medicine
Medication. *See* specific condition
Menopause, 226-236
    defined, 229
    exercise objectives, 226
    health promotion, 232
    hormone replacement therapy, 230-232, 233-235
    hot flashes, 229-230
    patient history, 226-228
    sexual health and, 229, 232
Migraine headaches, 58
    classification of, 61-62
    International Headache Society definition of, 69-70
    nonpharmacologic therapies, 63-64
    oral contraceptives and, 63
    pharmacologic therapy, 64-66
Mini-Mental Status Examination, 10, 26
Mood disorders. *See* Depression
Moore, Adam, 211-225

National Asthma Education Program, 185, 186, 188
National Center for Health Statistics, 159
National Diabetes Data Group, 75
National Institute of Mental Health (NIMH) Treatment of Depression Collaborative Research Program, 16-17
NIH Concensus Development Panel on Depression in Late Life, 7, 15
NIH Technology Assessment Panel, 38

Olefsky, Raffi, 27-45
Olfactory sensitivity, 3
Osler, William, vii

Polysomnography, 36-37
Primary care medicine, vii
Psychophysiologic insomnia, 34
Psychotherapy, 16-17
Pulmonary disease, 4

Restless legs syndrome, 34
Ross, Stewart, 109-122

Sleep:
    disorders, 34
    hygiene, 34, 35, 38
    logs, 41, 42, 43
    restriction, 38-39

See also American Sleep Disorders Association;
    Insomnia
Smoking cessation, 195-210
    biochemical measures of consumption, 204
    cold turkey, 202, 205, 210
    cough and, 205-206
    exercise objectives, 195
    guidelines for, 199-200
    management of, 201-203
    nicotine replacement, 203-204, 205
    patient history, 195-197
    relapse prevention, 206, 207-208
    tobacco use assessment, 198-199
    tobacco use history, 200-201
    withdrawal symptoms/weight gain, 203
St. George, Francine, 138-152

Stapleton, Shannon, 55-71
Suicide risk, 9, 217

Waugh, Nigel, 94-108
Webber, Liane, 176-194, 195-210
Weight loss, involuntary, 1-26
    dementia and, 9
    depression and, 5
    elderly population and, 3-4, 5
    evaluation of, 4-5
    exercise objectives, 1
    patient history, 1-3
    screening measures, 5-6
World Health Organization (WHO), 74, 140, 141,
    144, 145, 146

About the Author

Goutham Rao, M.D., C.M., C.C.F.P., is Clinical Assistant Professor, University of Pittsburgh Medical School. A graduate of McGill Medical School, Dr. Rao completed his residency training at the University of Toronto. His academic interests include undergraduate medical education, curriculum design, computers in medicine, and preventive health care.

Printed in the United States
By Bookmasters